AF252131

DISTRIBUTIONAL ASPECTS OF HUMAN FERTILITY:

A Global Comparative Study

THE INTERNATIONAL INSTITUTE FOR APPLIED SYSTEMS ANALYSIS

is a nongovernmental research institution, bringing together scientists from around the world to work on problems of common concern. Situated in Laxenburg, Austria, IIASA was founded in October 1972 by the academies of science and equivalent organizations of twelve countries. Its founders gave IIASA a unique position outside national, disciplinary, and institutional boundaries so that it might take the broadest possible view in pursuing its objectives:

To promote international cooperation in solving problems from social, economic, technological, and environmental change

To create a network of institutions in the national member organization countries and elsewhere for joint scientific research

To develop and formalize systems analysis and the sciences contributing to it, and promote the use of analytical techniques needed to evaluate and address complex problems

To inform policy advisors and decision makers about the potential application of the Institute's work to such problems

The Institute now has national member organizations in the following countries:

Austria
The Austrian Academy of Sciences

Bulgaria
The National Committee for Applied Systems Analysis and Management

Canada
The Canadian Committee for IIASA

Czechoslovakia
The Committee for IIASA of the Czechoslovak Socialist Republic

Finland
The Finnish Committee for IIASA

France
The French Association for the Development of Systems Analysis

German Democratic Republic
The Academy of Sciences of the German Democratic Republic

Federal Republic of Germany
Association for the Advancement of IIASA

Hungary
The Hungarian Committee for Applied Systems Analysis

Italy
The National Research Council

Japan
The Japan Committee for IIASA

Netherlands
The Foundation IIASA–Netherlands

Poland
The Polish Academy of Sciences

Sweden
The Swedish Council for Planning and Coordination of Research

Union of Soviet Socialist Republics
The Academy of Sciences of the Union of Soviet Socialist Republics

United States of America
The American Academy of Arts and Sciences

DISTRIBUTIONAL ASPECTS OF HUMAN FERTILITY:
A Global Comparative Study

A volume in the series
STUDIES IN POPULATION
edited by **H. H. Winsborough**

Wolfgang Lutz
International Institute for Applied Systems Analysis
Laxenburg, Austria

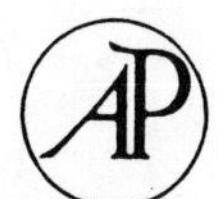

ACADEMIC PRESS
Harcourt Brace Jovanovich, Publishers
London San Diego New York Berkeley
Boston Sydney Tokyo Toronto

ACADEMIC PRESS LIMITED
24/28 Oval Road,
London NW1 7DX

United States Edition published by
ACADEMIC PRESS INC.
San Diego, CA 92101

British Library Cataloguing in Publication Data

Is available

ISBN 0-12-460470-6

Printed in Great Britain by
St Edmundsbury Press Ltd, Bury St Edmunds, Suffolk

Foreword

This book opens a new window on human fertility. Most of the literature, both popular and scholarly, deals with averages, as indicated by the observation that for long-term stationarity we need 2.1 children per woman at present low mortality rates. This could mean that 90% of women have two children and 10% have 3; it could alternatively mean that 30% have no children and 70% have 3. It could even mean that a few women have 5 to 10 children, and most have none. To enact policy that aims to raise or lower the birthrate it makes a great deal of difference which distribution applies, and on this the mean provides little information.

This question of distribution is conveniently discussed in this book in terms of parity progression: of women who have one child, what fraction goes on to have a second child; of those who have a second child, what fraction goes on to have a third; and so forth. We know that in all countries a high proportion of women try to give birth to at least two children; of those who try to bear two, what fraction goes on to have a third is in one sense the essence of the question of replacement fertility in the developed countries. One cannot imagine a policy succeeding without its main effect being to influence women to want three children rather than two.

Distribution is important for the interpretation of cohort and period fertility data. In the former, one follows statistically groups of women born at the same time through their childbearing careers; in the latter, one tries to draw conclusions from the childbearing behavior of a cross section of women observed in a particular calendar year or over a period of years. The cohort information discloses more about fertility than does the period data; however, the period data is more up to date, by about 30 years. To study thoroughly human fertility we need the averages and distributions of both.

Nathan Keyfitz
Leader
Population Program
International Institute for
Applied Systems Analysis

Preface

This study on distributional aspects of human reproduction has two major roots, the first coming from the tradition of research on heterogeneity dynamics in IIASA's Population Program. Recent work by my colleagues stimulated my focus on parity distributions instead of, and in addition to, the more familiar emphasis on mean family size. Although most of the work done by James Vaupel and Anatoli Yashin at IIASA treats hidden heterogeneity for non-repeatable events, such as mortality, their provocative results pointed to the next obvious challenge: an attempt to study heterogeneity in reproduction. A first logical step seemed to be a broad survey of observed reproductive heterogeneity and its implications.

This stimulus coincided with the other major root of this study, namely, my earlier interest in parity-specific fertility analysis under a period perspective – *parity* used here in the sense of the number of children already born (from the Latin *partus*, mean birth). The hypothesis was that, especially after the transition toward fertility control, parity should play a crucial role in determining fertility. Recently refined methods to estimate period parity-progression ratios and large data sets extracted from the World Fertility Survey could directly be used in this study.

Another root of this study is the notion of demographic dimensions. The fact that every demographic event can be examined with regard to a number of demographic dimensions (e.g., historical time, age, marital duration, etc.) is very useful for the definition of demographic rates and for disentangling various demographic effects. This concept seems to be especially useful for the analysis of distributional aspects. Finally, the belief that visual methods of displaying large data sets are often preferable to tabular forms for detecting major patterns and collaboration with James Vaupel on questions of fertility concentration, were important stimuli for this study.

The book discusses conceptual issues and provides a global survey of fertility distributions under both period and cohort perspectives. Various data sets were used. Data from 41 World Fertility Survey (WFS) files of the International Statistical Institute and 14 surveys conducted by WFS from Europe and the USA at the UN Economic Commission for Europe were merged together for the first time. Another unique data set comes from the Finnish population register and gives all vital events during 1984 for the population cross-classified by sex, age, marital status, duration in marital status, parity, and duration in parity. Together with additional sources, these two major data sets allow a thorough empirical treatment of the distributional aspects of fertility on a global scale.

The sequence of chapters has the following logic: starting with the general concept of demographic dimensions and illustrating them with examples from less- and more-developed countries, a logit model is developed in Chapter 1 to assess the relative effects of various dimensions on fertility. This perspective is multidimensional. Chapter 2 then focuses on distributions in respect to parity. Using a cohort perspective, variations in the (mostly completed) parity distributions among countries and among socioeconomic groups within countries are discussed. Chapter 3 looks at similar questions from a period perspective. This perspective refers to more recent fertility behavior, but poses many complex methodological problems. For this reason, a significant part of the chapter is devoted to methodologies used to estimate period parity-progression ratios. Chapter 4 summarizes the information given in the complete parity distribution using a single distributional indicator – a coefficient of concentration. Here, special attention is given to the changing relationship between the level and concentration of fertility. In the Epilogue an effort is made to point out that – in addition to the consequences of the level of fertility – distributional aspects of reproduction have important consequences on the individual, on society, and on the economy.

While planning and preparing this study many people contributed to it by providing comments, ideas, and practical help. I especially want to thank Gustav Feichtinger, Nathan Keyfitz, Mauri Nieminen, Thomas Pullum, James Vaupel, Douglas Wolf, Anatoli Yashin, Gerhard Bruckmann, Charles Calhoun, and Griffit Feeney. The able research assistance of Andreas Bakany and the skillful editorial help of Babette Wils are highly appreciated. Thanks, too, to the following members of the Publications Department at IIASA – Wendy Caron (Editor) and Anka James and Ewa Delpos (Graphic Artists). Last, but not least, the superb secretarial work of Susanne Stock is gratefully acknowledged.

Wolfgang Lutz
International Institute for
Applied Systems Analysis

Contents

Contents

CHAPTER 1

The Demographic Dimensions of Fertility

1.1. Introduction

A human birth may be perceived and registered in relation to a wide range of criteria and background variables, demographic and non-demographic. Demographic analysis traditionally considered the time at which the event took place (historical time) and the age of the mother (individual time) as the basic demographic dimensions of fertility. Other demographic covariates of fertility have received much less attention, and simultaneous consideration of several demographic dimensions has been very rare, indeed. In this study we want to introduce on a broader basis, discuss, and illustrate the general concept of measurement and analysis in a multidimensional space defined by specific demographic dimensions.[1] In the following sections we will first discuss individual demographic dimensions, then combinations of them.

1.2. Time

In demography the analytical dimension of time – historical time as well as individual age – is by far the most important of all background variables. Before going into specific considerations of the demographic time concept, we will do well to give some thought to alternative concepts of time.

The philosopher Kant (in "Transzendentale Ästetik," 1778, p. 46f) said most explicitly that there is only one time – absolute and objective. According to Kant, space and time are the basic concepts of our *pure intuition* and they make *synthetic a priori knowledge* possible. Opposing this Kantian doctrine – which was influenced by Plotinus, St. Thomas, Descartes, and others – is another tradition of thought expounded by philosophers such as Parmenides and also modern physicists such as Boltzmann and Heisenberg. They contend that time can only be subjective; some even call it an illusion.[2] Einstein's relativization of time is incompatible with Kant's notion of absolute time. However, as Popper (1972) stresses, a historian cannot accept the doctrine that time and change are illusions. Without having to accept the absolute objectiveness of time in a universal sense, demographers are likely to join historians in assuming that it is possible to measure change over time objectively, at least for human macro-environments on this planet.

The biological concepts of time and aging are also of certain interest to demography. When we accept the biological view that the life cycle of individuals is steered by genetically programmed processes of aging and that for different individuals these processes go at somewhat different speeds in terms of objective time (e.g., variance in the age of menarche), we may conclude that biological time should be our scale, especially for mortality analysis. However, because biological age is rather difficult to measure and there seems to be a strong correlation between biological age and intersubjective age measured in years, demographers usually do not bother with biological age.

The concept of social aging looks at age as it is perceived by the family, the community, or society. It has demographic implications especially for major transitions in the life cycle, such as age of entry into marriage or other union or age of retirement. In traditional societies social age correlated highly with biological age; in modern societies age as measured in years plays the dominant role. During the history of mankind, biological maturity and social maturity probably have never been so far apart as they are in our modern societies. Moreover, the age at retirement and the age of incapability of work are moving, on the average, further apart.

The demographic notion of individual time must finally be distinguished from that of personal perception, where 10 minutes may seem like an hour or three years may seem like one. Although under certain circumstances demographic behavior, such as the timing of marriage and births, may depend more on the individually perceived length of time than on the objectively measurable time elapsed, a study comparing individuals and grouping them into cohorts must be confined to measurable time – if for no other reasons than the fact that we have no unit to measure perceived time intersubjectively.

In demography we define individual or personal time as a clock that begins ticking at the birth of a human being and goes on in counting the (intersubjectively measurable) hours until the person dies. As other demographically relevant events occur, i.e., marriage, birth of a child, divorce or death of spouse, additional clocks start to run and count the time in the new status.

Independent of the individual clocks, historical time is measured across all individuals of all age groups, marriage durations, or open birth intervals. Historical time is the standard for the analysis of trends, evolutions, or periodic fluctuations on an aggregate level. Needless to say, historical time is also counted in objectively measurable time units of equal length. The fact that individual time (years of age or duration) and historical time (years of time) are measured by using the same unit is one of the deeper reasons for the analytical strength of demographic methodology. The homomorphism of these two time concepts allows demographers to construct synthetic cohorts and make period analysis comparable with cohort analysis.

All demographic processes over the life cycle of an individual occur within time – both individual and historical time. In this study we are concerned with the event of a birth. At the time of birth, individual time for every child is, by definition, zero, so we will study births with respect to the individual times of the parents.

At the time of a birth, several individual clocks are running for the parents. Generally, three such individual times or durations are considered to have some relevance for fertility: age, duration of marriage in case of marital fertility, and time since the last birth in case of two or more children. We will consider all three demographic dimensions of individual time in separate sections and estimate their relative impact on fertility.

1.3. Measurement

Before recording a birth with respect to any scaling of demographic dimensions, it must be unambiguously defined what is meant by a live birth.[3] Next, the country or region of birth is a decisive criterion. National boundaries determine under which system the birth will be registered. In existing registration systems the parents' nationality is mostly second in significance to the place of birth. Most statistical systems include births by foreigners within their national boundaries in their statistics of total births, although in some cases they might be shown under a separate heading.

Once the event of a birth is unambiguously defined and it is clear to which universe it belongs, for demographers *time* becomes by far the most important dimension under which this event is registered and studied.

In addition to the continuous demographic dimensions measured in time units, there are two major discrete demographic dimensions of fertility: marital status and parity. Several other discrete demographic dimensions could be constructed, such as the size of household or fecundity status, and an almost unlimited number of non-demographic variables (continuous or discrete) may be considered as being relevant for fertility.

One further perspective in demographic fertility analysis is whether to view the birth by the mother's characteristics or by the father's. Although a woman and a man are needed to create a new individual, demographic analysis so far has almost exclusively focused on the mother's characteristics and left out the father's altogether. The question of male fertility is almost never raised in conventional demography, but it often comes up in interdisciplinary discussions. There are several good reasons to focus on the mother instead of the father. First, it is the mother who actually carries out the birth, and in some cases the father cannot even be identified (recall the old Roman principle: *pater semper incertus*). Second, the age span during which individuals can have children is more clearly limited for women than for men, which is convenient for statistical analysis. Finally, demographers have little chance to study male fertility because of the lack of appropriate data. All these considerations, however, do not fully justify the complete neglect of men in fertility analyses. Later in this chapter we will make an attempt to measure and analyze male fertility.

In this chapter we will illustrate the distribution of fertility with respect to the major demographic dimensions. This will be done by the means of two- and three-dimensional line charts and by three-dimensional contour maps. The visual impression of the distribution of birth intensities is more intuitively understandable and informative than extensive tables and gives a clearer picture of the overall pattern. In each section, we will give examples from developed and from less-developed countries. In the last section the relative effects of the various demographic dimensions on fertility will be assessed quantitatively by means of logit regression models.

The remaining chapters of the book will focus on the distribution of births over various populations, i.e., on parity distributions. Consequently, parity will be the major demographic dimension of interest to us; others, such as age, will be taken into account only where this is necessary for the appropriate measurement of demographic processes. Non-demographic variables, such as mother's education or place of residence, will also be considered because they can contribute to the understanding of the process and might be used as a proxy for measuring heterogeneity in the population.

The measurement of events along demographic dimensions is generally the result of two factors: (1) demographic theory, i.e., a concept of the phenomenon to be measured and an *ex ante* expectation of which dimensions will be of explainatory value and what measurement scale would be appropriate; and (2) the availability of data and the mode of data collection. These two factors are not independent, and, as we will point out below, certain concepts of measurement and especially certain modes of temporal aggregation of the measured data fit to certain modes of data collection.

There are two major distinctive modes of temporal aggregation in demographic analysis: the cohort and period modes (e.g., Ryder, 1982). In terms of our distinction between individual and historical time, one point in historical time (or to be more precise, a short interval) creates a cohort by marking the beginning of individual times of all persons who belong to that cohort. Or, put the other way around, a cohort is a group of people with simultaneous individual time. In the period mode of temporal aggregation, different groups at different points of individual time are observed at one point (or interval) of historical time.

Cohort and period modes give different types of information, even if age specific period rates are aggregated to form a synthetic cohort that is isomorphic to a real cohort. Generally, they also come from different data sources: analyses in the cohort mode generally use census-type sources while period analyses use vital statistics with only the denominator from censuses. Ryder (1982) makes a very strong case for this distinction. He goes even further, saying that, in the analysis of surveys that share the structural characteristics (advantages and disadvantages) of censuses, measures for real cohorts are generally preferable to those for synthetic cohorts, which are appropriate for period analysis only. "The major problem with the exploitation of survey data for fertility measures has been the tendency to use the configuration of data provided by the survey as a surrogate for the kinds of data produced by registration system," (Ryder, 1982, p. 10). Following this logic the present study, which is largely based on the

WFS, will primarily use the real cohort approach to analyze the distributional aspects of reproduction.

Next to censuses, vital statistics, and surveys, one additional source of data existing, in only a few countries, is the complete computerized population register. In such a register each person has a number and all the attributes that are usually asked in a survey are attached to it. In addition, all vital events and changes in status are recorded on the person's file. This allows the analysis of event histories (usually only since the beginning of the computerized record). Such a population register makes the distinction between censuses and vital statistics obsolete because (at least in theory) everything can be derived from the register.

1.4. Data

One of the data sources used in this study, and especially in the rest of this chapter, is an extract from the population register of Finland. The data file consists of a cross classification of the complete Finnish population on January 1, 1984, by sex, age, marital status, duration in marital status, parity, and duration in parity. For each of the cells, the number of vital events during 1984 is given. Except for some technical problems of treating such a large data set and some questions of definition, such as adopted children and multiple births, this is an ideal data set for studying the demographic dimensions of fertility under a period perspective. Some special data sets from Austria, the FRG, the GDR, Finland, and the USA are also used.

The main data source of this study is the WFS. An attempt was made to combine and compare the large standardized set of data for 41 less-developed countries (LDCs) and the 13 recode files of industrialized countries (Europe plus the USA) that carried out surveys in various kinds of loose affiliation with the WFS. While the International Statistical Institute – with its WFS headquarters in London – tried to achieve a high degree of standardization and comparability among less-developed countries, the European surveys were much more heterogeneous and under the primary responsibility of the individual countries.[4] For this reason the recode files prepared by the United Nations Economic Commission for Europe (ECE) in Geneva are less detailed than the LDC files, especially for births beyond the third. As a consequence, the summary tables for all WFS countries in the following chapters and in the Appendices are less complete for the European countries. The author of the present study had the opportunity for research stays in both London and Geneva to extract the necessary tables from the standard recode files.

One of the great achievements of the WFS is its thorough documentation on sampling methods, coding, consistency checking, recoding, and assessment of the quality of data. Since several books and many technical reports and comparative studies have been published on these technical subjects, the strengths and weaknesses of the WFS are not discussed at this point.[5] Only where these questions become immediately relevant for our analysis will we consider them in detail. The objective of this study, however, is to examine the substantive findings from the WFS with respect to parity-specific fertility and distributional aspects of reproduction.

1.5. Age of Mother

As mentioned above, in traditional demographic analysis, the age of the mother has been considered the basic underlying covariate of human fertility. Aside from the fact that most data sources provide age as the sole or at least most important covariate of fertility, there is also good substantive reason for doing so. Age as measured in years seems to be a good proxy for biological age, and fertility is very dependent on biological age. Not only do menarche and menopause set bounds to the reproductive age span, but within this age span births are unevenly distributed, due in part to biological or *natural* reasons and in part to more or less conscious behavior with respect to the spacing of births or parity-specific fertility limitation.

The distinction between natural and behavioral limitations to fertility is crucial. According to Henry's (1961) definition, in a *natural* fertility regime, an additional birth does not depend on parity. The age-fertility curve is concave (see below). In controlled fertility, the converse is true. *Figure 1.1*, inspired by Bongaarts and Potter (1983) and taken from Lutz (1984), summarizes the major factors causing a decline of marital fertility with age. Technically, such social and economic factors that affect fertility are denoted intermediate variables (Davis and Blake, 1956), proximate determinants (Bongaarts, 1978), or simply instrumental variables (Ryder, 1982).

Figure 1.1 gives marital fertility curves for five populations, with very different reproductive patterns, and four sources of reduced fertility. There is a theoretical maximum fertility of one child per woman per year, which cannot be achieved in any population or subpopulation because of intrauterine mortality, postpartum amenorrhea, and a certain waiting time before conception. Married Hutterite women have the highest fertility studied so far in an existing population. Their fertility declines with increasing age because of increased infecundity and possibly higher intrauterine mortality for women of higher biological age. The fertility curve is concave, i.e., *natural.* Two other populations also exhibit concave marital fertility curves: Finnish rural communities in 1890 (see Pitkänen, 1982; Lutz, 1987a) and Dobe!Kung bushpeople (Howell, 1979). For these natural fertility populations, fertility is much lower than that of the Hutterite because of longer birth intervals that are likely to be the consequence of prolonged breast-feeding or abstinence. Although Finnish urban populations in 1920 had already passed the transition from natural to controlled fertility and show a clearly convex curve, their total marital fertility rate was still somewhat higher than that of the Dobe!Kung. The instrumental reasons for the additional decline in fertility, especially in higher age groups, marking the transition from *natural* to *controlled fertility* populations, are contraception and abortion. The recent marital fertility pattern of Austria at the bottom of the chart has essentially the shape of that of the Finnish towns in 1920, but at a much lower level

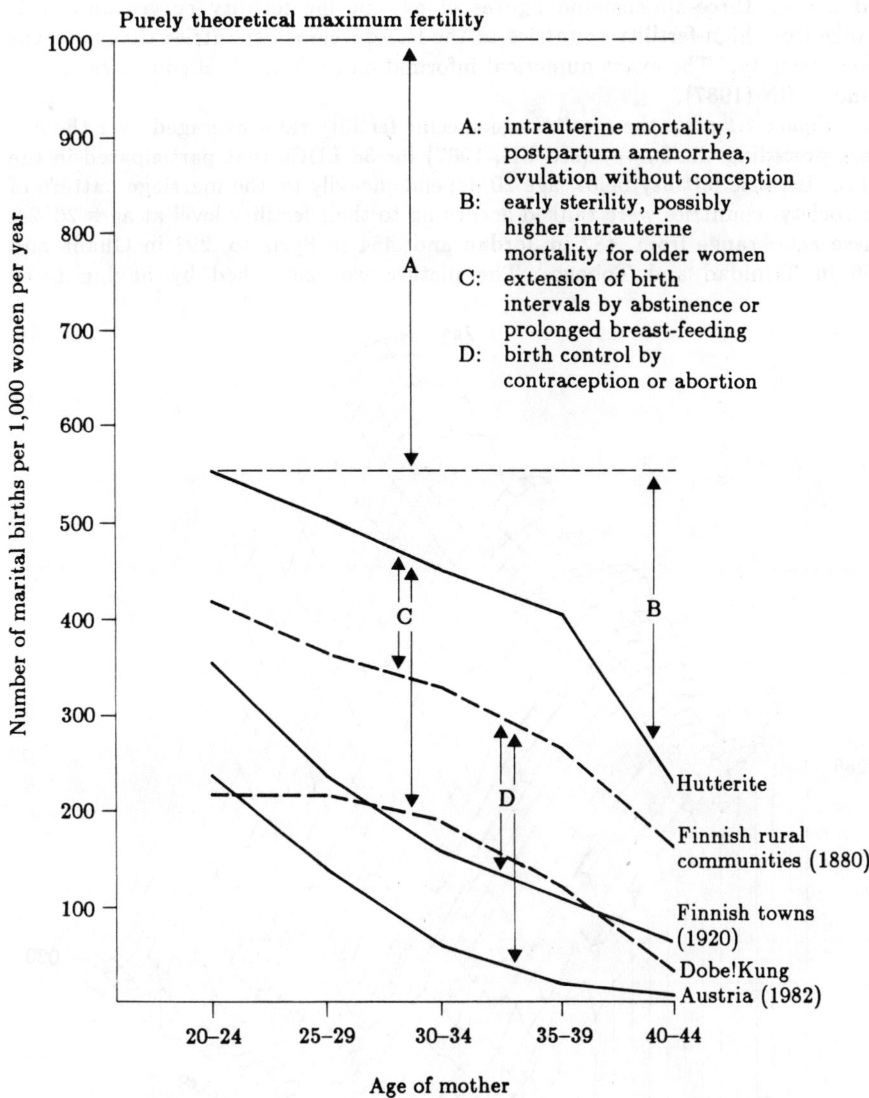

Figure 1.1. Causes of reduced marital fertility rates. (Source: Lutz, 1984).

owing to greater use of contraception or abortion. The age patterns of fertility of all the countries that will be analyzed in the following sections and chapters, whether industrialized or developing, will fall into the range between the two extreme cases discussed above: the Hutterite high and the recent Austrian low fertility pattern.

To observe fertility patterns in today's high-fertility countries, we will show and discuss three-dimensional figures of age-specific fertility curves and their change from high-fertility countries to the less-developed countries that have the lowest fertility. The exact numerical information on individual countries can be found in UN (1987).

Figure 1.2 plots the marital age-specific fertility rates averaged over the five years preceding the survey (see UN, 1987) for 38 LDCs that participated in the WFS. Because fertility below age 20 depends heavily on the marriage pattern of the society, countries were ranked according to their fertility level at ages 20–24. These rates range from .482 in Jordan and .454 in Syria to .292 in Ghana and .256 in Trinidad and Tobago. The picture was smoothed by having three

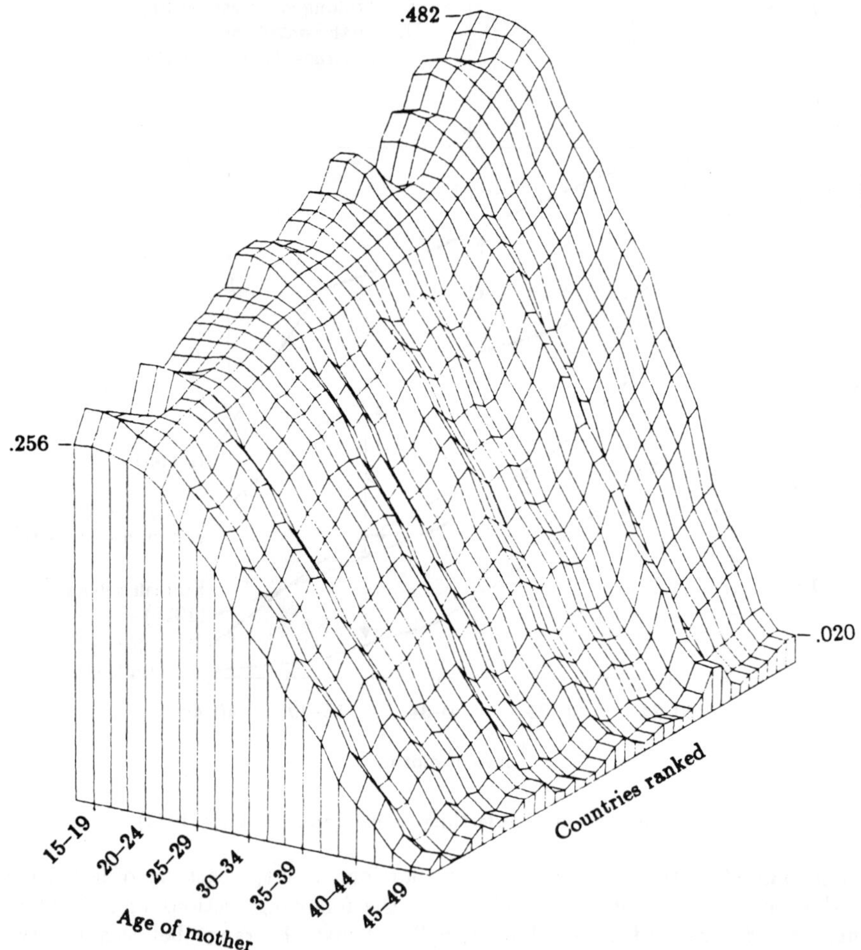

Figure 1.2. Marital age-specific fertility rates for 38 LDCs participating in the WFS ranked by fertility levels in the age group 20–24. (Source: UN, 1987.)

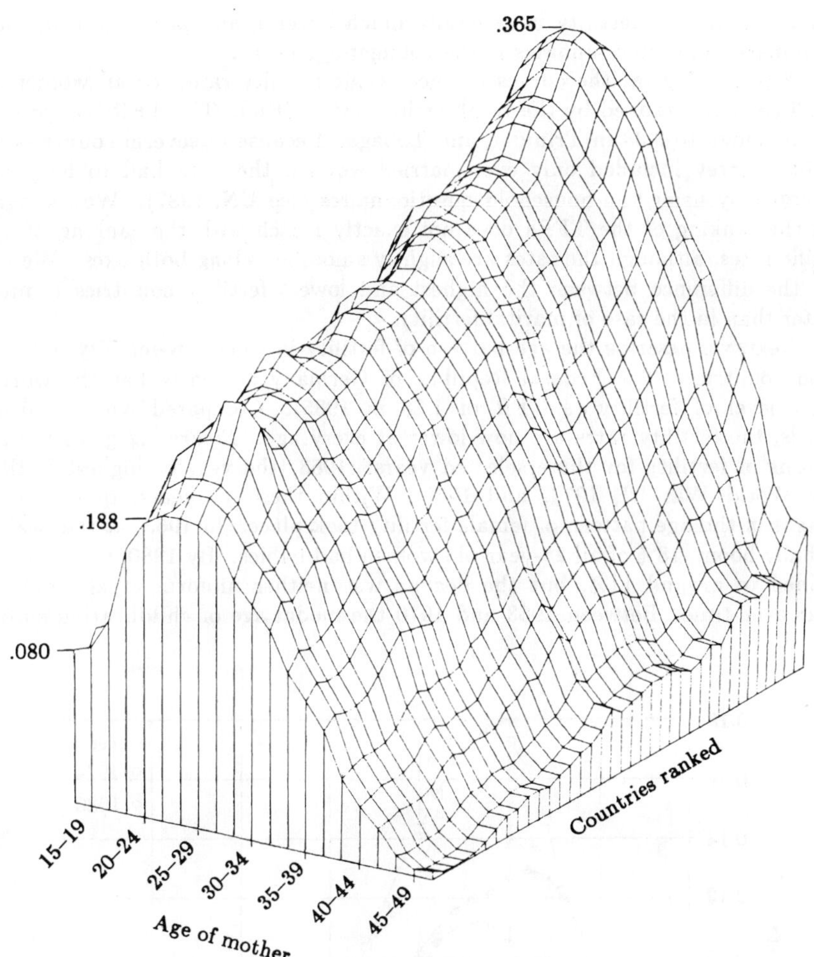

Figure 1.3 Age-specific fertility rates for 38 LDCs participating in the WFS ranked by TFR. (Source: UN, 1987.)

vertical lines stand for each five-year age group. As the figure indicates, at higher ages the ranking of the countries changes somewhat. For example, at age 40–45 Kenya has the highest marital fertility rate (.165), whereas Korea and Panama have the lowest (both .040). Here we see a difference in the shape of the curve (more or less concave) that is not expressed in the level of the fertility rate for ages 20–24.

Marital fertility rates of women below age 20 are strongly affected by selectivity due to differential marriage ages and a higher fertility of those who marry young. For age-specific fertility rates that refer to all women regardless of marital status, the fertility patterns look quite different for young ages. Until the age of highest fertility (mostly around 25), fertility increases with age. This is

because premarital fertility is generally much lower than marital fertility, and
the unmarried group dominates in the younger age range.

Figure 1.3 gives the curves of age-specific fertility rates for all women for
the 38 countries ranked by the total fertility rate (TFR). The TFRs range from
8.26 in Kenya to 3.38 in Trinidad and Tobago. Because in several countries the
fertility survey included only ever-married women, the data had to be partly
estimated by using the household questionnaires (see UN, 1987). We see again
that the ranking of the TFRs does not exactly match with the ranking of age-
specific rates, although the rates are slightly smoothed along both axes. We find
that the difference between the highest and lowest fertility countries is much
greater than in the case of marital fertility.

Next, we describe the age pattern of fertility in some low-fertility industrialized countries. The Federal Republic of Germany currently has the world's
lowest level of fertility (a TFR of 1.28 in 1985). Compared with historical
records, the fertility rates are now lower at every age. *Figure 1.4* gives the age
patterns of fertility for three selected years: 1963 (the year of highest fertility
after World War II), 1974, and 1980. Within these 17 years, quite serious
changes in the age pattern of female fertility took place. In 1963, at the peak of
the baby boom, 18% of all 25-year-old women had babies. By 1980, this rate had
declined to around 11%, but the decline was neither uniform at all ages nor
linear over time. Between 1963 and 1970 the modal age of childbearing shifted

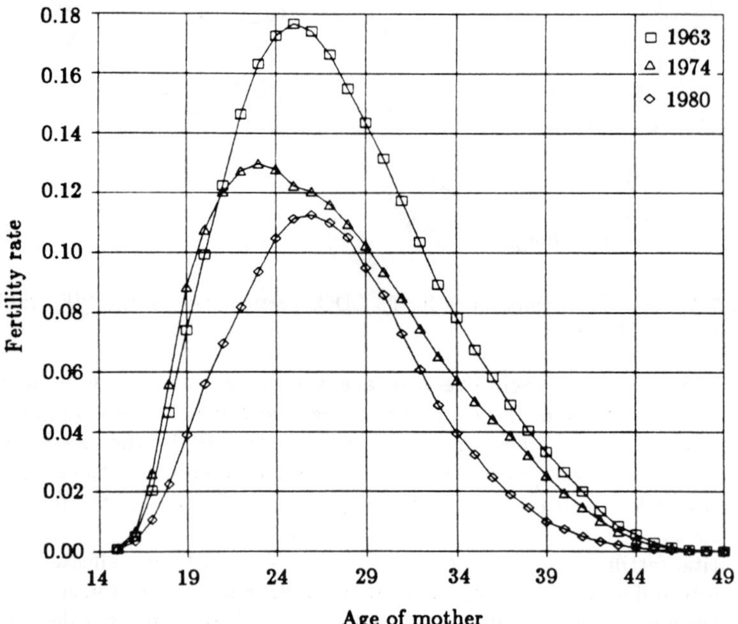

Figure 1.4. Age-specific period fertility rates in the FRG for 1963, 1974, and 1980.

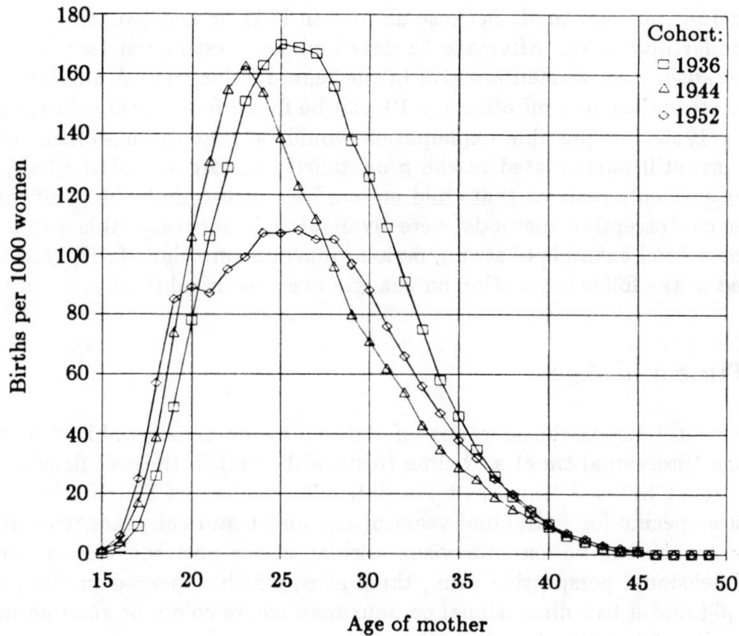

Figure 1.5. Age-specific fertility rates for three selected cohorts in the FRG.

down from 25 to 23 years, and fertility below age 21 in 1970 was even higher than in 1963 despite a dramatic decline at all other ages. After 1970, the modal age increased again and reached 26 in 1980. During these 10 years, fertility decreased at every age and especially at younger ages, making the 1980 pattern more even and more similar in shape to the 1963 pattern, although at a significantly lower level.

Thus, the age pattern of period fertility depends very heavily on period changes in the timing of birth. One might ask if the emerging shape of the age-specific fertility curve is more sensitive to such period changes or if it resembles the cohort pattern. *Figure 1.5* gives the cohort age pattern of fertility for three selected cohorts in the FRG. At first glance the cohort rates show even less regularity than the period pattern. For the cohort of women that was born in 1936 and reached their prime childbearing ages at the peak of the baby boom, the shape of the curve is very similar to the period pattern of 1963. At the peak fertility ages, the period and cohort rates almost coincide because they largely refer to the same women. Under age 24 and above age 30, the difference between the period and cohort rates is more visible because of changes in the fertility pattern. The younger cohort of 1944 shows the same shift toward higher fertility at young ages and reduced fertility above age 24 that we observed in the period data.

The cohort of 1952, however, exhibits a rather strange and irregular age pattern of fertility: a very fast increase in fertility until age 19, followed by a slow, stepwise increase to the highest fertility ages 24 to 28. During these five years there is no clear mode because all women in their mid-twenties have about the same fertility level. After age 28 data had to be estimated (see Birg, *et al.*, 1984) because these women are still in the reproductive age. A similar pattern, with the strong leveling off after age 19, can be found for several cohorts born in the early 1950s. A possible explaination would be that those women, while in their teens, still participated in the pronatalistic atmosphere of the baby boom and then suddenly realized that children had become less desirable, and that new effective contraceptive methods were available. If accurate, this explaination would be a good example of strong period influences on cohort fertility, a subject discussed in the following section on changes over historical time.

1.6. Time and Age

For the simultaneous consideration of the two major demographic time dimensions, age (individual time) and time (historical time), a three-dimensional perspective must be used to present the data. To depict the distribution of birth intensities specific for individual years of age and historical years, two different types of graphs can be used for visual display of the pattern: the conventional three-dimensional perspective using three axes, which appeared in the previous section [6]; and a two-dimensional contour map where colors or shading indicate the intensity of fertility at each age in each year.

Both types of presentation have advantages and disadvantages. Contour maps, which are widely used in depicting spatial patterns, can be used to present any surface that is defined over two dimensions on a metric scale (see Vaupel *et al.*, 1987). In contrast to the conventional 3–D plot, where part of the information is usually hidden behind the *mountain* and it is difficult to trace back the exact numerical location of any given point, the contour map always displays the complete array of data and makes it easy to identify each point in terms of its coordinates, as on a topological map. For longer time-series covering relatively strong fluctuations, however, the contour maps become too complex to discern major patterns at a glance. For such cases, the conventional 3–D plot is more informative.

As an example of such a long-term perspective, *Figure 1.6* gives the trends in age-specific fertility in Finland over more than two centuries. We can readily see from this figure the major phases of Finnish fertility history: a period of high premodern fertility levels with some short-term fluctuations until about 1910, when fertility entered a steep secular decline. In Finland the baby boom reached its peak right after World War II in 1947. Since then, fertility has been declining, although less steeply in recent years. Another surprising feature of early Finnish fertility trends is clearly visible from the graph: between 1776 and 1810, overall fertility declined significantly in Finland. This is surprising because it predated the often-cited early fertility decline in France at the beginning of the nineteenth century. Lutz and Pitkänen (1987) and Lutz (1987a, 1987b) demonstrate that this early decline in Finland was due to a change in the marriage pattern (later and less frequent marriage) rather than to a change in marital fertility, which was the reason for the early decline in France. Grossly speaking,

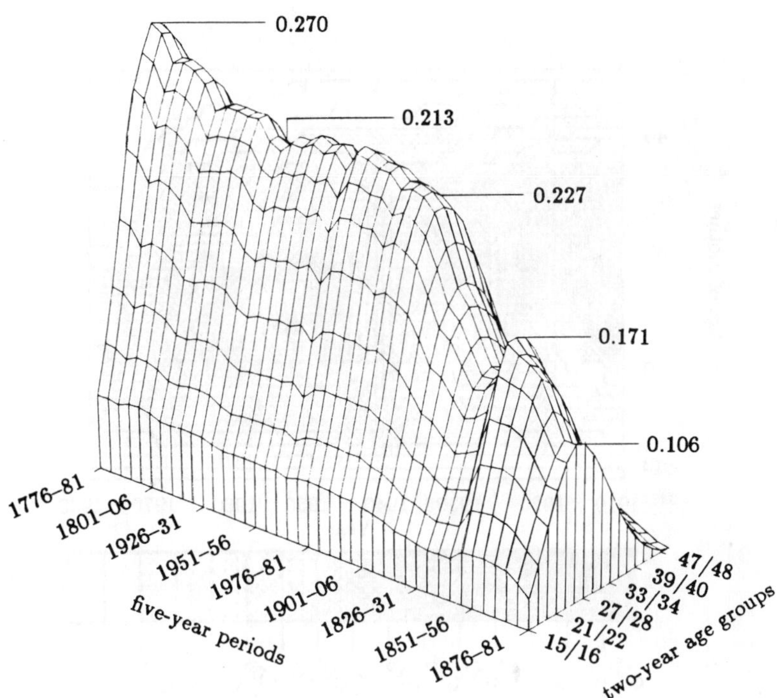

Figure 1.6. 3–D plot of age-specific fertility rates from 1776 to 1981 in Finland. (Source: Lutz, 1987b.)

during the second half of the eighteenth century, Finland moved from a pattern of early and frequent marriage to what Hajnal (1965) called the *European marriage pattern.* *Figure 1.6* also gives some hints of a declining modal age of childbearing since the onset of the modern fertility transition around 1910. Such details, however, are more clearly identifiable on the contour map than on the somewhat smoothed 3–D plot.

Figure 1.7 gives the contour map perspective of age-specific Finnish fertility trends since 1910.[7] In this graph we clearly recognize the fertility-depressing effects of the two world wars. We also see the tail of the great fertility transition that resulted in reduced fertility at all ages, but most dramatically at ages above 35. Immediately after World War II, the fertility of women in their twenties increased almost to the level of 1910. Women over 30, however, hardly took part in the postwar baby boom: fertility at higher ages shows an almost monotonically declining trend over those 70 years of Finnish fertility history. *Figure 1.7* also indicates that women in their early twenties kept the high fertility levels for a longer period of time than women in their late twenties, a fact that resulted in a decrease of the mean age at birth until the early 1970s. Looking at cohort lines that, as in a Lexis diagram, follow along the diagonals (in *Figure 1.7* the angle of cohort lines is steeper than 45° because the two axes have different scales), we

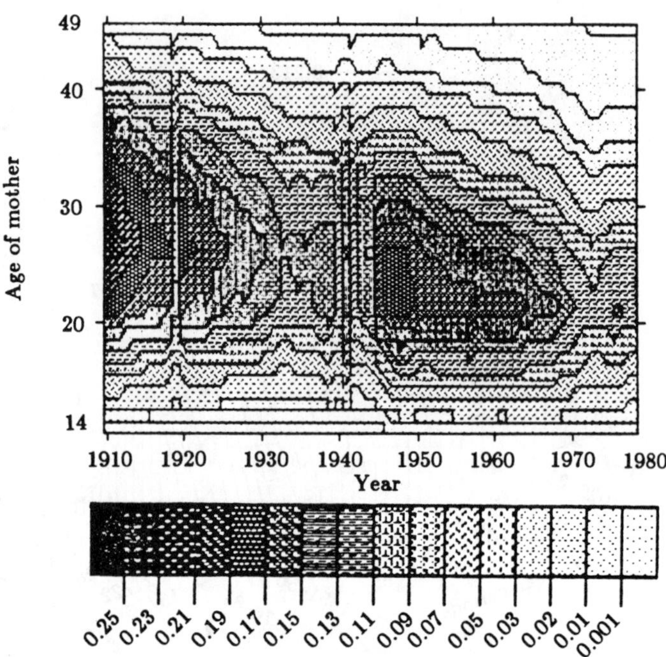

Figure 1.7. Shaded contour map of Finnish age-specific fertility rates, 1910–1980. (The categories of shading will be the same for all other contour maps in this chapter.)

can also see that the baby boom in part compensated for very low fertility at earlier times and ages and that the women who participated in the peak of the boom had significantly lower fertility at ages above 30 than earlier cohorts. This indicates for the Finnish case that period fluctuations were stronger than cohort fluctuations.

In the Germanies, the trends were quite different, as the contour maps of age-specific fertility trends in East and West Germany show. One finds that the Federal Republic of Germany experienced a clear and pronounced baby boom in the early 1960s (see *Figure 1.8*). After 1970, fertility decreased at all ages and the modal age of birth also increased, a fact we already noted in the previous section on age patterns. In the German Democratic Republic (see *Figure 1.9*), the trend was completely different. From 1950 until very recently, fertility of women in their early twenties remained at levels that in the FRG were only reached during the baby boom. Above age 28, however, the fertility patterns were rather similar in both Germanies. In the GDR, fertility levels are more responsive to political measures. In 1974, for instance, the period TFR dropped dramatically due to a package of social laws that included liberalization of abortion. Shortly thereafter, however, the fertility rate recovered, again due to new legislation that helped young families (see Büttner *et al.*, 1987).

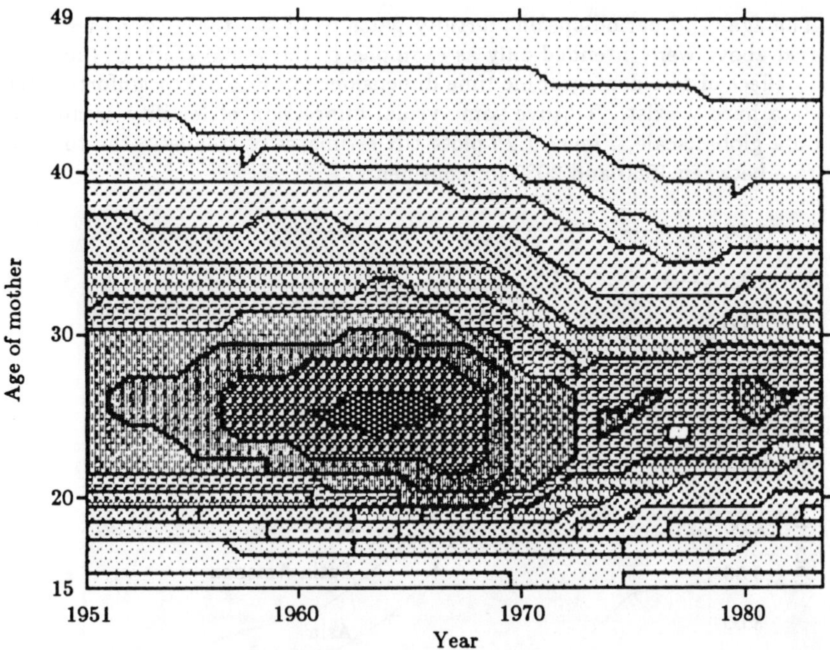

Figure 1.8. Shaded contour map of age-specific fertility rates in the FRG, 1951–1984.

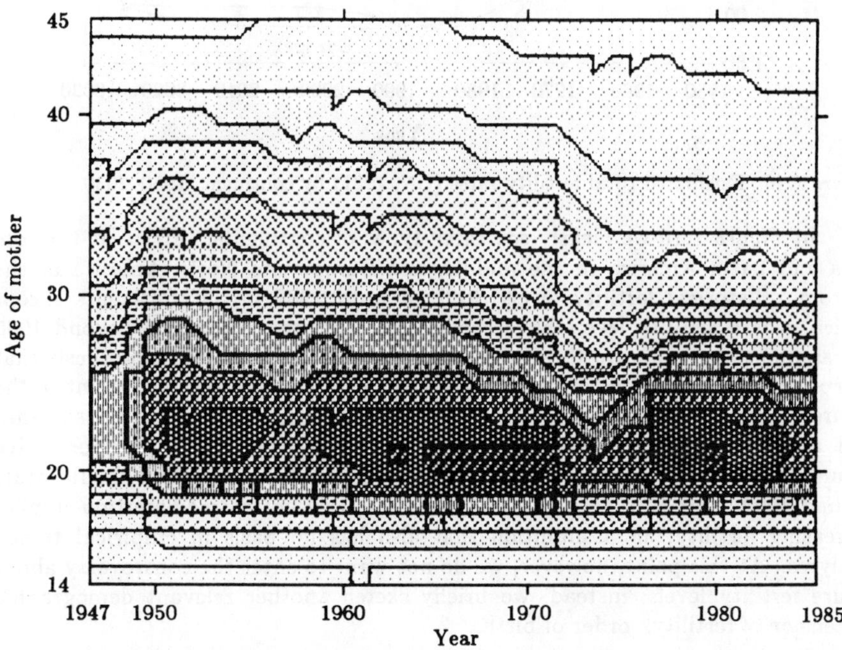

Figure 1.9. Shaded contour map of age-specific fertility rates in the GDR, 1947–1985.

The age- and period-specific fertility patterns of the three countries briefly discussed above were intended only as examples of the visual study of the simultaneous effect of two demographic time dimensions.[8] For LDCs, unfortunately, such data hardly exist. To give some visual impression of fertility trends over time on a global scale, *Figure 1.10* plots UN estimates of trends in the total fertility rate between 1950 and 2030 for continents.

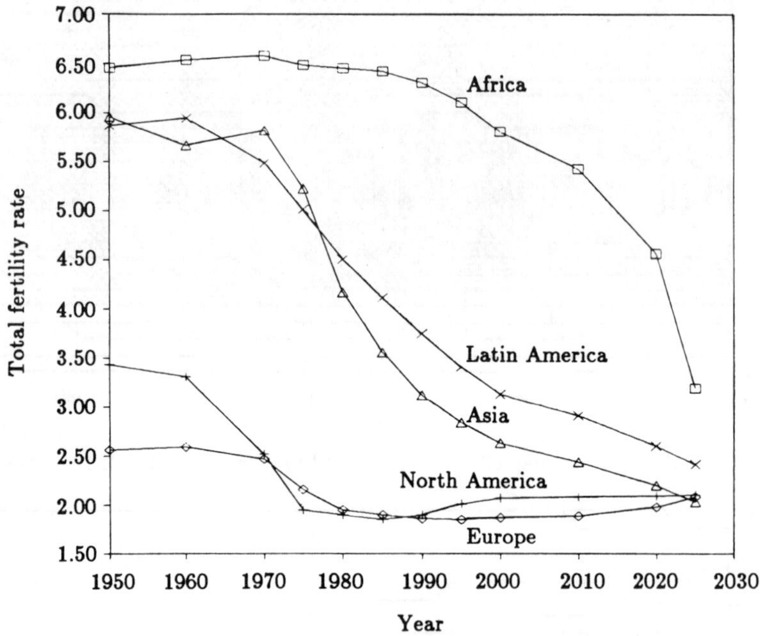

Figure 1.10. Estimated total fertility rates (UN, 1987) by continent, 1950–2030.

In *Figure 1.10* we clearly see three types of continents: Africa at the top, Asia and Latin America in the middle, and Europe and North America at the bottom. Historical fertility levels declined until 1980 in all continents except Africa, where fertility levels have shown little change. All trends beyond 1980 are assumptions made by the United Nations and based on the hypothesis that all countries are heading toward replacement level at some assumed point in the future. For Asia and Latin America, this means the continuation of a trend that had already begun by 1980. For Africa, however, this means the normative assumption of a dramatic change in reproductive behavior that should start around 1990. For Europe and North America, this normative assertion implies increasing fertility, an assumption that also has no basis in empirical trends analyses. At this point, however, we do not want to enter the controversy about future fertility levels; instead, we briefly sketch another relevant demographic dimension of fertility: order of birth.

1.7. Order of Birth, Parity

If reproductive behavior is within the calculus of conscious choice (Coale, 1974) and is controlled in the way that the birth of an additional child depends on the number of children already born (Henry, 1961), then the order of birth is by definition the most important demographic dimension within the reproductive age span. Even fertility shows some dependence on parity, partly because of the strong empirical association between age (declining fecundability) and parity and partly because of an assumed increase in the likelihood of sterility with parity. But even when disregarding parity as a determinant of additional births, order-specific fertility analysis is worthwhile because it shows the consequences of existing fertility patterns on the distribution of reproduction and the concentration of childbearing among women in a given population. At this point we will briefly introduce parity as a third demographic dimension, in addition to age and time. (We will treat it in more depth in Chapters 2 and 3.)

There often seems to be a fundamental confusion about the nature of order-specific rates. Generally, order-specific rates may be calculated using one of two different denominators. If the numerator includes all births of given order i, age a, and time t and the denominator all women at parity $i-1$, of age a, time t, then the result is a real parity-specific rate that could be used as input, e.g., for a life-table approach to parity progression. A summation of such rates over age or parity, however, does not make any sense, because the rates have different denominators, a fact that allows neither the computation of synthetic cohorts in analogy to the total fertility rate nor the calculation of age-specific rates over all orders of birth. If, however, the denominator includes all women at a given age and time, regardless of parity, the resulting rate (often called a reduced rate) is one that can be summed up over age or parity but may not be used for the analysis of parity progression.

Figures 1.11(a–d) present shaded contour maps for age-, period-, and order-specific reduced fertility rates in the United States. The figures give the reduced rates for first-, second-, third-, and fourth-order births, respectively. The data come from Heuser (1984) and were first presented in this way by Vaupel *et al.*, (1987). Since the denominators include all women, regardless of parity, the figures could be superimposed on each other and a summation would yield the combined fertility rates of orders 1 to 4.

At first glance, the figures show that fertility trends in the US between 1917 and 1980 differed significantly with respect to birth order. First births, i.e., births to women of parity zero, show very low degrees of fluctuation. It was only during the fertility increase immediately following World War II that first births played a major role in the general fertility trend. From that time until around 1970, the high intensity of first births around age 20 continued with no clearly pronounced peak at the height of the baby boom (around 1960). This peak, however, is very clear and pronounced for the fertility of women at parities 1 and 2. The intensities of second and third births for women in their twenties was even much higher around 1960 than in the first decades of the century. This is not true, however, for births of orders 4 to 6 (not given here) where the rates

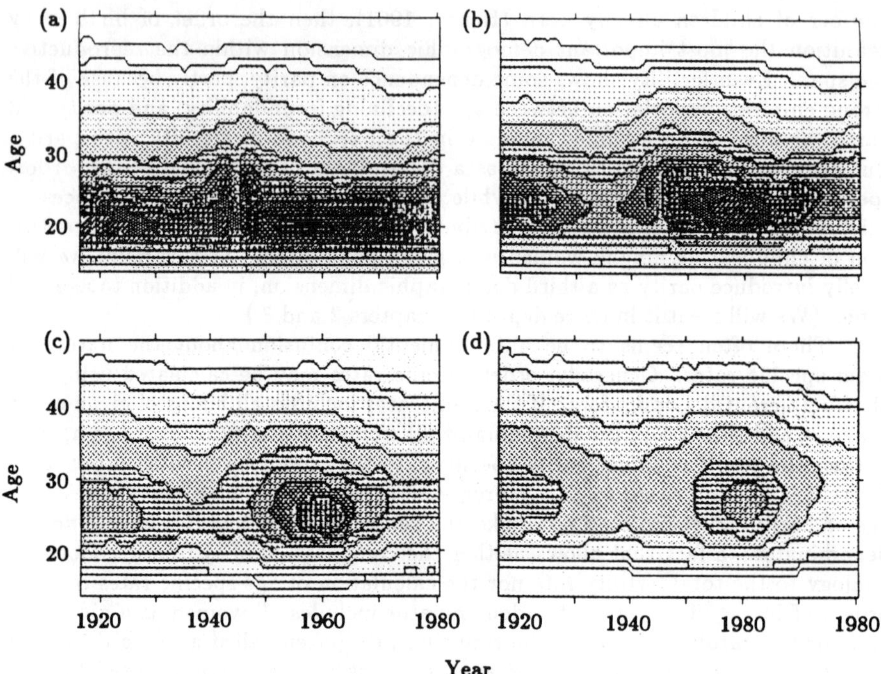

Figure 1.11. Shaded contour maps of US age-specific fertility rates 1917–1980 for births of order 1 (*a*), 2 (*b*), 3 (*c*), and 4 (*d*). (Source: Vaupel *et al.*, 1987.)

were higher around 1920 than around 1960. This confirms the often-stated assumption that the very high levels of period total fertility observed around 1960 (peaking in 1957 with a TFR of 3.7) can be attributed mainly to a higher incidence of second- and third-order births and only marginally to births of higher orders.

For high-fertility LDCs, similar time-series of age- and parity-specific fertility rates are not available, but period rates for the 1970s may be calculated from the WFS information. *Figure 1.12* presents the three-dimensional map of period parity-specific fertility rates for Kenya, the country with the highest current level of period fertility measured. Data come from the WFS and pertain to the third year before the survey. One axis of the contour map gives the continuous dimension of age while the other axis gives the discrete dimension of birth order, ranked from 1 to 15. The vertical axis refers to the age- and order-specific fertility rate. This graph is based on real order-specific rates where the denominator

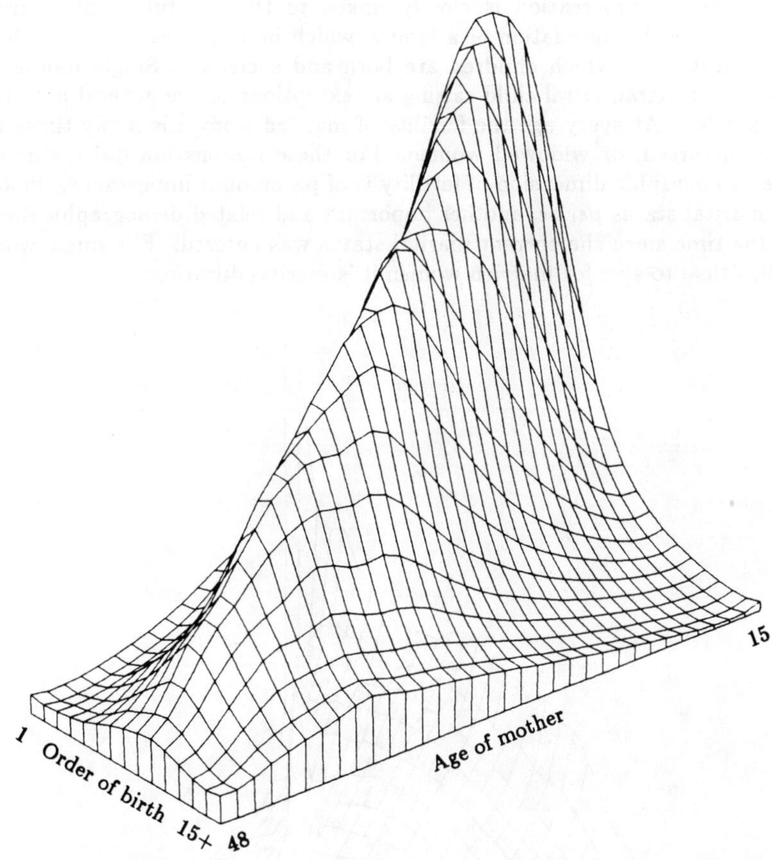

Figure 1.12. 3–D plot of age- and parity-specific fertility rates in Kenya. (Source: WFS.)

includes only women at risk of giving birth to the next order. The pattern – slightly smoothed to eliminate irregularities owing to small numbers of women in certain categories – is typical for an almost completely natural fertility situation. The graph clearly shows the strong positive correlation between age and order of birth. The reproductive pattern of the population is very homogeneous: most women follow the mainstream from a young age and low birth order to an older age and higher order. At age 48, this mainstream ends around the parities 9 and 10. The decline of the ridge with age and parity is a consequence of women dropping out of the reproductive process, most likely for involuntary biological reasons.

1.8. Duration of Marriage

In most societies procreation is closely linked to the institution of marriage.
Marriage means the foundation of a family, which in almost every society is the
major institution in which children are born and socialized. Single mothers or
other forms of extramarital child raising are exceptions to the general pattern in
most countries. At every age the fertility of married women is many times that
of single, divorced, or widowed women. For these reasons marital status as a
discrete demographic dimension of fertility is of paramount importance. In addition to marital status *per se*, another important and related demographic dimension is the time since the current marital status was entered. For single women
this is identical to age; for married women it is marital duration.

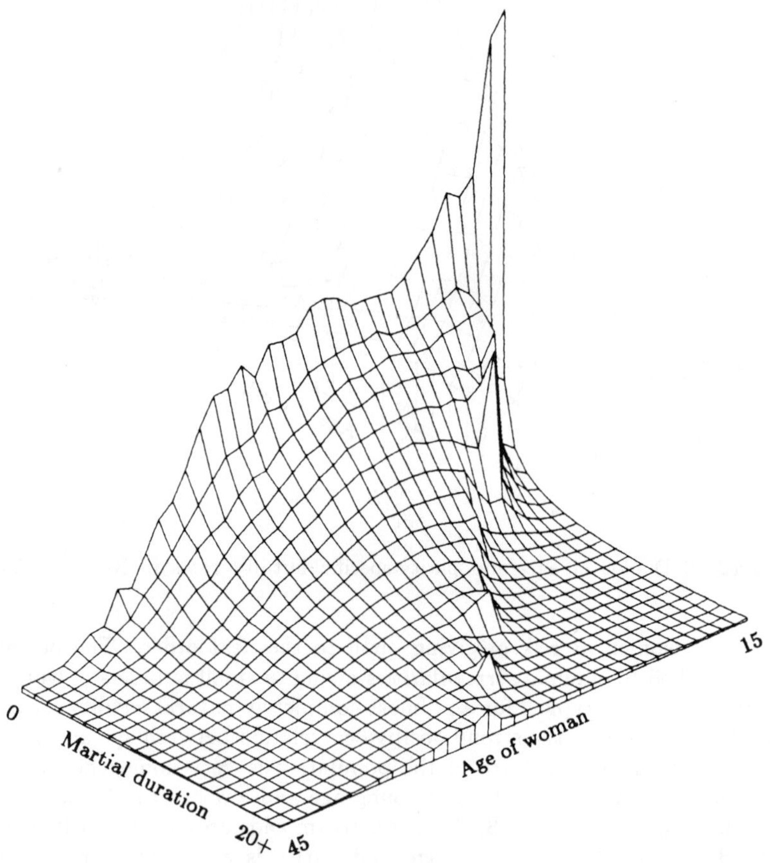

Figure 1.13. 3–D plot of female fertility rates specific for age and marital duration for
married Finnish women in 1984.

Why do we expect fertility to vary significantly according to marital duration? In all populations we may expect lower fecundability from women who have been married for a long time, on the one hand, and from those in the first years of marriage if their age at marriage is very low (i.e., 12 or 13), on the other. In societies with voluntary fertility control, however, the duration of marriage has a much more important direct effect on fertility. We know empirically that most couples in a modern society marry and have the few children that are intended in a relatively short range of years. Consequently, within the range of the prime childbearing ages we might reasonably expect marital duration to exert a more important influence on fertility than age – a notion that we will assess quantitatively in the last section of this chapter. Here, we give only a descriptive visual impression of the three-dimensional association among age, marital duration, and fertility.

Figures 1.13 and *1.14* are based on age-specific data for the married female population of Finland in 1984. The contour map in *Figure 1.14* gives an unsmoothed picture of the age- and duration-specific marital fertility rates, whereas the 3–D plot in *Figure 1.13* is slightly smoothed. There are two parts of the figures where the rates are zero. The triangle in the upper-left corner of the

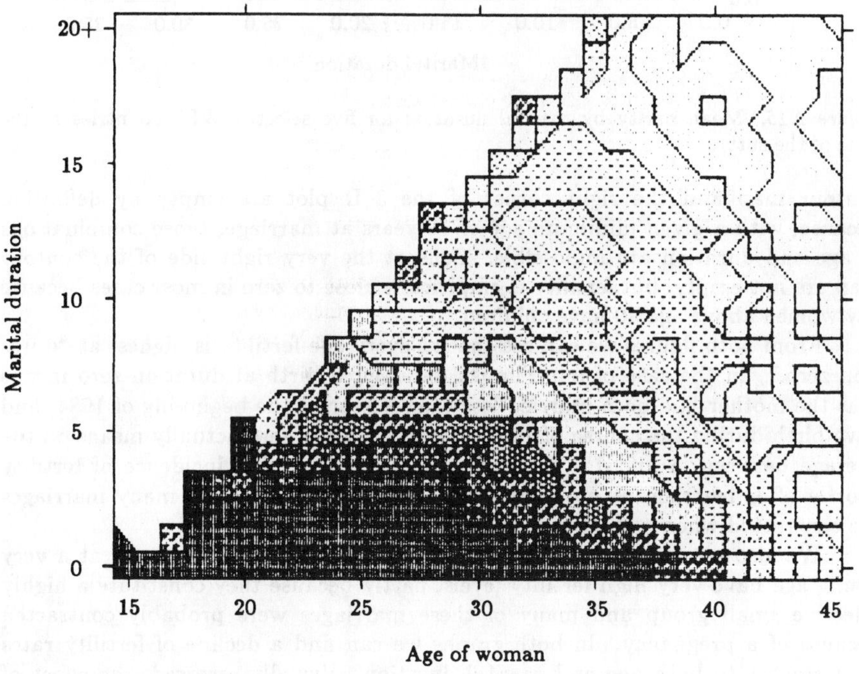

Figure 1.14. Shaded contour map of female fertility rates specific for age and marital duration for married Finnish women in 1984.

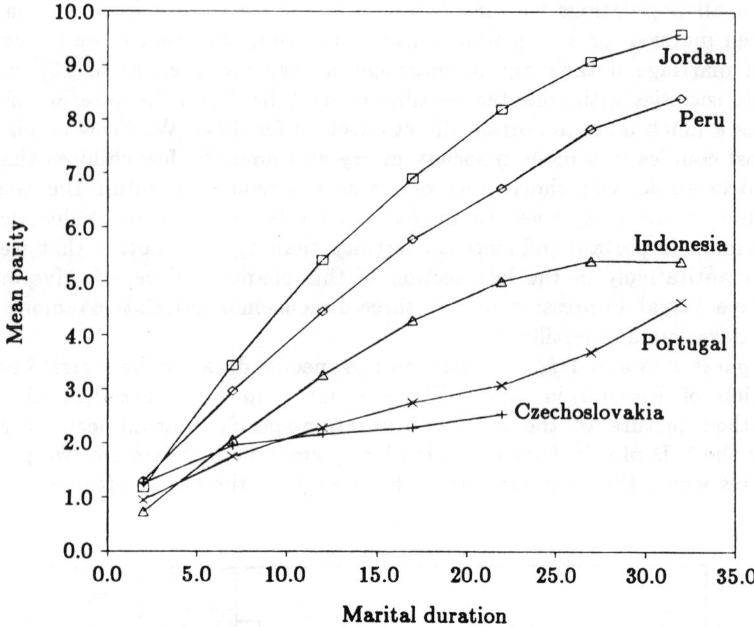

Figure 1.15. Mean parity by marital duration for five selected WFS countries at the time of the survey.

contour map and the right corner of the 3–D plot are empty by definition because, with a given minimum age of 15 years at marriage, those combinations of age and duration are impossible. Cells at the very right side of the contour map are not empty, but fertility is empirically close to zero in most cases because few women above age 40 have children.

From both figures we can see that at every age fertility is highest at "duration zero." In the case of our Finnish data set, a birth at duration zero means that the mother had been married less than a year at the beginning of 1984 and gave birth during the course of 1984. Thus, duration zero actually means on the average between .5 and 1.5 years of marriage. This high incidence of fertility shortly after marriage is not surprising when we consider how many marriages are contracted when a child is already on the way.

We also see from *Figures 1.13* and *1.14* that women who marry at a very young age have very high fertility levels, partly because they constitute a highly selective small group and many of these marriages were probably contracted because of a pregnancy. In both graphs we can find a decline of fertility rates with respect to both age and marital duration. Visually assessed, the effect of duration seems to be very strong during the prime childbearing ages where fertility at a given duration hardly varies with age; at higher ages and longer marital durations age seems to play a more important role. The quantitative analysis at the end will give us more exact information on this.

Figure 1.15 illustrates the effect of marital duration from a different perspective. It shows the cumulated fertility rate of synthetic marital duration cohorts in five selected countries participating in the WFS. The effect of age is not considered explicitly in this kind of presentation, but it is indirectly indicated through the given mean age at marriage. The concave shape of the curves in the near to natural fertility countries, Jordan and Peru, is due to declining fecundability with increasing age or higher parity or both. All curves increase monotonically. This is mathematically necessary for real cohorts only; if fertility fluctuates drastically, synthetic cohorts might show some discontinuities. From the shape of the curves and their end point in *Figure 1.15*, both the quantum aspect (i.e., level of fertility) and the speed of reproduction can be inferred: the end point to the right gives the average completed parity for the highest marital duration cohort, whereas the shape of the curve indicates how births are distributed over the years of marriage. A more detailed analysis of this kind for a larger set of countries will be conducted in Section 2.3.

1.9. Duration Since Last Birth

Another clock of individual time starts to run at the demographic event of a birth itself: the duration since that birth or the (open) birth interval. Unlike marital duration, which has no direct physiological effect on fertility, duration since last birth has both strong physiological and behavioral effects. Obviously, in a controlled fertility situation the behavioral components play the major role, whereas under a natural fertility regime physiological aspects are dominant. But even in a *perfect contraceptive society* important physiological components of the birth interval remain: the period of gestation can hardly be changed intentionally, and a short period of postpartum infecundability always remains. As a result, birth intervals shorter than 10 months are virtually impossible. Another important physiological component of the birth interval, especially in traditional societies, is the fertility inhibiting effect of breast-feeding. In the case of the Dobe!Kung bushpeople, long birth intervals through prolonged breast-feeding are the major reason for the low fertility under a regime that is still natural according to Henry's definition.

Abstinence by or separation of the parents for some period after birth is a traditional behavioral component of the birth interval. In modern societies deliberate spacing of births plays an important role. The spacing decisions are mostly governed by questions of the individual family life cycle, female career patterns, and psychological considerations of what birth intervals might be best for the children's mental development. In all societies birth intervals of more than seven years are rare exceptions, and even intervals of more than five years are unusual especially in high-fertility countries. This observation led to the measures of the quantum of fertility that are based on the duration since last birth to substitute for parity-progression ratios. One such measure is the *quintum* (see Hobcraft and McDonald, 1984), i.e., the proportion of women with additional births within five years after the birth of a given order. In low-fertility societies these measures become highly problematic because of the large

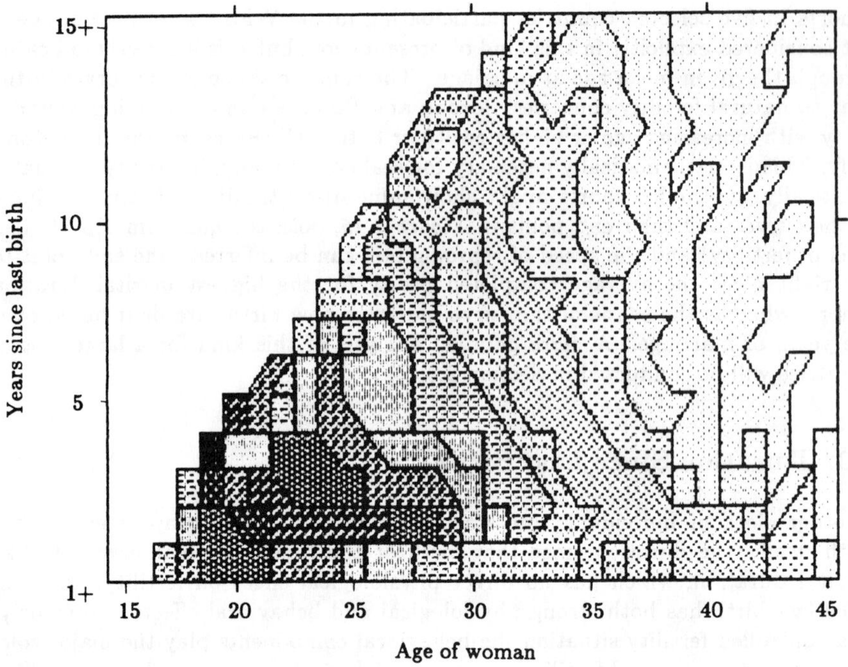

Figure 1.16. Shaded contour map of fertility rates specific for age and duration since last birth for all Finnish women with parity one or higher in 1984.

numbers of birth intervals longer than five years. Here, methods that estimate the quantum aspect of period fertility via parity-specific fertility rates (see Chapter 3) seem to be more appropriate.

This section will briefly illustrate some effects of the demographic fertility dimension duration since last birth, using the 1984 data from the Finnish population register. *Figures 1.16* and *1.17* give the distributions of fertility over the two-dimensional plane defined by age and time since last birth (*Figure 1.16*) and by marital duration and time since last birth (*Figure 1.17*). From the contour map we see that fertility is highly concentrated within a relatively short span of birth intervals. The peak fertility rates clearly appear for birth intervals between two and four years and within the age span of 20 to 30.[9] From this point fertility declines along both dimensions. The decrease that appears in the upper right corner is more symmetric than in the case of age and marital duration (see *Figure 1.14*). The pattern with respect to marital duration and the birth interval (see *Figure 1.17*) is quite similar except that very short marital durations seem to be associated with high fertility even at long birth intervals. These rates in the right corner of the 3–D graph pertain to the relatively few women who have had their last birth before their current marriage. These women are mostly divorcees and single mothers who, after remarrying, want to

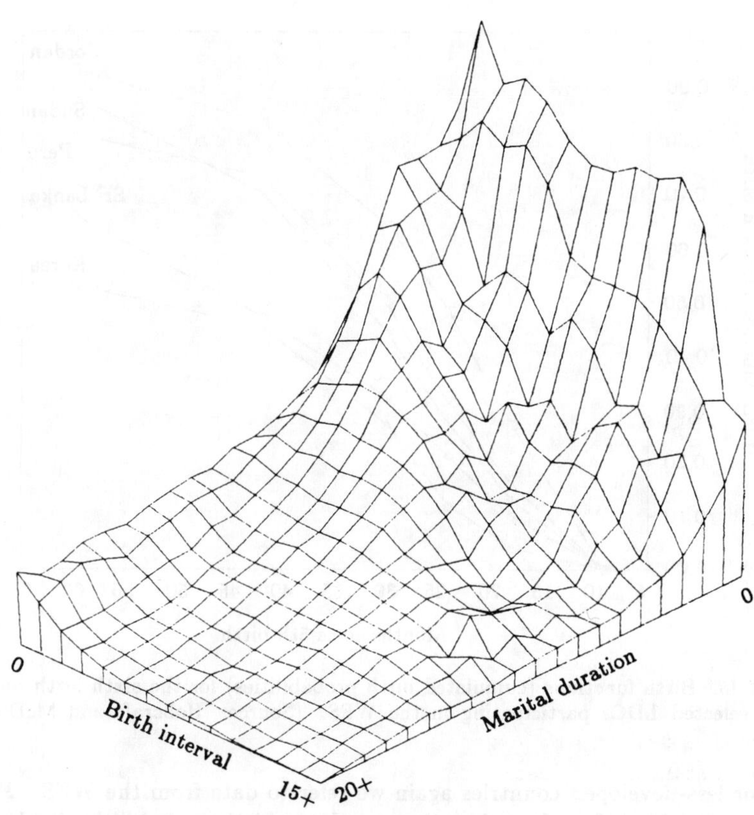

Figure 1.17. 3–D plot of fertility rates specific for marital duration and birth interval for all married Finnish women with parity one or higher.

have another child with their new partners very soon (or might even marry because of a pregnancy).

The majority of women, however, follows the regular pattern from high fertility at low marital durations and short birth intervals to low fertility in the shallow corner of *Figure 1.17.* If fertility rates were weighted by the number of women in the cells, the irregularities to the right would almost disappear. Another interesting irregularity is the fact that even at very high marital durations the probability of having an additional birth is moderately high at very short durations since last birth. In other words, if families have children at high marital durations they are likely to space them very close to each other. This phenomenon is owing to the small group of high-fertility women who continue to have babies.

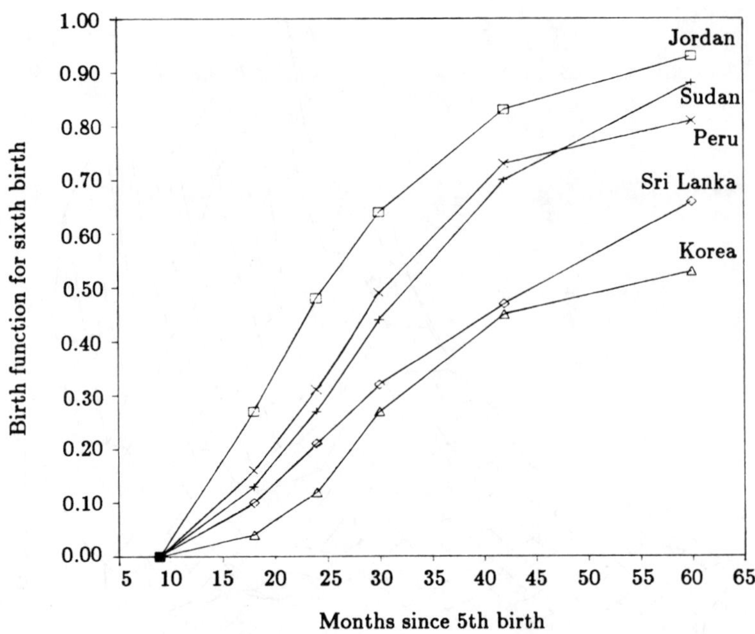

Figure 1.18. Birth functions (cumulated birth probabilities) for the sixth birth interval for five selected LDCs participating in the WFS. (Source: Hobcraft and McDonald, 1984.)

For less-developed countries again we refer to data from the WFS. *Figure 1.18* gives the birth functions, i.e., the cumulated birth probabilities in the first 60 months of the sixth birth interval. The figure indicates that at short durations since the fifth birth, functions for very high-fertility countries are already high while others remain lower from the beginning. Sometimes, there can be crossovers in the birth functions, e.g., in the case where Sudan passes Peru about four years after the fifth birth. South Korea starts out much slower than Sri Lanka in the first two years after birth but in 3.5 years reaches almost the same cumulated probability of an additional birth as Sri Lanka. As discussed above, the level of the birth function 60 months after the last birth gives some hint on the parity-progression ratio, which would be around .9 in Jordan and .5 in South Korea. However, only few countries show a leveling off in the birth function that would justify the use of the *quintum* of fertility as a proxy for the parity-progression ratio. Especially in Peru and Sri Lanka the slope of the curve between 42 and 60 months after the births is almost as steep as that of shorter durations since the last birth.

1.10. Father's Characteristics

One of the most basic facts in life is that two persons, a woman and a man, are always needed to give life to a new person. The reasons demographic analysis has been exclusively concerned with the mother's characteristics were discussed in Section 1.2. The lack of data on the father and father's individual time, e.g., age and marital duration, is also a major constraint. An exception is the data from the Finnish population register. It includes men and, hence, may be used for the analysis of male fertility.

Figure 1.19 gives the age-specific fertility rates for all men and women in Finland in 1984. The shape of the male curve is very similar to that of the

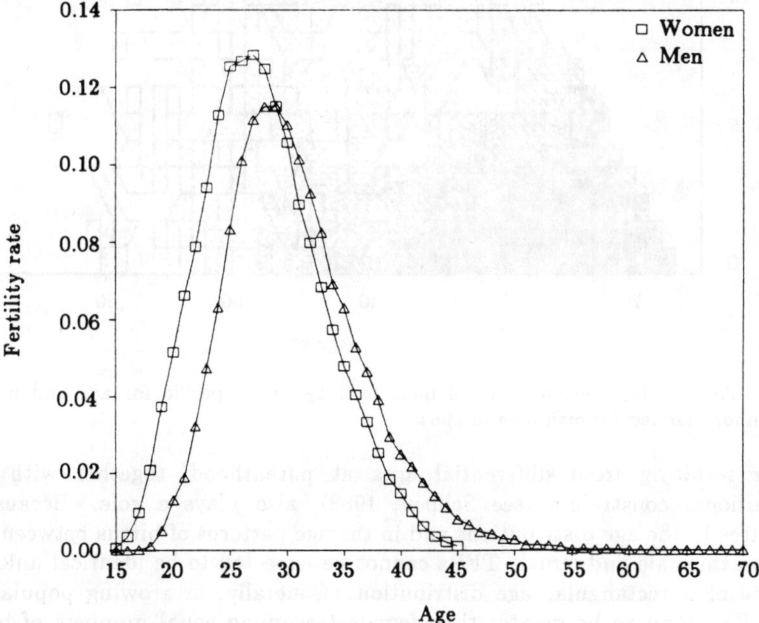

Figure 1.19. Male and female age-specific fertility rates in Finland, 1984.

female curve of fertility. Peak fertility rates are somewhat lower than those of women, and the curve is shifted to the right by about 3 to 4 years. Because the number of births linked to fathers is about 6% less than the number of births born to women in Finland in 1984, the male fertility rates are somewhat biased downward. Illegitimate births where the father is not declared and, in some cases, births where the father is abroad account for this discrepancy. The percentage of births without information on the father is about the same in several other European countries (see UN *Demographic Yearbook*, 1975).

A summation of all age-specific fertility rates yields a female total fertility rate (TFR) of 1.70 as opposed to a male TFR of 1.52. Although part of this discrepancy can be explained by the 6% of births with unknown fathers, the *birth*

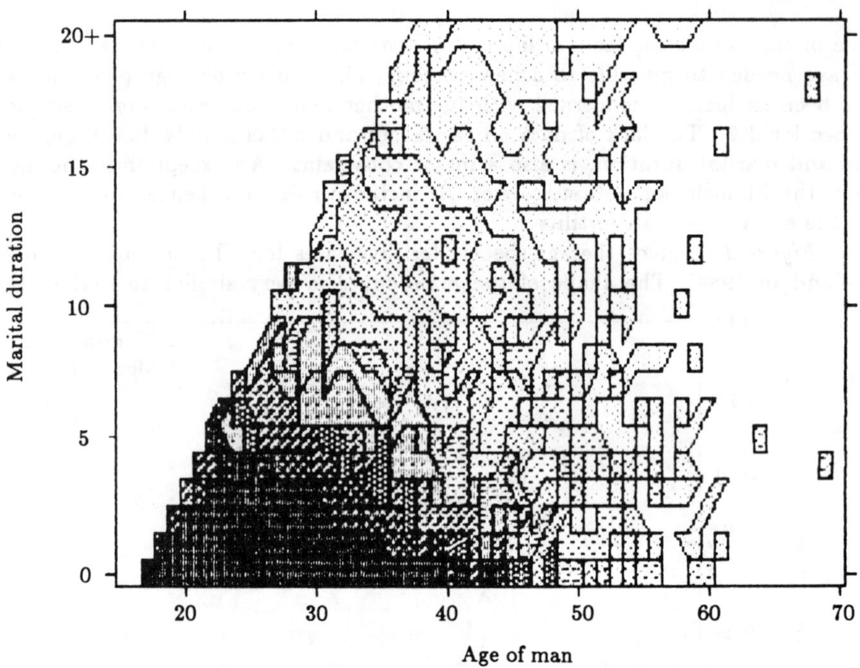

Figure 1.20. Shaded contour map of male fertility rates specific for age and marital duration for married Finnish men in 1984.

squeeze resulting from differential ages at parenthood, together with age-distributional constraints (see Schoen, 1988), also plays a role. Because of differences in the age distributions and in the age patterns of births between men and women, male and female TFRs cannot be expected to be identical unless in the case of a rectangular age distribution. Generally, in growing populations male TFRs tend to be greater than female (assuming equal numbers of births registered for men and women), whereas in shrinking populations the TFRs are of comparable size or the female is higher than the male (see Schoen, 1988).

From *Figure 1.19* we also see that above age 40 male fertility declines less sharply than female fertility, and the highest age at which sizable fertility rates can be measured is around 55. Although it is physiologically possible to become a father over the age of 55, empirical fertility rates are almost equal to zero.

Figures 1.20 and *1.21* illustrate the two-dimensional distributions of marital male fertility over age and marital duration. Again, the pattern is not significantly different from that of female fertility, it is only stretched out along the age dimension and shifted a few years to the right (compare with *Figures 1.13* and *1.14*). The figures indicate that men who have children over age 45 are mostly men that had recently married, i.e., have short durations of marriage. For married couples the marital durations for men and women are identical, so no difference between men and women should appear with respect to marital

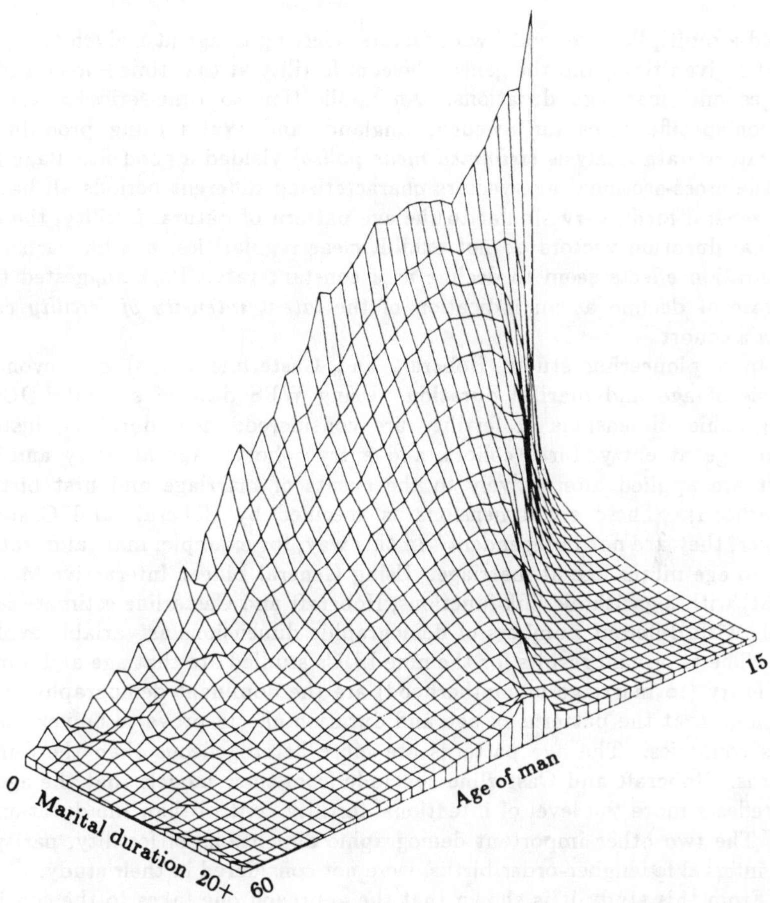

Figure 1.21. 3–D plot of male fertility rates specific for age and marital duration for married Finnish men in 1984.

duration. Hence, the marginal distribution with respect to marital duration is the same, and the interest of our analysis lies in the differential distribution of a given duration-specific fertility over age. The following section gives a quantitative assessment of the effects of demographic dimensions and sheds more light on this issue.

1.11. Estimating the Relative Effects of the Demographic Dimensions of Fertility

1.11.1. Logit models for female fertility

Demographers have demonstrated only recently the independent influences of both age and marital duration on fertility rates (Page, 1977; Gilks, 1979). Page applied a multiplicative model with factors referring to age at a given time, duration at a given time, and the general level of fertility at that time – averaged over all ages and marriage durations. An application to time-series of age- and duration-specific rates for Sweden, England, and Wales using procedures of exploratory data analysis (*trimmed mean polish*) yielded a good fit. Page found that the cross-sectional age vectors characterizing different periods all have the same general form, very similar to the age pattern of natural fertility; the cross-sectional duration vectors do not exhibit clear regularities, but for each cohort the duration effects seem to decline at a constant rate. Page suggested taking this rate of decline as an indication of the *latent intensity of fertility control* within a cohort.

In a pioneering study, Hobcraft and Casterline (1983) go beyond the analysis of age and marital duration. Using WFS data of several LDCs, six demographic dimensions of fertility are considered: age, duration, historical period, age at entry, birth cohort, and entry cohort. Age at entry and entry cohort are applied alternatively to the events of marriage and first birth (or motherhood). These six dimensions as specified by Hobcraft and Casterline; however, they are not independent. In this way, for example, marital duration is equal to age minus age-at-marriage. Using General Linear Interactive Modeling (GLIM) with logarithmic link functions, Hobcraft and Casterline estimate several models with different numbers of demographic dimensions as variable explainations. The two main results for the nine LDCs studied are that age and duration since entry (to marriage or motherhood) are the dominant demographic dimensions, and that the patterns of age and duration effects prove to be very similar across countries. The age patterns are more heterogeneous than the duration patterns. Hobcraft and Casterline conclude from their models that the age pattern reflects more the level of intentional fertility control than the duration pattern. The two other important demographic dimensions of fertility, parity and birth interval for higher-order births, were not considered in their study.

From this study it is shown that the approach one takes to the consideration of simultaneous effects of several demographic dimensions is highly dependent on the structure of available data. While Page used time-series data from official vital registration and Hobcraft and Casterline used retrospective data from sample surveys, this model will be based on the Finnish population register observing the events over one calendar year. This setting is not appropriate for cohort analysis, and past events such as the age at marriage could only be inferred. For this reason a clear period approach is taken considering independent demographic dimensions as they are measured at the beginning of 1984. The three continuous demographic dimensions of fertility that will be studied are age, marital duration, and duration since last birth. The models were calculated for all women and men and also separately for women of specific parities.

The models were all fitted using GLIM (release 3.77) with a logistic link function between the specific birth probability and the independent variables of age, marital duration, and birth interval that were entered in the form of dummy variables to allow the analysis of effects specific for single years of individual time.[10]   An appropriate measure for the performance of the model and its goodness of fit is the scaled deviance.[11]

Because of limited space it is only possible to present selected results from the numerous models. The parity-specific models are especially complex to discuss, but they can be summarized by stating that for lower-order births the results are quite similar to the total, whereas for higher-order births the patterns for age and duration shift in the expected direction toward higher ages and longer durations. Rather than introduce too many numerical results, we will emphasize and interpret the conversion of the resulting parameters to meaningful probabilities.

Table 1.1 gives the resulting parameter estimates for women for four different models. The values presented are those resulting from the estimation procedure and are still on the log (odds) scale. The first column lists the three demographic dimensions considered. In each model the dummy variable of the first category (e.g., age 15) was omitted, its value is given by the constant; all other parameters give the deviation from the constant. The second column (*Model Ia-c*) gives the results from different and completely independent runs where only one dimension was considered. In other words, the effects given for age in column 2 come from a model in which age was the only explanatory variable of fertility rates, similarly for marital duration and duration since last birth. The column head also indicates to which universe of women the model was applied. Column 3 (*Model II*) gives the result of a model where age and duration were considered simultaneously. In columns 4 and 5 the two other possible combinations of age plus birth interval and duration plus birth interval are given.[12] In columns 3 through 5 the constant always stands for the combination of the two lowest categories, e.g., age 15 at duration zero in *Model III*.

For models including birth intervals, only women with at least one child were selected and birth intervals of 0 were omitted because of coding problems with the data set. For models including marital duration, the analysis was restricted to married women. When only age was considered all Finnish women between ages 15 and 49 were included. To compare more thoroughly the estimates of the simultaneous effects of two dimensions (*Models II* to *IV* based alternatively on the populations of all women and all married women) and the estimates for a one-dimensional setup (*Model Ia-c*), column 2 gives the coefficients for the two universes of married women and all women.

Although some patterns can be readily detected from the table, most of the interpretation needs a combination and transformation of parameters. To calculate the probability of birth, e.g., for women aged 20 at marital duration 3 (*Model II*), one adds together the constant and the parameters of age 20 and duration 3. Because this is still the logarithm of the odds ratio, further algebraic transformation is needed to get the probability, which is .235 in this example. The following figures present a selected series of probabilities for one dimension when controlling for another.

Table 1.1. Relative effects of age, marital duration, and year since last birth on the fertility of Finnish women in 1984 (coefficients from a logit model).

	Each effect considered separately (Model Ia)		Combined effects		
			Age and marital duration (Model II)	Age and year since last birth (Model III)	Marital duration and year since last birth (Model IV)
Age					
	All	Married	Married	All	Married
Scaled deviance	9750	13847	627	2200	3630
Constant	-0.6931	7.226	9.227	-0.6931	
16	-0.4855	-6.938	-8.678	-0.2393	
17	-0.9014	-7.462	-9.292	-0.4618	
18	-0.5315	-7.544	-9.255	-0.1120	
19	-0.5699	-7.585	-9.199	-0.06310	
20	-0.6323	-7.902	-9.455	-0.09005	
21	-0.6570	-8.020	-9.503	-0.07245	
22	-0.7190	-8.184	-9.601	-0.1010	
23	-0.8009	-8.244	-9.597	-0.1442	
24	-0.8093	-8.283	-9.555	-0.1290	
25	-0.8736	-8.324	-9.508	-0.1676	
26	-0.9854	-8.470	-9.547	-0.2490	
27	-1.060	-8.568	-9.544	-0.2917	
28	-1.147	-8.682	-9.550	-0.3384	
29	-1.269	-8.829	-9.578	-0.4203	
30	-1.351	-8.966	-9.599	-0.4597	
31	-1.569	-9.201	-9.717	-0.6208	
32	-1.703	-9.347	-9.752	-0.6989	
33	-1.869	-9.548	-9.834	-0.8030	
34	-2.050	-9.748	-9.938	-0.9208	
35	-2.272	-9.954	-10.03	-1.072	
36	-2.443	-10.12	-10.10	-1.166	
37	-2.664	-10.36	-10.23	-1.315	
38	-2.941	-10.65	-10.44	-1.506	
39	-3.320	-10.98	-10.69	-1.796	
40	-3.603	-11.24	-10.84	-1.998	
41	-4.041	-11.59	-11.13	-2.364	
42	-4.574	-12.09	-11.55	-2.805	
43	-5.326	-12.61	-12.02	-3.487	
44	-5.866	-13.08	-12.43	-3.937	
45	-7.267	-13.72	-13.04	-5.277	
46	-7.806	-14.36	-13.64	-5.749	
47	-9.334	-15.50	-14.75	-7.229	
48	-12.31	-20.04	-22.24	-12.03	
49	-11.90	-19.92	-22.12	-11.61	
50	-11.79	-19.73	-21.94	-11.43	

1.11.2. Interpretation of the logit coefficients

Figure 1.22 plots the age-specific birth probabilities for married women in Finland in 1984, controlling for marital duration, based on results of *Model II*. The figure clearly shows that lower marital duration means higher birth probabilities

Table 1.1. Continued.

Marital duration	Each effect considered separately (Model Ib)	Combined effects		
		Age and marital duration (Model II)	Age and year since last birth (Model III)	Marital duration and year since last birth (Model IV)
	Married	Married		Married
Scaled deviance	8439			
Constant	-0.4301	–		-0.08762
1	-0.5942	-0.5971		-0.7084
2	-0.7086	-0.6881		-0.5188
3	-0.8117	-0.7795		-0.6101
4	-1.020	-0.9692		-0.7825
5	-1.221	-1.156		-0.9454
6	-1.468	-1.383		-1.189
7	-1.638	-1.530		-1.336
8	-1.864	-1.715		-1.523
9	-2.019	-1.819		-1.630
10	-2.213	-1.958		-1.781
11	-2.402	-2.082		-1.927
12	-2.537	-2.149		-1.996
13	-2.738	-2.266		-2.132
14	-2.917	-2.354		-2.237
15	-3.191	-2.513		-2.429
16	-3.515	-2.707		-2.624
17	-3.693	-2.736		-2.703
18	-3.996	-2.854		-2.882
19	-4.450	-3.077		-3.179
20+	-5.719	-3.095		-4.009

Years since last birth[a]	(Model Ic)		(Model II)	(Model III)	(Model IV)
	All	Married		All	Married
Scaled deviance	13124	16496			
Constant	-1.156	-1.041		–	–
2	-0.9619	-0.9124		-0.9459	-0.8727
3	-0.6928	-0.6152		-0.5961	-0.4379
4	-0.9495	-0.8650		-0.7661	-0.5062
5	-1.206	-1.127		-0.9271	-0.5834
6	-1.543	-1.483		-1.168	-0.7685
7	-1.718	-1.674		-1.255	-0.8103
8	-1.903	-1.857		-1.345	-0.8689
9	-2.147	-2.097		-1.484	-1.002
10	-2.414	-2.388		-1.639	-1.179
11	-2.564	-2.495		-1.671	-1.182
12	-2.833	-2.796		-1.809	-1.362
13	-3.006	-3.002		-1.840	-1.454
14	-3.266	-3.257		-1.938	-1.580
15	-3.644	-3.646		-2.135	-1.845

[a]Only women with parity 1 or more.

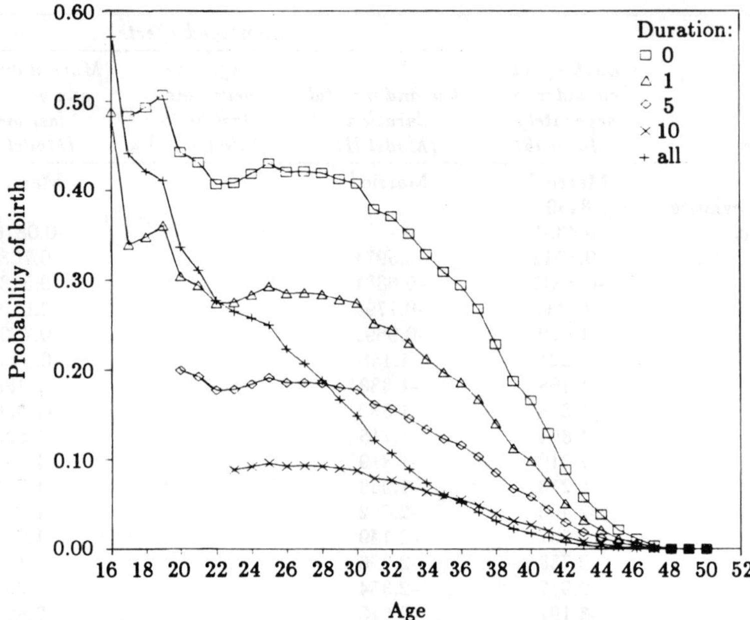

Figure 1.22. Estimated probabilities of age-specific female fertility for selected marital durations in 1984.

at all ages. The decline seems to be steepest between durations zero and one. *Figure 1.23* demonstrates that for durations one to four the decline is also somewhat slower than for the higher durations up to about eight years. Below age 20 the pattern is irregular because the number of women married at that age is very small and selective. To a demographer the most exciting finding from this graph is that the curve of age-specific fertility at low marital durations and especially at duration zero is concave to the origin such as that in a completely natural fertility population without fertility control. And, indeed, it is very plausible that even in a modern society in which contraceptives are easily accessible, fertility within the first years of marriage is practically uncontrolled even for women above age 35. The figure shows that newly married women in their late thirties have significantly higher fertility rates than other married women at the same age. This high fertility rate appearing at low durations even for older women shows that marriage and childbearing are closely related even in an industrialized society with low fertility levels.

To illustrate the difference between the general pattern for age-specific marital fertility and that for women with short marital durations, *Figure 1.22* also plots the age pattern for women of all marital durations. The figure shows that the rate of decrease with age is initially steeper for all married women, and the line actually crosses the curves duration. The statistical reason for these

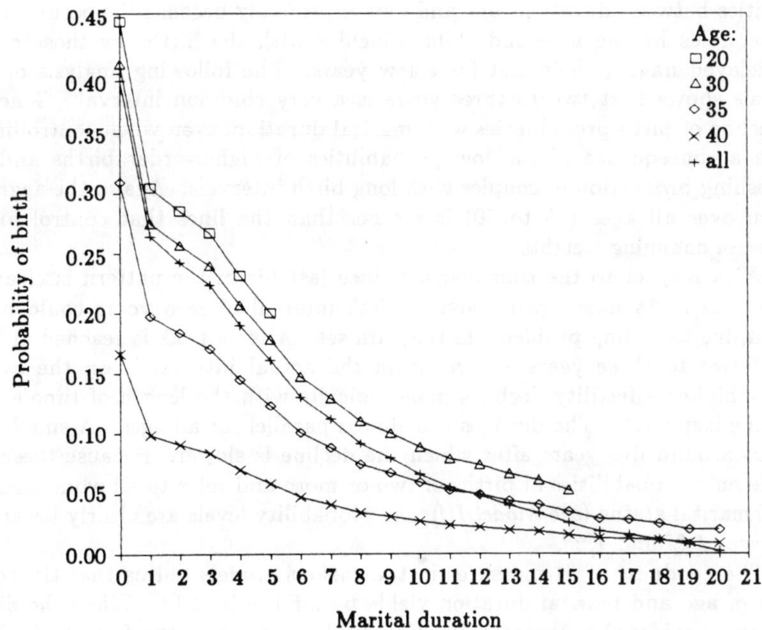

Figure 1.23. Estimated probabilities of marital duration-specific female fertility for selected age groups.

crossovers lies in the change of weights with age: women in their early twenties with short marital duration and therefore high fertility dominate the picture, whereas, there are few newly wed women in their late thirties, and their relatively high fertility has little impact on the total level. From this it can be concluded that marital duration has a very significant impact on fertility. If the lines that control for duration were horizontal then the picture would be completely dominated by duration and an age effect appearing in the aggregate distribution including all durations would be an artifact caused only by the change in the marital duration composition of the population. As we see, this is almost the case between ages 20 and 30. After that, however, fertility declines as age increases, even at fixed marital durations.

Figure 1.23 turns the perspective around and looks at the fertility patterns along the dimension of marital duration when controlling for age. A distinct pattern seems to apply for all ages: fertility is by far the highest at duration zero (here again duration zero actually means a duration that is on average .5 to 1.5 years), declines sharply at duration one, and then shows a monotonic decline that is steepest between durations three and eight. This pattern is more pronounced at younger ages. It is not difficult to speculate on the reasons for this pattern. In Finland – as in many other European countries – marriages are often contracted because the woman is already pregnant; also, many conceptions probably take place shortly after marriage. Hence, the high level at duration zero and the decline to duration one is plausible; the slower decline in birth intensities between durations one and four is probably because the occurrences of those couples having a second child coincides with the births by those couples who delayed having their first for a few years. The following analysis of birth intervals shows that two to three years is a very common interval. Generally, the decline of birth probabilities with marital duration, even when controlling for age, is a consequence of the low probabilities of higher-order births and of a diminishing proportion of couples with long birth intervals. Again, the aggregate pattern over all ages (15 to 50) is steeper than the lines that control for age because of changing weights.

With respect to the time elapsed since last birth, the pattern is clear (see *Figure 1.24*). As mentioned above a birth interval of zero years could not be studied due to coding problems in the data set. After a peak is reached at intervals of two to three years – here again the actual interval is on the average slightly higher – fertility declines monotonically with the length of time elapsed since the last birth. The declines are almost parallel for all ages. A small notch appears around five years after which the decline is slower. Because these data include only probabilities of births of two or more and refer to all women regardless of marital status (see *Model III*), the probability levels are clearly lower than in *Figures 1.22* and *1.23*.

The goodness of fit measures in the various models tell us that the combination of age and marital duration yields by far the best fit. When the dimensions are considered separately duration explains more of the fertility variation than age. The explainatory effect of age, however, is improved when treating the population of all women with at least parity one; conversely the explaination of marital duration weakens somewhat when restricting the population to all married women with at least parity one. This is obviously because of the especially strong association between marriage and first birth, a dominant feature of the fertility pattern.

1.11.3. Logit models for male fertility

Table 1.2 gives the results of the logit model as described above for assessing the relative effects of age and marital duration for Finnish men in 1984. The pattern of the table for men is very similar to that for women (see *Table 1.1, Model II*), only stretched along the age dimension. *Figure 1.25* gives the male birth probabilities by age controlling for marital duration. It shows that the initial irregularities occurring at a young age last up to age 21 for men. The few men who were married before age 20 had an even higher fertility than the very young women. Around age 25 an insignificant local minimum appears that is hard to explain and might be because of some period fluctuations. Over age 27 fertility declines at all durations until birth probabilities are close to zero beyond age 55. An interesting detail is that between age 50 and 55 the steep decline in fertility of men at duration zero seems to come to a short hold, indicating that the men who have children at that age are to a large extent newly wed.

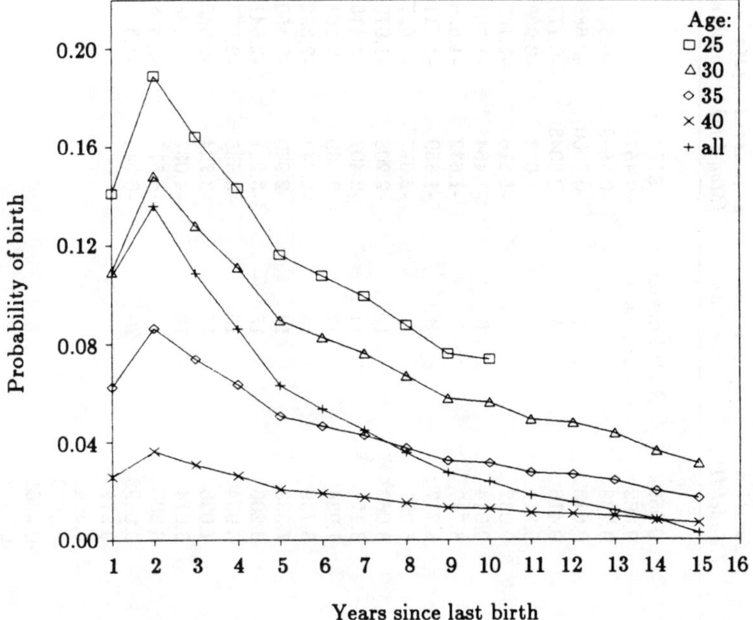

Figure 1.24. Estimated probabilities of female fertility specific for time since last birth for selected age groups.

1.11.4. Conclusion

All the models of male and female fertility were separately tested for significance, and chi-square tests were applied to the differences in scaled deviance with the given difference in degrees of freedom. The results were compared, and may be summarized in the following way: for every model presented the reduction in deviance owing to the inclusion of a second dimension into a model that already included another dimension was highly significant (at a probability level of .995). In other words, the Finnish data give extremely strong evidence that there is a real effect of marital duration on fertility in addition to age, of birth interval in addition to age, of duration in addition to birth interval, of age in addition to marital duration, etc. This test, however, only concerns the complete dimensions including all ages, all durations, and all intervals. It does not give us information about the relative importance of dimensions restricted to partial age spans, selected duration spans, etc. There is no reason not to conduct such tests, although in practice it would require innumerable models that need to be fitted, a task that goes beyond the objective here. On the basis of the presentation of estimated patterns of probabilities (see *Figures 1.13* to *1.25*), however, one can make inferences on the change of relative importance at various ages or durations. One such example is fertility at duration zero (see *Figure 1.23*) between the ages 20 and 30 remains virtually constant with respect to age.

Table 1.2. Relative effects of age and marital duration on the fertility of married Finnish men in 1984 (coefficients from logit model).

Age	Only age considered (Model Ia)	Combined effects of age and marital duration (Model II)	Age continued	Only age considered (Model Ia)	Combined effects of age and marital duration (Model II)	Marital duration	Only marital duration considered (Model Ib)	(Model II) continued
Scaled deviance	17916	953	41	8.569	9.959	Scaled deviance	8770	–
Constant	-12.11	-11.06	42	8.326	9.862	Constant	-0.4574	–
16	–	–	43	8.090	9.728	1	-0.5859	-0.5913
17	20.37	20.32	44	7.852	9.6132	2	-0.7000	-0.6883
18	11.89	11.06	45	7.546	9.416	3	-0.8043	-0.7775
19	11.97	11.18	46	7.374	9.311	4	-1.013	-0.9682
20	11.64	10.96	47	6.991	9.032	5	-1.216	-1.152
21	11.40	10.77	48	6.872	9.014	6	-1.464	-1.381
22	11.36	10.79	49	6.565	8.749	7	-1.632	-1.526
23	11.28	10.77	50	6.451	8.717	8	-1.859	-1.711
24	11.16	10.69	51	5.749	8.027	9	-2.017	-1.827
25	11.14	10.75	52	5.688	8.062	10	-2.208	-1.970
26	11.12	10.81	53	5.720	8.127	11	-2.407	-2.115
27	11.01	10.79	54	5.425	7.924	12	-2.539	-2.191
28	10.88	10.76	55	4.246	6.739	13	-2.743	-2.332
29	10.76	10.75	56	4.768	7.338	14	-2.930	-2.450
30	10.61	10.71	57	3.627	6.206	15	-3.211	-2.641
31	10.44	10.67	58	4.321	6.954	16	-3.538	-2.877
32	10.28	10.62	59	4.379	7.026	17	-3.724	-2.955
33	10.11	10.57	60	3.403	6.074	18	-4.037	-3.146
34	9.887	10.46	61	3.495	6.200	19	-4.513	-3.498
35	9.750	10.45	62	-0.6654	-0.6893	20+	-6.641	-4.304
36	9.542	10.35	63	-0.5523	-0.5727			
37	9.386	10.30	64	2.512	5.304			
38	9.187	10.23	65	-0.2426	-0.2613			
39	8.882	10.03	66	-0.3076	-0.3261			
40	8.697	9.971	67	-0.1046	-0.1043			
			68	2.759	5.562			
			69	2.744	5.559			

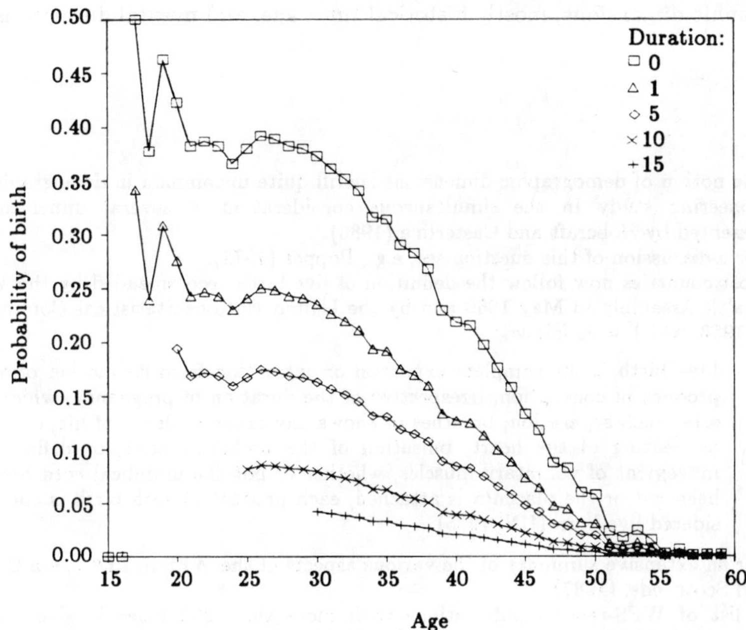

Figure 1.25. Estimated probabilities of male age-specific fertility for selected marital durations.

1.12. Summary

To speak of demographic dimensions is still uncommon among demographers. Few authors (e.g., Hobcraft and Casterline, 1983) have explicitly referred to this notion. We believe that the rather general concept of seeing a demographic event registered in a space defined by various demographic and non-demographic dimensions is very helpful to understand the basic philosophy of the approach of measurement one uses and to recognize it as one possibility. It seems to be a concept that is also wide enough to cover all the demographic approaches taken so far and could help to clarify more difficult questions such as the age-period-cohort question.

Aside from the conceptual issue, this chapter attempted to give a short substantive empirical survey of the major demographic dimensions of fertility in developing and industrialized societies. The empirical material had to be highly selective, but, in trying to pick out both typical and atypical cases, it is to be hoped that most of the range of fertility variations existing today could be covered.

In some ways fertility is distributed along each of the demographic dimensions. The rest of this study, however, is primarily concerned with the dimension parity, its distributions, and its consequences. The following three chapters will focus primarily on parity distribution, but at every point of the analysis – even for the definition of what is to be explained – more information about other demographic dimensions, mostly historical time, age, and marital duration is still needed.

Notes

[1]   The notion of demographic dimensions is still quite uncommon in demography. A pioneering study in the simultaneous consideration of several dimensions is presented by Hobcraft and Casterline (1983).

[2]   For a discussion of this question see, e.g., Popper (1972).

[3]   Most countries now follow the definition of live birth recommended by the World Health Assembly in May 1950 and by the United Nations Statistical Commission in 1953, which is as follows:

> Live birth is the complete expulsion or extraction from its mother of a product of conception, irrespective of the duration of pregnancy, which after such separation, breathes or shows any other evidence of life, such as beating of the heart, pulsation of the umbilical cord, or definite movement of voluntary muscles, whether or not the umbilical cord has been cut or the placenta is attached; each product of such birth is considered live-born (UN, 1955).

[4]   For an extensive summary of the various aspects of the WFS in LDCs, see Cleland and Scott, eds. (1987).

[5]   A list of WFS-related publications with more than 200 titles is given in the Appendix of Cleland and Scott, eds. (1987).

[6]   The 3–D plots given in this study are axometry and not genuine 3–D perspectives since the lines of the skirt do not get closer as the image retreats into the distance. For our purpose of identifying major patterns, however, this is not a problem.

[7]   This graph is based on annual information for five-year age groups. Single-year age groups were calculated by interpolation. (Source: Lutz, 1987b.)

[8]   A more comprehensive comparison of eight countries for which longer time-series of age-specific data are available is given in Lutz and Yashin (1987).

[9]   As with age and marital duration, a birth interval measured as, for example, 2 at the beginning of 1984, could indicate an actual birth interval of between 2.0 to almost 4.0 years by the time a child is born in 1984. Because of a coding problem in the data set, we do not have unambiguous information on birth interval zero, which was left out for this reason.

[10]   For the logistic link function a binomial error structure taking the exposure as an offset and using a maximum likelihood approach is known as iterative weighted least squares. For more information about the mathematics of this type of model and about GLIM in general, see Payne (1985).

[11]   Because the deviations of the data points from those predicted by the model must be weighted according to both the size of the denominators and the values fitted by the model, several cycles are required using the old estimates to obtain better ones. After the process has converged to a given degree of accuracy, the deviance, which is an appropriate function of the weighted residuals, indicates how good a fit the model gives. The scaled deviance is particularly useful to compare models because we know (see Kendall and Stuart, 1967) that the difference between deviances follows (asymptotically) a chi-squared distribution with the difference between the degrees of freedom as the degrees-of-freedom parameter.

[12] A simultaneous consideration of all three dimensions was not conducted because it would be excessive in terms of computer space and time, and the results would be extremely difficult to interpret.

CHAPTER 2

The Quantum and Tempo of Cohort Fertility: A Comparative View of 55 WFS Countries

2.1. Methodological Considerations

In an analysis of completed fertility patterns only women who are beyond their reproductive age may be considered. For these women the fertility history reported in the survey is not truncated by the interview. The only assumptions to be made concern the accuracy of the information given in the interview and the absence of selectivity with respect to fertility. Such records of women beyond reproductive age allow a very detailed analysis of the tempo and quantum of fertility in birth cohorts.

This section focuses on the quantum aspect and does not include an explicit time dimension. The implicit aspect of time lies in the fact that the process of female marital fertility is assumed to begin at the time of marriage and to last until sometime between the ages 40–49. For the lack of data on non-marital fertility in many WFS-countries this chapter only looks at the reproductive patterns of women who had married by the age of 40. Hence, it includes information on premarital fertility, but it does not give data on the fertility of women who never married.

Empirically, the basic source of information is the tabulation of the number of children ever born. These data on the quantum aspect of reproduction can be easily transformed into tables of successive parity-progression ratios. In this study the information has been arranged on the quantum of completed cohort fertility in a tabular form homomorphic to a life table, where parity is the indexing variable. These tables are straightforward, useful to the description of parity progression, and contain almost all important information. The data to construct the tables for each country in the WFS are given in Appendix A, and the text summarizes and discusses them. However, first a brief explanation of their presentation will be given.

Using Kenya's parity-progression table as an example, (see *Table 2.1*), it is easy to see the way in which it is analogous to an ordinary life table. Age is replaced by parity as the indexing variable; survival from one age to another becomes parity progression; the survival probabilities become parity-progression ratios, denoted here as $p(i)$. The complementary probability, i.e., the probability of dying in the normal life table, becomes the probability of remaining at a certain parity, i.e., dropping out of the process of parity progression. The element common to the approach of the fertility table based on parity and the ordinary life table is that they both refer to the probability that a person will leave the process at a certain stage (age or parity).

Table 2.1. Parity-progression table for Kenya.

Parity i	Parity-progression ratio $p(i)$	Number of women reaching parity $l(i)$	Women remaining at parity (i) $d(i)$	Total fertility rate for parity (i) and above $F(i)$
0	.9684	1000	31	7.74
1	.9751	968	24	6.77
2	.9753	944	23	5.83
3	.9657	920	31	4.91
4	.9628	889	33	4.02
5	.9341	856	56	3.16
6	.8937	799	85	2.36
7	.8347	714	118	1.65
8	.7541	596	146	1.05
9	.6555	449	155	.60
10	.5510	294	132	.31
11	.5185	162	78	.14
12	.4375	84	47	.06
13	.3878	36	22	.02
14	.3158	14	9	.01
15+		4	4	

Assuming a radix $l(0)$ of 1,000 women marrying, the $l(i)$ column gives the number of women in the fertility table that had at least i births:

$$l(i+1) = l(i)\, p(i). \tag{2.1}$$

In further analogy to the ordinary life table is $d(i)$, which gives the number of women dropping out of the process of reproduction at parity i, i.e., women who have completed parity i. Therefore, $d(i)$ is defined by

$$d(i) = l(i) - l(i+1) \quad \text{or} \tag{2.2}$$

$$d(i) = l(i)[1 - p(i)]. \tag{2.3}$$

Dividing $d(i)$ by the radix yields the completed parity distribution. It is not shown in the table because the transformation is trivial. Dividing $l(i)$ by the radix $l(0)$ results in a quantity $f(i)$, which Ryder (1982) calls the total fertility rate for births of order i:

$$f(i) = l(i)/l(0). \tag{2.4}$$

A summation over all parities then yields

$$F = \sum_{i=1}^{m} f(i), \tag{2.5}$$

with m being the highest parity considered. Thus, F is the total fertility rate considering births of all orders or simply the mean number of children born to the cohort. More generally, $F(i)$ is the total fertility rate beyond i or the mean number of children to be born beyond parity i. It is defined by

$$F(i) = \sum_{x=i+1}^{m} f(x). \tag{2.6}$$

In terms of the ordinary life table the $F(i)$ function corresponds to $T(x)$ divided by the radix, where $F(0)$ [equal to F according to (2.5)] is analogous to life expectancy at birth. The analogy to life expectancy at any other age is in our case the mean number of additional children once a certain parity i is achieved. It can be derived as

$$E(i) = F(i)/f(i). \tag{2.7}$$

Section 2.2 of this chapter discusses parity-progression tables for ever-married women between the ages of 40 and 49 at the time of the survey. By including these women in the calculation of the tables, a slight underestimate of completed fertility is introduced because some of the women may still bear children after the time of the interview. As a consequence the values of $F(0)$ are slightly lower than the number of children ever born to women between ages of 45 and 49 given in other tables. However, this disadvantage is regarded as minor in comparison with the gain in the number of women available for the calculation and detailed description of parity-progression ratios.

Parity-progression tables can also be broken down according to selected socioeconomic variables. Several WFS cross-national summaries introduce two dichotomies: place of residence (urban or rural) and mother's education (some education or no education). In some countries the educational categories are slightly different, as will be indicated. Generally, this results in five tables per country, in which the first fertility table refers to the total cohort.[1] The parity-progression differences by residence and education are also discussed and compared across countries in the second section.

Section 2.3 provides a detailed picture of the timing of fertility for cohorts of women who have already completed their reproductive career. A first crude description of the timing aspect is given by the set of mean ages of mothers at births of order i, denoted here by $x(i)$. A second description is the mean interval between births. For calculating the mean interval between any two births (e.g.. from the first to the second birth) in a population, it is not legitimate, however, to take the differences between the two mean ages of those births directly. This is because the $x(i)$'s also include births of women that will not experience an additional birth (i.e., a birth of order $i+1$). To yield the correct interval one must differentiate between the mean ages at birth of order i for women who experience additional births and those with completed parity i.

To derive the correct interval between any two births, a complete breakdown of the mean ages at birth of order i by completed parity j is needed. Such tables are provided in Appendix B for 41 countries participating in the WFS. These quantities are denoted by $x(i \cdot j)$, which stands for age at birth of order i conditional upon completed parity j. The crude mean age at birth of order i, $x(i)$, can then be interpreted as a weighted average (see Chiang and van den Berg, 1982) of the $x(i \cdot j)$'s:

$$x(i) = \sum_{j=i}^{m} \frac{d(j)}{l(i)} \, x(i \cdot j), \tag{2.8}$$

where the $d(i)$ and $l(i)$ functions are as defined above and m is the highest parity considered. The weights are the probabilities that a woman in parity i will end up with j children. The correct formula for the birth interval, denoted $t(i)$, between births of order i and $i+1$ then becomes

$$t(i) = \sum_{j=i+1}^{m} \frac{d(j)}{l(i+1)} \, [x(i+1 \cdot j) - x(i \cdot j)] \tag{2.9}$$

(see Feichtinger and Lutz, 1983). The difference between the correct interval and the unweighted interval calculated by $x(i+1) - x(i)$ is very substantial (i.e, many years) at higher parities because of the declining parity-progression ratios.

In addition to providing a detailed descriptive picture of the tempo of fertility in a cohort, the $x(i \cdot j)$ values are also important input data to more refined measures of family life cycle analysis. For instance, the mean age at the birth of the last child – denoted by $x(1) + e(1)$ (see Feichtinger, 1978) – can be calculated as a weighted average of the conditional mean ages $x(i \cdot j)$, giving the age at ith birth, if the ith birth was the last one:

$$x(1) + e(1) = \sum_{i=1}^{m} \frac{d(i)}{l(1)} \, x(i \cdot i), \tag{2.10}$$

where $e(1)$ is mean duration from birth of order 1 to family completion. More generally, the mean duration $e(i)$ from births of order i to completion of the family is

$$e(i) = \sum_{j=1}^{m} \frac{d(j)}{l(i)} \, [x(j \cdot i) - x(i \cdot j)] \tag{2.11}$$

or more simply according to (2.8):

$$e(i) = \sum_{j=1}^{m} \frac{d(j)}{l(i)} \, x(j \cdot i) - x(i). \tag{2.12}$$

Then, $x(i) + e(i)$ is the mean age at last birth for women with i or more births. Obviously, $e(i)$ becomes zero if the ith birth is the last birth.

Section 2.4 treats the tabulation of parity at the time of the survey (current parity; see data in Appendix C) for cohorts whose reproductive career is not yet completed and provides figures that combine the aspects of tempo and quantum of fertility. A comparatively low mean number of children for women surveyed between the ages 20 and 24 in a certain country may indicate either that the number of children eventually born to women of this cohort is lower in that country (quantum) or that births of the same order occur at a higher age (tempo). In most cases the figures probably represent a combination of these two aspects.

The percentage distributions over all parities, given for various cohorts, allow a more detailed analysis than the mean parities. When comparing these percentage distributions across age and marital-duration groups, one must recognize cohort effects, i.e., differential fertility patterns for different cohorts. Because in most countries cohort fertility has been steady or declining recently, unusually higher percentage parity at low parities for older cohorts are rare. As a consequence of reductions in the proportions of sterile women over time owing to better nutrition and medical advances, the percentages of childless women, however, are higher among older cohorts in some instances. For example, in Cameroon the proportion of women with current parity zero increased to 8.6% for married women 15 to 19 years, to 13.6% for those married 25 to 29 years, and to 22.5% for women married 30 years or more. For current parity distributions the effect of decreasing cohort fertility cannot be disentangled from the expected increase of cumulated fertility with age. However, even with the cohort effects the distributions provide a crude indication of the tempo and quantum of more recent fertility.

2.2. The Quantum Aspect of Completed Cohort Fertility

2.2.1. Parity-progression ratios

Of the functions introduced in the fertility table, the parity-progression ratios, $p(i)$, show the most irregularity and sensitivity among and within populations. They largely represent the behavioral component in the fertility table. The other fertility-table functions, i.e., $l(i)$, $d(i)$, and $F(i)$, follow directly or indirectly from these transition probabilities from one parity status to the next. Although in our retrospective data set parity-progression ratios had to be calculated from the distribution of completed family sizes, $d(i)$, it was originally the parity-progression ratios that produced these distributions.

Because of the largely behavioral determination of the transitions to higher parity categories, the pattern of parity-progression ratios is hard to describe by any standard function. The $f(i)$ and $l(i)$ functions must by definition decrease monotonically, the integral under the $d(i)$ function must equal $l(0)$; but for the parity-progression ratios there is no restriction other than that the values must lie between zero and one. Unlike its counterpart in mortality analysis – the force of mortality function – the $p(i)$ function is very hard to describe by a parameteric model because its shape is biologically determined only in the case of completely natural fertility. In other cases it is subject to the implicit or explicit decisions made by the couples. The major biological components in it are the proportional increases in infecundity with age and with parity and menopause.

Keeping in mind the great potential for irregularities in the parity-progression ratios, it is surprising to see how regular they are in less-developed countries: the cohorts of ever-married women with completed parity show almost monotonically declining parity-progression ratios from a maximum at parity zero to a minimum at the highest parity. There are a few exceptions. In some countries (e.g., Cameroon) the parity-progression ratios at parity zero are smaller than those at parity one, and in a relatively large number of countries the ratios level off or even increase at high parities. In part these irregularities may be because of the small survey sample in those categories, but a comparison with industrialized countries where this phenomenon is much stronger suggests that it may be an accurate reflection due to the heterogeneity in the population: there is one small group of women with extremely high fertility that, beyond a certain parity, dominates the picture.

Figure 2.1 shows a sample of different shapes of the parity-progression functions in five countries with different fertility levels. After Jordan, Kenya has the second highest cohort fertility among all WFS countries. There, parity-progression ratios stay above .96 until parity four. Parity increases from zero to one in Kenya and Cameroon. In other words, in Kenya and Cameroon the probability of a birth is higher for women who already had one birth and thus have proved their fecundity than for women who are still childless. This is true mainly for eastern and central Africa and is probably due to the high incidence of infecundity resulting from venereal disease and malnutrition. Between parities five and ten the parity-progression ratios in Kenya and Cameroon decrease

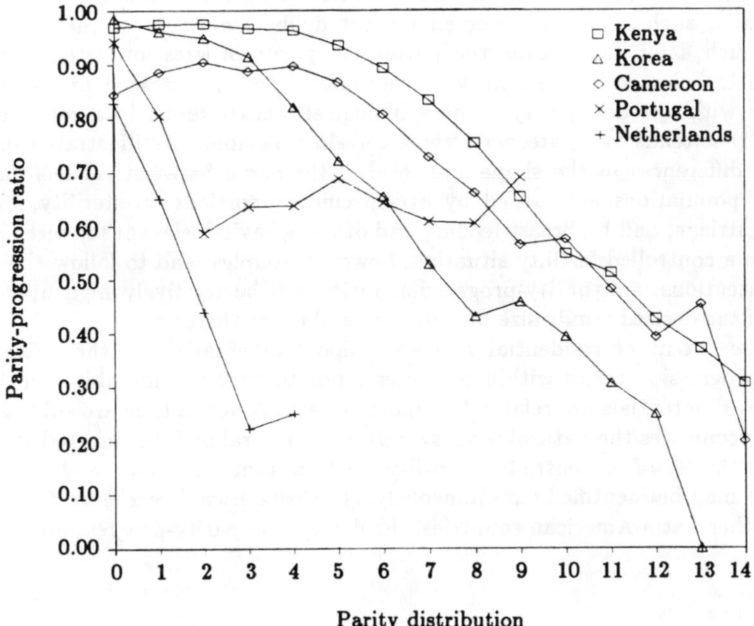

Figure 2.1. Parity-progression ratios for cohorts of ever-married women aged 40 to 49 in Kenya, Republic of Korea, Cameroon, Portugal, and the Netherlands.

at accelerating speeds. After parity ten the pattern is more irregular but generally declining.

The pattern for Korea is quite different: a slow and almost linear decline between parities zero and four followed by a steeper but also linear decline between parities four and eight and parities nine and thirteen, except for a slight increase between parities eight and nine.

Typical patterns of parity-progression ratios for low-fertility industrialized countries are shown by Portugal and the Netherlands. This pattern is characterized by a steep decline in parity-progression ratios until parity two, after which the curve levels off or even increases. Only in the Netherlands do the parity-progression ratios show a steep progression from parity two to three, but a slight increase to parity four.[2] An increase in parity-progression ratios at higher parities can be observed in many low fertility countries and is due to a few high-fertility women.

What is the reason for this dramatic shift in the pattern of parity-progression ratios from high-fertility countries to low-fertility countries? Theoretically, a decline in fertility can happen in many different ways ranging from a proportional decline of each parity of the typical LDC curve to a stepwise function with high progression ratios up to a certain threshold parity and low ratios thereafter. The observed pattern of change, however, becomes plausible in terms of the paradigm of natural versus controlled fertility. In a natural fertility population, such as Kenya, women do not deliberately control their fertility. Under such a fertility regime the pattern of parity-progression ratios depends only on the change in the ability to reproduce and an increased prevalence of sterility with age and parity. These biological factors result in a monotonous decline that tends to be steeper after a certain threshold. As illustrated in *Figure 1.1* differences in the shape and level of the curve between various natural fertility populations are caused by age-specific proportions on sterility, by age upon marriage, and by breast-feeding and other behavior relevant for birth intervals. In a controlled fertility situation, however, couples tend to follow their fertility intentions, and parity-progression ratios will be relatively high up to the mode of the desired family size distribution and lower thereafter.

The extent of residential and educational differentials in the pattern of parity-progression ratios within countries tends to vary considerably. In Africa and Asia differentials are relatively minor; in Latin America they are substantial. In some countries the natural fertility pattern (for rural and uneducated women) and the onset of a controlled fertility pattern (among urban and educated women) may be identified simultaneously. In Costa Rica (see *Figure 2.2*), as in many other Latin American countries, the decrease in parity-progression ratios is

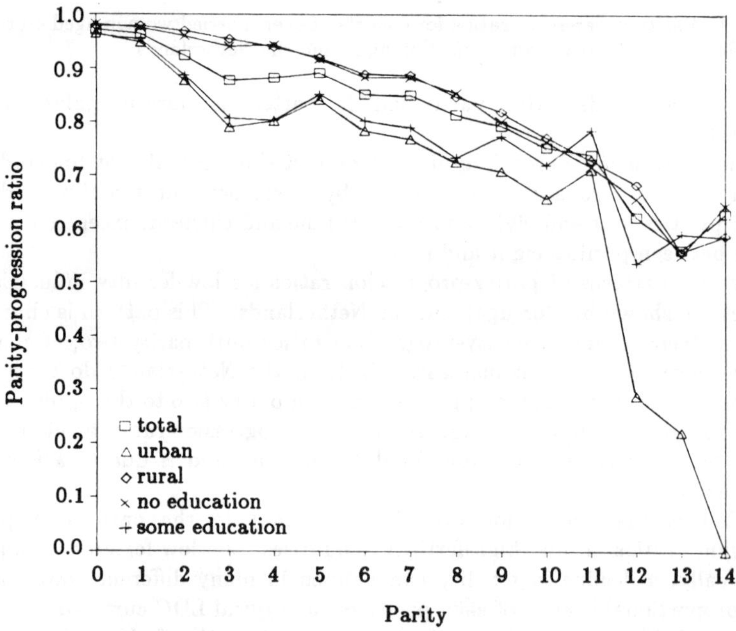

Figure 2.2. Parity-progression ratios for subpopulations in Costa Rica by place of residence and level of education.

relatively slow and – at least for rural and uneducated women – almost linear up to parity ten. Urban women and women with more education by contrast, have quite a distinct pattern with a fast decline until parity three followed by an increase and further slow declines. This can already be seen as the beginning of the pattern of the $p(i)$ function that is typical for low-fertility countries, although in Costa Rica it is still at a rather high level of fertility.

In Europe differentials in the level of parity-progression ratios beyond parity three are also marked. The general pattern is a fast decline, followed by a leveling off (*Figure 2.3*).

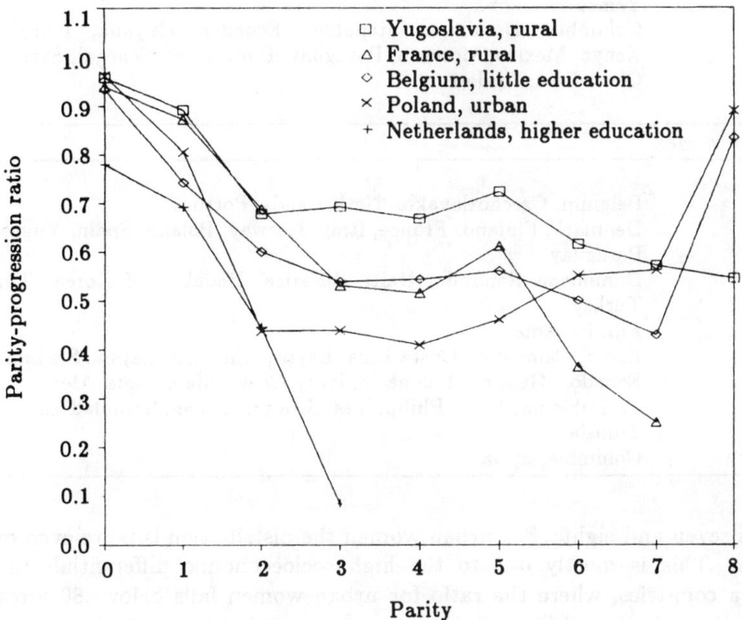

Figure 2.3. Parity-progression ratios for selected subpopulations in Europe: rural Yugoslavian women, rural French women, Belgian women with little education, urban Polish women, and Dutch women with higher education.

Although graphs are good methods to highlight general patterns, more succinct indices are needed to compare other countries. A *prima facie* study suggested that in a great number of countries a level of .80 in the decline of the parity-progression ratios might be considered a threshold, because the pace of decline increases after this level is achieved. This level can be used to rank countries according to the parity at which their parity-progression ratios fall below .80. *Table 2.2* ranks total and urban female populations between the ages of 40 and 49. The total female population is distributed into two groups: the low-fertility countries are heavily concentrated at parity two, whereas the high-fertility countries range between five and nine with a heavy concentration at

Table 2.2. List of countries according to the parity at which the cohorts of ever-married women with completed parity reach parity-progression ratios below .80.

A: Total

---

(1)	Belgium, Netherlands
(2)	Czechoslovakia, Denmark, Finland, France, Great Britain, Italy, Norway, Poland, Portugal, Spain, United States, Yugoslavia
(5)	Republic of Korea, Panama
(6)	Ghana, Haiti, Indonesia, Lesotho, Nepal, Nigeria, Sri Lanka, Trinidad and Tobago
(7)	Bangladesh, Benin, Cameroon, Egypt, Fiji, Jamaica, Malaysia, Mauritania, Pakistan, Peru, Sudan, Thailand, Tunisia, Turkey, Venezuela, Yemen
(8)	Columbia, Dominican Republic, Ecuador, Guyana, Ivory Coast, Kenya, Mexico, Morocco, Paraguay, Philippines, Senegal, Syria
(9)	Costa Rica, Jordan

B: Urban women

---

(1)	Belgium, Czechoslovakia, Netherlands, Portugal
(2)	Denmark, Finland, France, Italy, Norway, Poland, Spain, Yugoslavia
(3)	Paraguay
(4)	Dominican Republic, Haiti, Jamaica, Republic of Korea, Thailand, Turkey
(5)	Fiji, Panama
(6)	Benin, Cameroon, Costa Rica, Egypt, Ghana, Malaysia, Sri Lanka
(7)	Ecuador, Guyana, Indonesia, Ivory Coast, Mauritania, Mexico, Morocco, Pakistan, Peru, Philippines, Senegal, Sudan, Trinidad and Tobago, Tunisia
(8)	Columbia, Syria

---

parities seven and eight. For urban women the distribution is more even over all parities. This is mostly due to the high socioeconomic differentials in Latin America countries, where the ratio for urban women falls below .80 already at parities three, four, and five.

A comparison between the above list and the distribution of average completed family sizes, $F(0)$, *Table 2.5*, reveals that a later decline in parity-progression ratios does not necessarily mean a higher mean number of children. This is because average completed parity also depends on the shape of the curve of parity-progression ratios before and after our chosen value of .80. In Costa Rica, for instance, the parity-progression ratio remains higher than .80 until parity nine, but many other countries have higher fertility levels. Generally, however, for less-developed countries the empirical correspondence between the ranking in *Table 2.2* and average completed fertility is quite good because the shapes of the progression ratio curves are similar. For the more-developed countries the ranking according to the critical point of .80 is less informative. The reason for this is the homogeneous, sharp decline at low parities to below .80 and the high variance at higher parities.

It was mentioned above that in modern contraceptive societies the vast majority of the population limits their fertility to three children. In these societies numerically small but high-fertility groups of women may dominate the picture after parity four. For these women the probability of having a fifth or sixth or higher-order birth child are relatively constant. This specific feature of heterogeneity in reproduction is only apparent in the analysis of conditional birth probabilities, i.e., parity-progression ratios. The other functions of the fertility table consider the relative weight of these high-fertility women, which tends to be rather small. This results in a more uniform picture for all other table functions.

2.2.2. Explanation of the $l(i)$ and $d(i)$ columns

The $l(i)$ column in the fertility table gives the number of women in a cohort of 1,000 who are still in the process of parity progression at parity i. A graph of this column shows that the curve of $l(i)$ declines by definition from 1,000 to 0 for every country. Differentials in the fertility pattern can be seen from the extent to which the curve is convex or concave.

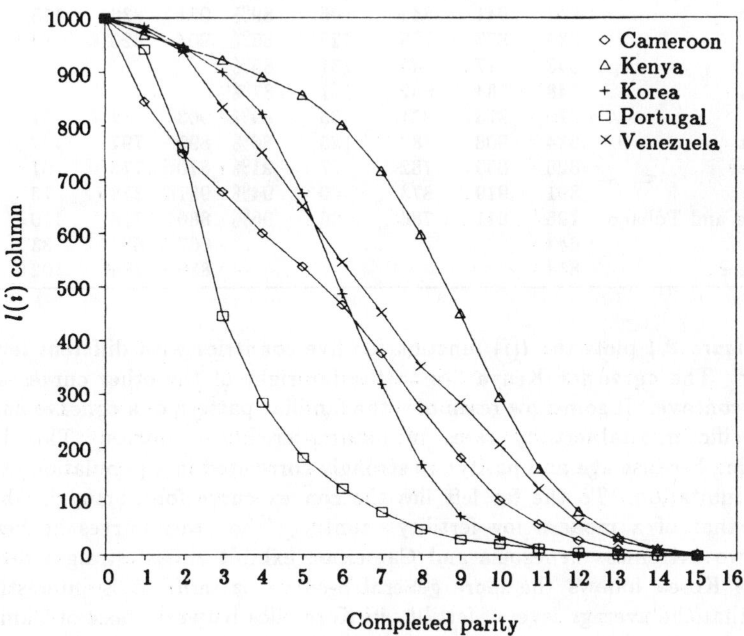

Figure 2.4. A graphic representation of the $l(i)$ column for Portugal, Kenya, Cameroon, Venezuela, and Korea.

Table 2.3. Number of women (out of 1,000) that reached at least parity three, $L(3)$, according to residence and education.

| | | Residence | | | | Education | | | |
	Total	Rural	Urban	Differ-ence	Rel. diff.	Low	High	Differ-ence	Rel. diff.
AFRICA									
Benin	880	889	848	41	95%				
Cameroon	676	693	588	105	84%				
Egypt	884	891	875	16	98%	899	860	39	95%
Ghana	906	922	859	63	93%	910	879	31	96%
Ivory Coast	866	869	853	16	98%				
Kenya	922					909	958	−49	105%
Lesotho	782					758	794	−36	104%
Mauritania	834	853	803	50	94%	830	837	−7	100%
Morocco	854	881	806	75	91%				
Nigeria	801								
Senegal	882	895	847	48	94%				
Sudan	807	792	845	−54	106%				
Tunisia	913	923	903	19	97%				
AMERICAS									
Colombia	878	901	863	38	95%	900	833	68	92%
Costa Rica	865	928	802	127	86%	918	814	105	88%
Dominican Republic	832	906	768	138	84%	847	804	43	94%
Ecuador	897	941	845	96	89%	951	836	115	87%
Guyana	835	877	755	122	86%	904	820	84	90%
Haiti	843	877	746	131	85%				
Jamaica	748	784	682	101	87%				
Mexico	870	925	831	95	89%	903	852	51	94%
Panama	834	908	782	125	86%	899	797	102	88%
Paraguay	826	859	782	77	91%	870	773	97	88%
Peru	891	919	873	46	94%	931	858	73	92%
Trinidad and Tobago	796	811	786	25	96%	886	776	110	87%
USA	644					667	634	33	95%
Venezuela	834					885	784	102	88%

Figure 2.4 plots the $l(i)$ function for five countries with different levels of fertility. The curve for Kenya lies to the far right of the other curves and is clearly concave. It somehow resembles the familiar pattern of a concave curve of age-specific marital-fertility rates in natural-fertility countries. This is not surprising because age and parity are strongly correlated in a population without family limitation. To the far left lies the convex curve for Portugal, which is clearly that of a modern low-fertility country. The other curves lie between these two extremes. Venezuela and Cameroon exhibit almost straight declines, whereas Korea follows the more general S-curve pattern. It is interesting to notice that the average level of fertility in Korea lies between those of Cameroon and Venezuela, although at lower parities it has levels above those two and at higher parities below.

Tables 2.3 and *2.4* give global overviews of inter- and intra-country differentials in the $l(i)$ function. *Table 2.3* shows the proportion of women that

Table 2.3. Continued.

	Total	Residence		Differ-ence	Rel. diff.	Education		Differ-ence	Rel. diff.
		Rural	Urban			Low	High		
ASIA and PACIFIC									
Bangladesh	907					904	913	−9	101%
Fiji	854	868	826	42	95%	879	837	42	95%
Indonesia	765	767	755	12	98%	754	814	−59	107%
Jordan	947					952	930	21	97%
Korea, Republic of	898	930	869	61	93%	913	885	28	96%
Malaysia	852	858	836	22	97%	869	822	47	94%
Nepal	847								
Pakistan	900	909	871	38	95%				
Philippines	901	911	877	34	96%	927	889	38	95%
Sri Lanka	835	845	780	65	92%	863	821	42	95%
Syria	927	934	921	12	98%	932	894	38	95%
Thailand	878	888	813	75	91%	879	874	5	99%
Turkey	879	941	802	139	85%	937	779	159	83%
Yemen	916								
EUROPE									
Belgium	423	434	421	13	97%	416	425	−9	102%
Czechoslovakia	348	471	297	174	63%	487	292	195	59%
Denmark	453	656	391	265	59%	497	366	131	73%
Finland	471	573	387	186	67%	537	389	148	72%
France	474	564	435	129	77%	500	428	72	85%
Great Britain	448					462	444	18	96%
Italy	385	403	362	41	89%	418	287	131	68%
Netherlands	237	429	164	265	38%	231	240	−9	103%
Norway	556	594	505	89	85%	656	519	137	79%
Poland	472	678	338	340	49%	594	276	318	46%
Portugal	447	519	295	224	57%	549	315	234	57%
Spain	485	626	578	48	92%	583	614	−31	105%
Yugoslavia	484	579	399	180	68%	515	148	367	28%

had a third child. On the national level the values range from 95% in Jordan to as low as 24% in the Netherlands. The range is even wider for residential and educational subpopulations.

Norway and Spain were the only European countries where more than 50% of urban women had a third child. In rural areas, however, two-thirds of the European countries showed proportions of over 50%. Similar differentials appear with respect to education – with the exception of Belgium and the Netherlands where a higher proportion of better-educated women had a third child. The relative extent of educational and residential differentials in Europe is quite irregular. Usually the residential differentials were greater. In four countries, most prominently in Yugoslavia, educational differentials were stronger.

With regard to less-developed countries, socioeconomic differentials are highest in Latin America. In several African countries as well as in Bangladesh and Indonesia (both Islamic), educated women had higher probabilities of having

Table 2.4. Number of women (out of 1,000) that reached at least parity seven, $L(7)$, according to residence and education.

| | | Residence | | | | Education | | | |
	Total	Rural	Urban	Differ-ence	Rel. diff.	Low	High	Differ-ence	Rel. diff.
AFRICA									
Benin	494	506	453	53	89%				
Cameroon	375	401	238	163	59%				
Egypt	539	604	459	145	75%	568	492	76	86%
Ghana	510	524	469	55	89%	523	443	80	84%
Ivory Coast	586	593	556	36	93%				
Kenya	715					704	748	−44	106%
Lesotho	358					328	374	−47	114%
Mauritania	457	453	462	−9	102%	422	484	−61	114%
Morocco	613	649	527	122	81%				
Nigeria	378								
Senegal	610	625	575	50	91%				
Sudan	497	500	487	13	97%				
Tunisia	559	586	529	57	90%				
AMERICAS									
Colombia	531	599	489	110	81%	585	419	166	71%
Costa Rica	508	682	335	347	49%	660	361	299	54%
Dominican Republic	460	626	316	311	50%	538	306	233	56%
Ecuador	535	633	411	222	64%	658	388	270	58%
Guyana	510	577	377	200	65%	601	489	111	81%
Haiti	428	471	289	182	61%				
Jamaica	410	497	252	245	50%				
Mexico	558	684	467	217	68%	650	507	143	77%
Panama	383	556	261	295	46%	570	281	289	49%
Paraguay	460	619	258	360	41%	615	274	341	44%
Peru	524	651	437	214	67%	680	393	287	57%
Trinidad and Tobago	364	434	319	115	73%	479	340	139	71%
Venezuela	451					596	312	284	52%
ASIA and PACIFIC									
Bangladesh	602					593	652	−58	109%
Fiji	502	560	391	169	69%	549	468	81	85%
Indonesia	366	361	389	−27	107%	358	398	−40	111%
Jordan	760					826	569	256	68%
Korea, Republic of	318	450	193	257	42%	437	224	213	51%
Malaysia	460	496	379	117	76%	490	405	85	82%
Nepal	404								
Pakistan	607	610	590	21	96%				
Philippines	553	611	427	183	69%	694	497	196	71%
Sri Lanka	400	423	296	126	70%	495	356	139	71%
Syria	660	692	629	63	90%	700	439	261	62%
Thailand	489	527	284	243	53%	510	473	37	92%
Turkey	427	554	260	295	46%	556	202	354	36%
Yemen	530								

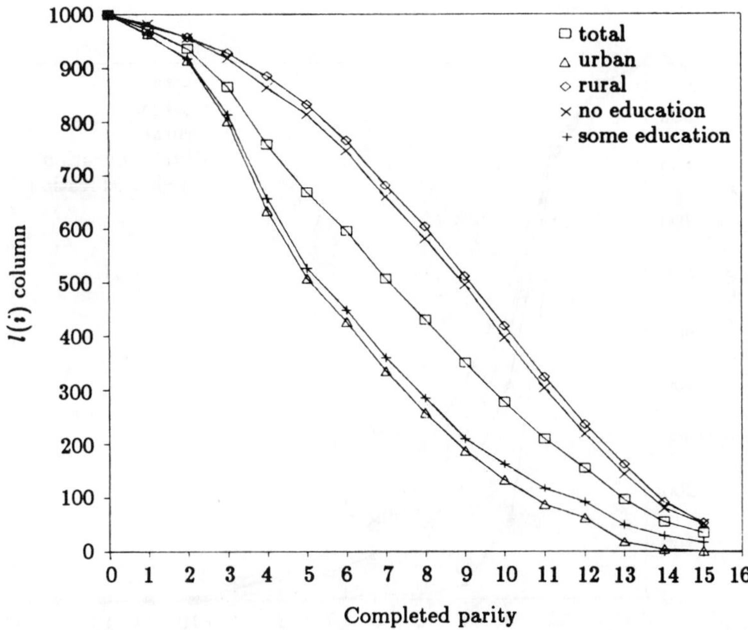

Figure 2.5. Socioeconomic differentials in the $l(i)$ column for Costa Rica.

a third child. With respect to place of residence all countries (except for the Sudan) show higher proportions of rural women with a third child. Among the 40 less-developed countries studied, there are only five countries – namely, Cameroon, Lesotho, Jamaica, Trinidad and Tobago, and Indonesia– where less than 80% of the women had a third child. In Cameroon the percentage is only 67%, which comes rather close to the highest European values. The reason lies in the relatively high proportion of childless and low-parity women in Cameroon.

Table 2.4 gives comparable figures for the proportions of women that had a seventh child. Low-fertility countries with extremely small proportions were not included in the table. Within the LDCs, national levels range from a high of 76% in Jordan to lows of 32% in Korea and 36 to 37% in Lesotho, Indonesia, Cameroon, and Nigeria.

Differentials in the proportions of women with a seventh birth with respect to residence and education are substantial in most countries and greater than the differentials with respect to third births. In all cases except for Kenya, Lesotho, Mauritania, and Indonesia, differentials go into the expected directions with higher fertility in rural areas and for women without schooling. In these four countries the differentials are lower. Without going into a more detailed country-specific analysis, one might assume that in these countries the reproductive behavior of educated and urban women was still traditional, and higher socioeconomic status resulted in higher fecundability – probably combined with

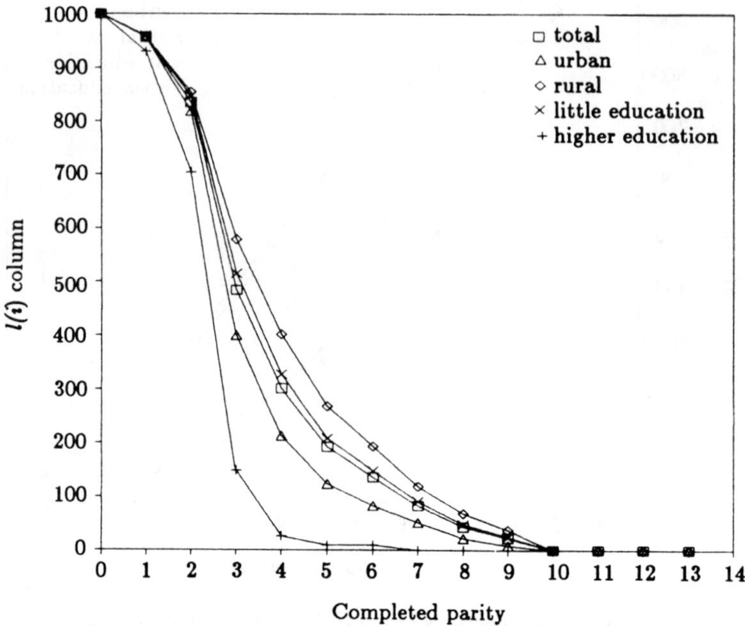

Figure 2.6. Socioeconomic differentials in the $l(i)$ column for Yugoslavia.

less breast-feeding. Another, separate reason for the unexpected fertility differentials might be based on the differential quality of reporting, with educated women giving more complete birth histories. After all, these figures refer to women whose prime childbearing years were about 20 years earlier. If a similar bias were also assumed for all other countries, this would mean even higher socioeconomic differentials than those observed in the survey.

Generally, socioeconomic differentials with respect to the frequency of a seventh child are highest in Latin America. Absolute and relative differences are highest in Paraguay, Costa Rica, the Dominican Republic, and Panama for both place of residence and mother's education. The rural figures tend to be twice that of the urban in many cases. The relative importance of the residential and educational differentials varies from Central America and the Caribbean, where urban-rural differentials tend to be higher in South America and where education for women seems to be more important. The Asian countries tend to take an intermediate position between South America and Africa. Turkey, Korea, and Thailand stand out as exceptions with very high differentials. Concerning the relative importance of the differentials, the pattern is very irregular in Asia. In Syria, for instance, the difference with respect to education is four times that of the residence, whereas in Thailand the urban-rural differential is many times higher than the educational one. In Africa differentials tend to be moderate.

Figures 2.5 and *2.6* show the extent of socioeconomic differentials for the complete sets of $l(i)$ values in two selected countries, Costa Rica and Yugoslavia. In Costa Rica (*Figure 2.5*) the figures for the total population decline in a linear fashion after parity two, while the differentials are especially pronounced: the pattern for rural, uneducated women shows the concave natural-fertility shape, whereas for urban, educated women the shape is clearly convex. This was clearly demonstrated in *Figure 2.2*. The figure also indicates that in Costa Rica residential differentials are somewhat more significant that educational ones.

In Yugoslavia (*Figure 2.6*) curves for the total and all subgroups in the population are convex, indicating controlled fertility. Within this regime of controlled fertility there are significant differentials. The women with higher education exhibit a pattern of reproduction that is similar to that of highly industrialized Western countries. The $l(i)$ functions for rural women and women with little education decline more slowly and resemble the $l(i)$ curves of some lower-fertility subpopulations in less-developed countries. In the villages of Yugoslavia, 40% of all married women still had four or more children by age 40 to 45.

The steepness of decline in the $l(i)$ column as expressed by first differences is given in the $d(i)$ column that is plotted for some selected countries in *Figure 2.7*. This curve is derived from the $l(i)$ column and clearly shows the shape of the distribution.

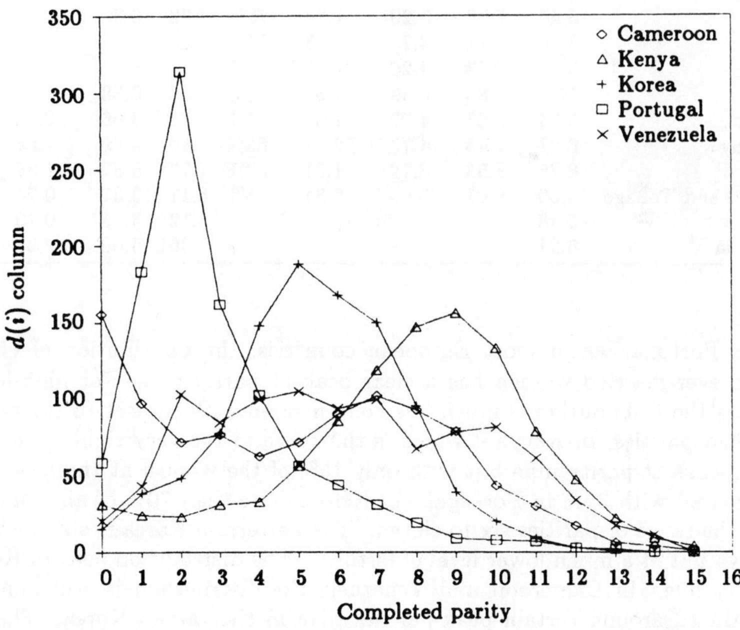

Figure 2.7. Completed parity distributions in the $d(i)$ column for Portugal, Kenya, Cameroon, Venezuela, and Korea.

Table 2.5. Total fertility rate at parity zero and above, $F(0)$, (the mean parity for all women) according to residence and education.

| | | Residence | | | | Education | | | |
	Total	Rural	Urban	Differ-ence	Rel diff.	Low	High	Differ-ence	Rel. diff.
AFRICA									
Benin	6.14	6.22	5.83	0.39	93%				
Cameroon	4.91	5.12	3.88	1.24	75%				
Egypt	6.64	6.97	6.22	0.75	89%	6.81	6.36	0.45	93%
Ghana	6.38	6.56	5.86	0.70	89%	6.47	5.96	0.51	92%
Ivory Coast	6.78	6.83	6.49	0.34	94%				
Kenya	7.73					7.60	8.09	−0.48	106%
Lesotho	5.22					5.00	5.32	−0.32	106%
Mauritania	6.01	6.02	5.93	0.09	98%	5.91	6.05	−0.14	102%
Morocco	7.08	7.23	6.30	0.93	87%				
Nigeria	5.41								
Senegal	6.92	7.02	6.69	0.34	95%				
Sudan	6.00	5.96	6.07	−0.11	101%				
Tunisia	6.78	6.90	6.62	0.28	95%				
AMERICAS									
Colombia	6.90	7.60	6.48	1.12	85%	7.35	5.93	1.41	80%
Costa Rica	6.92	8.44	5.34	3.10	63%	8.22	5.65	2.57	68%
Dominican Republic	6.39	7.74	5.23	2.51	67%	6.85	5.45	1.40	79%
Ecuador	6.98	7.78	5.93	1.85	76%	7.99	5.71	2.28	71%
Guyana	6.46	7.08	5.20	1.88	73%	7.32	6.30	1.02	86%
Haiti	5.80	6.11	4.73	1.38	77%				
Jamaica	5.51	6.13	4.26	1.87	69%				
Mexico	7.03	7.89	6.39	1.50	80%	7.66	6.68	0.98	87%
Panama	5.74	6.87	4.92	1.95	71%	7.11	4.96	2.15	69%
Paraguay	6.27	7.45	4.73	2.71	63%	7.40	5.89	1.88	75%
Peru	6.76	7.53	6.22	1.31	82%	7.78	5.89	1.88	75%
Trinidad and Tobago	5.50	6.01	5.16	0.84	86%	6.11	5.37	0.74	87%
USA	3.48					4.12	3.33	0.79	81%
Venezuela	6.21					7.36	5.09	2.27	69%

In Portugal, as in most European countries, the distribution of children born to ever-married women has a clear peak at parity two. For high-fertility countries the distribution is much less concentrated with respect to the range of completed parities. In Kenya – which is the curve to the very right – the distribution peaks at parity nine but with only 15% of the women at the peak parity as compared with 31% in Portugal. In Kenya more than 70% of all women are within the range of parities six to eleven. The pattern in Korea is similar to that in Kenya but at a much lower level of fertility. The distribution peak in Korea is at parity five. In Cameroon and Venezuela the distribution is still much less concentrated around certain peak parities than in Kenya and Korea. There are no clear modes in the distributions, the mean being somewhere around six.

Table 2.5. Continued.

		Residence		Differ-ence	Rel. diff.	Education		Differ-ence	Rel. diff.
	Total	Rural	Urban			Low	High		
ASIA and PACIFIC									
Bangladesh	6.95					6.92	7.13	−0.20	102%
Fiji	6.31	6.65	5.58	1.07	83%	6.63	5.99	0.64	90%
Indonesia	5.25	5.25	5.30	−0.05	101%	5.17	5.64	−0.47	109%
Jordan	8.66					9.10	7.27	1.83	79%
Korea, Republic of	5.42	6.13	4.75	1.38	77%	5.96	4.97	1.00	83%
Malaysia	6.13	6.29	5.65	0.64	89%	6.34	5.70	0.64	89%
Nepal	5.65								
Pakistan	6.91	6.91	6.76	0.15	97%				
Philippines	6.86	7.24	5.99	1.25	82%	7.73	6.50	1.23	84%
Sri Lanka	5.73	5.88	5.09	0.79	86%	6.44	5.40	1.04	83%
Syria	7.66	7.80	7.53	0.27	96%	7.95	6.21	1.74	78%
Thailand	6.36	6.63	5.00	1.63	75%	6.35	6.27	0.07	98%
Turkey	6.08	7.05	4.80	2.25	68%	6.99	4.49	2.50	64%
Yemen	6.65								
EUROPE									
Belgium	2.56	2.63	2.54	0.09	97%	2.52	2.51	0.01	99%
Czechoslovakia	2.34	2.69	2.20	0.49	82%	2.65	2.20	0.45	83%
Denmark	2.55	2.93	2.43	0.50	83%	2.62	2.41	0.21	92%
Finland	2.67	3.00	2.40	0.60	80%	2.93	2.34	0.59	80%
France	2.69	2.92	2.59	0.33	89%	2.87	2.37	0.50	83%
Great Britain	2.60					2.80	2.50	0.30	89%
Italy	2.38	2.40	2.31	0.09	96%	2.50	2.01	0.49	80%
Netherlands	1.67	1.95	1.56	0.39	80%	1.85	1.58	0.27	85%
Norway	2.78	2.89	2.64	0.25	91%	3.16	2.64	0.52	84%
Poland	2.78	3.44	2.35	1.09	68%	3.13	2.16	0.97	69%
Portugal	2.95	3.29	2.25	1.04	68%	3.49	2.25	1.24	64%
Spain	3.10	3.28	3.07	0.21	94%	3.06	3.16	−0.10	103%
Yugoslavia	3.05	3.48	2.67	0.81	77%	3.17	1.83	1.34	58%

2.2.3. Total fertility rates at various parities

The previous sections identified the general pattern of the specific parity-progression processes and compared various populations. The first moments of the completed parity distributions, i.e., the mean completed parities have not yet been discussed. *Figure 2.7* shows the distribution of the $d(i)$column and gives some information about the mode and the dispersion of the distribution, but not about total fertility. This section looks at the total fertility rates at parity i and above, $F(i)$, as they were defined in Section 2.1.1.

Table 2.5 gives the values of $F(0)$ for all 54 WFS countries. $F(0)$ equals the mean number of children born by all women in the cohort considered and is analogous to the cohort total fertility rate. The cohorts are all ever-married women between the ages of 40 to 45. The mean parities for the national cohorts range from 8.66 in Jordan to 2.67 in the Netherlands. Four other countries,

Table 2.6. Total fertility rate at parity three and above, $F(3)$, according of residence and education.

		Residence		Differ-ence	Rel. diff	Education		Differ-ence	Rel. diff.
	Total	Rural	Urban			Low	High		
AFRICA									
Benin	3.35	3.41	3.08	0.33	90%				
Cameroon	2.64	2.81	1.75	1.07	62%				
Egypt	3.86	4.19	3.45	0.74	82%	4.01	3.62	0.39	90%
Ghana	3.54	3.69	3.10	0.59	83%	3.63	3.15	0.49	86%
Ivory Coast	4.05	4.10	3.77	0.33	91%				
Kenya	4.90					4.80	5.18	−0.38	107%
Lesotho	2.61					2.43	2.70	−0.26	110%
Mauritania	3.32	3.29	3.31	−0.02	100%	3.22	3.35	−0.14	104%
Morocco	4.41	4.50	3.72	0.77	82%				
Nigeria	2.81								
Senegal	4.15	4.23	3.98	0.25	94%				
Sudan	3.39	3.38	3.39	−0.01	100%				
Tunisia	3.96	4.08	3.81	0.27	93%				
AMERICAS									
Colombia	4.12	4.78	3.72	1.06	77%	4.53	3.22	1.31	71%
Costa Rica	4.14	5.57	2.65	2.92	47%	5.36	2.95	2.40	55%
Dominican Republic	3.72	4.92	2.68	2.24	54%	4.17	2.80	1.37	67%
Ecuador	4.14	4.88	3.17	1.72	64%	5.08	2.97	2.12	58%
Guyana	3.80	4.33	2.71	1.61	62%	4.51	3.66	0.84	81%
Haiti	3.08	3.34	2.16	1.18	64%				
Jamaica	2.99	3.55	1.87	1.69	52%				
Mexico	4.27	5.05	3.69	1.36	73%	4.85	3.94	0.91	81%
Panama	3.01	4.03	2.28	1.75	56%	4.28	2.29	1.98	53%
Paraguay	3.56	4.70	2.07	2.62	44%	4.63	2.24	2.39	48%
Peru	3.95	4.70	3.42	1.28	72%	4.92	3.12	1.79	63%
Trinidad and Tobago	2.88	3.37	2.57	0.81	76%	3.35	2.78	0.57	82%
USA	1.02					1.66	0.87	0.79	52%
Venezuela	3.46					4.54	2.41	2.12	53%

namely, Kenya, Morocco, Mexico, and Syria, have total fertility rates of more than 7.0 children. More than half of all the less-developed countries have fertility rates between 6.0 and 7.0. Ten LDCs lie between 5.0 and 6.0, and only Cameroon has a figure below 5.0 (4.91). Among the low-fertility countries, only the USA, Spain, and Yugoslavia have completed fertility above 4.0. The values for all other countries, except Holland, range from 3.0 to 4.0.

Table 2.6 presents the corresponding data for $F(3)$, i.e., the mean number of children still to be born by women who have three children. This value ranges from 5.77 in Jordan to 0.30 in the Netherlands. Because of heterogeneity in the population, the $F(3)$ ranking of the countries from highest to lowest, is similar but not identical to the $F(0)$ ranking from highest to lowest: women that already had three children have different reproductive patterns than all women, i.e., starting at parity 0. This difference is expected to be higher in low-fertility

Table 2.6. Continued.

		Residence				Education			
	Total	Rural	Urban	Differ-ence	Rel. diff.	Low	High	Differ-ence	Rel. diff.
ASIA and PACIFIC									
Bangladesh	4.12					4.10	4.26	−0.16	103%
Fiji	3.60	3.92	2.90	1.02	73%	3.88	3.31	0.57	85%
Indonesia	2.70	2.69	2.79	−0.10	103%	2.64	3.00	−0.35	113%
Jordan	5.77					6.21	4.40	1.81	70%
Korea, Republic of	2.59	3.25	1.96	1.28	60%	3.13	2.15	0.98	68%
Malaysia	3.39	3.55	2.91	0.63	82%	3.58	2.99	0.58	83%
Nepal	2.92								
Pakistan	4.11	4.08	4.04	0.04	98%				
Philippines	4.04	4.41	3.19	1.21	72%	4.88	3.69	1.19	75%
Sri Lanka	3.02	3.16	2.44	0.73	77%	3.68	2.72	0.96	73%
Syria	4.82	4.92	4.72	0.20	95%	5.09	3.45	1.64	67%
Thailand	3.57	3.83	2.29	1.54	59%	3.57	3.49	0.08	82%
Turkey	3.28	4.16	2.10	2.07	50%	4.10	1.82	2.28	44%
Yemen	3.80								
EUROPE									
Belgium	0.49	0.47	0.50	−0.03	106%	0.48	0.44	0.04	92%
Czechoslovakia	0.21	0.30	0.19	0.11	63%	0.27	0.16	0.11	59%
Denmark	0.32	0.45	0.28	0.17	62%	0.39	0.17	0.22	44%
Finland	0.44	0.61	0.30	0.31	49%	0.61	0.23	0.38	38%
France	0.50	0.55	0.45	0.10	82%	0.64	0.24	0.40	38%
Great Britain	0.39					0.54	0.33	0.21	61%
Italy	0.28	0.27	0.26	0.01	96%	0.35	0.08	0.27	23%
Netherlands[a]									
Norway	0.39	0.46	0.34	0.12	74%	0.42	0.09	0.33	21%
Poland	0.51	0.83	0.27	0.56	33%	0.69	0.17	0.52	25%
Portugal	0.81	1.02	0.34	0.68	33%	1.18	0.31	0.87	26%
Spain	0.68	0.78	0.65	0.13	83%	0.65	0.68	−0.03	105%
Yugoslavia	0.78	1.09	0.50	0.59	46%	0.84	0.06	0.78	7%

[a]Since only in the Netherlands the marriage cohorts of 1963–1973 were interviewed, the sample is too selective and had very few higher-order births.

countries where the proportion of women dropping out between parities zero and three is large.

The pattern of residential and educational differentials in *Tables 2.5* and *2.6* is quite similar to the pattern discussed earlier for $l(i)$. A comparison between the two tables shows that generally the absolute differences between urban and rural or educated and uneducated women are lower for $F(3)$. This is no surprise because the values for $F(3)$ must be lower than those for $F(0)$ in all cases. However, the relative differences in $F(i)$, i.e., urban fertility as a percentage of rural fertility, increase for higher i. This is true for high-fertility countries as well as for low-fertility countries. It implies that socioeconomic differentials in fertility are concentrated in fertility beyond parity three, and not in very low-order births.

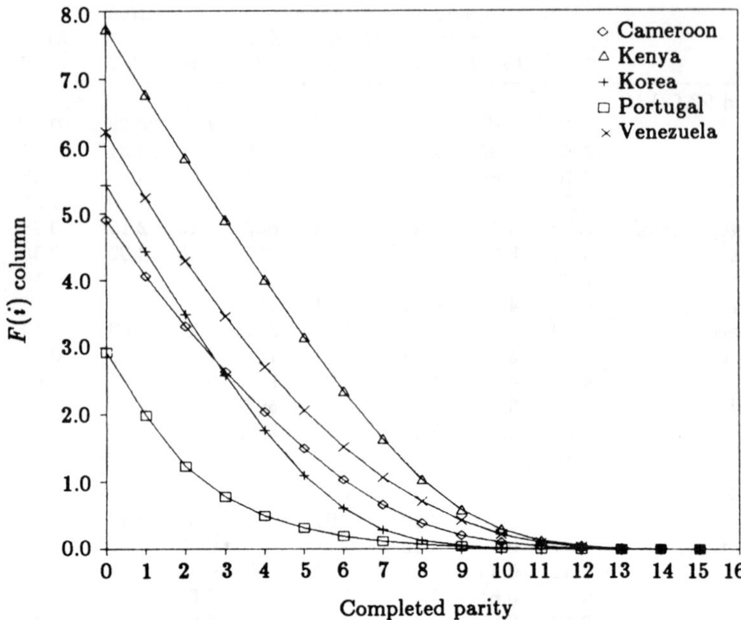

Figure 2.8. Cohort total fertility rates at parities i and above, $F(i)$ column, for Portugal, Kenya, Cameroon, Venezuela, and Republic of Korea.

Graphically, the $F(i)$ function gives a very smooth picture (see *Figure 2.8*) because at each parity $F(i)$ must decline by somewhat less than 1.0. The flattening of the curves at higher parities corresponds to the decline in the parity-progression ratios that start beyond a certain threshold. If all parity-progression ratios were equal, the line would be straight. For many less-developed countries – e.g., for Kenya between parities zero and seven – this is nearly the case. The curves for Cameroon and Venezuela are shown because the crossing of the curves indicates an interesting change in the relative ranking of countries. It is mainly the unusual fertility pattern in Cameroon – high childless proportions and completed parities one and two, and subsequent higher fertility – that causes this crossover. Such crossovers occur if one country, at a similar average level of fertility, has a higher degree of internal heterogeneity than the other country.

This description of the quantum aspect of cohort fertility sketches only some general patterns and selected specific features of the rich empirical material given in *Tables 2.2* through *2.5* and in Appendix A. As previously mentioned, the unbiased study of the quantum of cohort dertility is only possible for women beyond reproductive age. Therefore, most births included in this part of the analysis occurred 15 or more years before the survey, which might make the findings less interesting to people concerned about present and future fertility. Nevertheless, points of central concern in the study of declining fertility in less-developed countries are the age and the parity in which women stopped reproducing. The onset of family limitation, which in fact is parity-specific fertility control, can best be studied in the later phases of childbearing, i.e., when women are nearing the end of their reproductive years. For this reason, Section 2.3, which looks at the timing aspect of completed cohort fertility, addresses the topic of when women stop having additional children. The last section, 2.4, also includes more recent information on the fertility of women who are still in the process of reproduction.

2.3. The Tempo of Completed Cohort Fertility

2.3.1. Retrospective and prospective views

The previous section on the quantum of completed cohort fertility provides a detailed picture of the level of fertility among women who are already beyond reproductive age and of their distribution over all possible completed family sizes. This section studies the timing of the sequence of births that finally resulted in the observed completed parity. This analysis also gives some indirect evidence on why fertility differentials exist from a more formal perspective. Because the reproductive span of women is limited, women who have their first child at an older age or who wait a relatively long interval between births reduce the possible maximum number of children they may have.

Obviously the analysis of the timing of completed cohort fertility is primarily retrospective because only women who have already born all their children have completed fertility. Whenever a prospective view of the data is taken, i.e., fertility is interpreted as a dynamic process of progression from one parity to the next with different birth intervals or even as the continuous choice made by women to have a child, it is quite different from the usual prospective view because the individual outcomes of this dynamic process are already known. For heterogeneity analysis, however, the view of the process we must take here is very useful. A real prospective analysis deals with unknown or hidden heterogeneity since the completed highest parity of the women is still not known and only a certain fraction of their reproduction can be studied. But with a retrospective data set one can consider what is known about the women's past heterogeneity with respect to completed fertility and can study their earlier reproductive behavior with the background knowledge of their ultimate family size.

2.3.2. Mean ages at births of certain orders

For the 40 less-developed countries (and Portugal) included in the WFS, Appendix A provides detailed information on the mean ages at births of all orders (mostly 1 to 15) broken down by the woman's completed parity. These tables are the basis for all further mean ages presented in this section. The usual mean age at birth of a given order i is calculated from period data and includes women of all categories of completed parity i or above. This crude mean age, $x(i)$, can be calculated as a weighted average of the mean ages at birth of order i given completed parity j, $x(i \cdot j)$, the weights coming from the completed parity distribution including only women with i or more births [see formula (2.8) in Section 2.1]. This crude mean is isomorphic to the mean age observed in period data of a real population, assuming that mortality between the mean age and age 40 through 49 does not depend on the number of additional births during that age span.

Table 2.7 presents the crude mean ages for births of orders one to nine in the 41 countries included in Appendix B. The mean age at first birth is probably largely a function of the marriage pattern in the country concerned. The crude mean age at first birth is lowest in Bangladesh with 17.6 years followed by Senegal with 18.6 years. The highest mean age at first birth for a less-developed country is 22.9 years in Yemen. In Portugal it is 24.2 years, reflecting the general European pattern.

For second- and third-order births a similar ranking appears although the differentials between countries diminish. The rankings of countries in which marriages occur at a later age seem to catch up with a higher speed of fertility. For births of order five several countries already have lower mean ages than Bangladesh, namely, Costa Rica, Egypt, Guyana, Jordan, Morocco, Panama, and Trinidad and Tobago. The mean age for the fifth birth is lowest in Jordan with only 27.2 years. Because we know that Jordan will have the highest average completed parity of all countries, this is not surprising because a lower speed of fertility would not result in such high quantum levels.

The rank order of countries changes again for births of order nine. The lowest mean ages for the ninth birth appear in Central America, with the youngest age in Costa Rica (33.0 years) followed by Trinidad and Tobago, Venezuela, and Panama. We find the highest mean ages in Korea with 38.6 years of age, followed by Lesotho, Haiti, and Benin; Yemen and Portugal have lower mean ages for the ninth birth.

Figure 2.9 illustrates the relationship between the average national fertility level, $F(0)$, and the mean ages at births of orders one, five, and nine. Since the mean ages at first birth vary according to different marriage patterns, the eventual mean completed family size does not play a major role. For fifth births it is already more apparent that high-fertility countries generally have lower mean ages than low-fertility countries. The reason for this is purely mathematical: to achieve higher fertility within a limited age span, the birth intervals must be shorter and, therefore, the mean ages at higher-order births lower. For ninth births the range of mean ages is wider than for births of order five. However, the regression line is hardly steeper than for fifth births because in many countries the weight in which women with nine or more births get on the national average is already relatively small.

Table 2.8 gives the mean ages at births of certain orders for two subpopulations of women: women with completed parity below and above eight. The rank of the countries is similar to that in *Table 2.7*: Bangladesh has the lowest mean age at first birth for both high- (16.8 years) and low- (18.8 years) fertility women. The high-fertility women in five other countries have mean ages at first birth between 17 and 18, namely, Egypt, Indonesia, Mauritania, Panama, and

Table 2.7. Mean ages at births of order i.

Country	\multicolumn{9}{c}{Order of birth}								
	1	2	3	4	5	6	7	8	9
AFRICA									
Benin	20.5	23.2	25.7	28.1	30.3	32.4	34.6	36.6	38.1
Cameroon	21.2	23.6	25.9	28.2	30.2	32.2	34.0	35.7	36.9
Egypt	19.4	21.4	23.4	25.4	27.4	29.2	31.0	30.9	33.9
Ghana	20.4	23.1	25.9	28.5	30.7	32.9	34.8	36.5	38.2
Ivory Coast	19.8	22.5	24.9	27.2	29.6	31.6	33.6	35.4	37.0
Kenya	20.0	22.3	24.7	27.0	29.2	31.4	33.4	35.1	36.8
Lesotho	21.1	24.1	26.9	29.5	31.7	33.6	35.6	37.1	38.5
Mauritania	20.2	23.0	25.5	27.7	29.4	30.9	32.8	34.5	35.6
Morocco	19.4	21.5	23.5	25.5	27.6	29.6	31.7	33.3	35.0
Nigeria	21.5	24.2	24.2	28.6	30.5	32.0	33.3	34.6	35.5
Senegal	18.6	21.6	24.1	26.6	29.0	31.2	33.2	35.2	37.0
Sudan	20.4	22.7	25.1	27.2	29.1	30.6	32.2	34.0	35.4
Tunisia	21.4	23.4	25.5	27.7	29.7	31.6	33.3	34.8	36.2
AMERICAS									
Colombia	21.3	23.4	25.3	27.2	28.7	30.2	31.5	33.1	34.2
Costa Rica	21.1	22.9	24.6	26.3	27.8	29.2	30.4	31.8	33.0
Dominican Republic	20.3	22.6	24.8	26.8	28.6	30.4	32.0	33.1	34.4
Ecuador	20.8	22.9	25.1	27.1	28.9	30.4	32.0	33.5	34.9
Guyana	19.9	22.2	24.1	26.0	27.8	31.1	32.9	34.7	36.7
Haiti	22.3	24.9	27.2	29.4	31.3	33.3	34.9	36.7	38.2
Jamaica	21.0	23.9	25.9	28.0	29.8	31.5	33.0	34.3	35.4
Mexico	20.6	22.7	24.7	26.7	28.6	30.5	32.2	33.8	35.3
Panama	19.7	21.8	23.9	25.8	27.5	29.2	30.8	32.5	33.8
Paraguay	21.0	23.4	25.8	28.0	29.4	31.2	32.8	34.4	36.1
Peru	20.9	23.3	25.6	27.6	29.4	31.1	32.7	34.2	35.6
Trinidad and Tobago	20.2	22.5	24.4	26.1	27.8	29.3	30.9	32.4	33.7
Venezuela	20.5	22.6	24.7	26.3	28.1	29.9	31.2	32.7	33.8
ASIA and PACIFIC									
Bangladesh	17.6	20.3	23.0	25.5	27.9	30.2	32.2	34.0	35.2
Fiji	19.8	22.1	24.3	26.3	28.0	29.8	31.5	33.1	34.6
Indonesia	19.8	22.6	25.2	27.4	29.5	31.4	33.1	34.6	35.8
Jordan	19.3	21.2	23.1	25.3	27.2	28.9	30.8	32.5	34.0
Korea, Republic of	20.6	23.5	26.2	28.8	31.2	33.3	35.3	37.2	38.6
Malaysia	19.9	22.3	24.5	26.7	28.6	30.5	32.2	33.8	35.2
Nepal	21.2	23.9	26.6	28.9	31.0	32.8	34.4	36.0	37.2
Pakistan	18.9	21.5	23.9	26.3	28.6	30.8	32.7	34.5	36.0
Philippines	21.7	23.7	25.8	27.9	29.8	31.6	33.3	34.8	36.5
Sri Lanka	20.6	22.9	25.1	27.2	29.2	31.0	32.7	34.1	35.6
Syria	21.2	23.1	25.2	27.2	29.2	31.3	32.9	34.4	35.9
Thailand	21.7	24.0	26.1	28.2	30.3	32.1	33.8	35.4	36.5
Turkey	20.0	22.1	24.6	26.4	28.4	30.2	31.7	33.1	34.3
Yemen	22.9	25.2	27.5	29.6	31.6	33.0	34.5	36.0	37.8
EUROPE									
Portugal	24.2	26.9	29.7	31.1	32.6	33.9	35.6	36.9	37.9

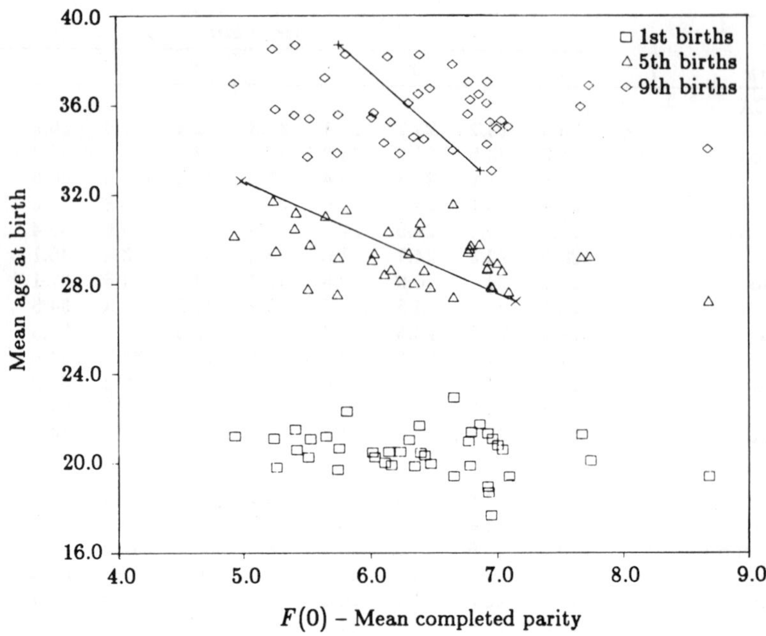

Figure 2.9. Cross-national association between mean ages at birth of selected orders and the average national fertility level, $F(0)$.

Senegal. Yemen and Portugal have the highest mean ages for low-fertility women.

A point of great interest in *Table 2.8*, however, is not the ranking of countries according to the absolute mean ages but the extent of internal heterogeneity in the distribution of mean ages. The smallest differences in the mean ages at births of a first or third child between women with completed parity less than eight and those with completed parity greater than eight can be found in Turkey. In other words, in Turkey the age of initiation of childbearing is least associated with completed fertility. Heterogeneity among young women is very low in Turkey, followed by Bangladesh, Benin, and Korea. Reproductive heterogeneity among young women is highest in Yemen (with almost a five-year difference in the means), Mauritania, Nigeria, and the Philippines. In these countries young women obviously start bearing children very early and seem to predetermine their completed family size.

Figure 2.10 gives a visual presentation of the association between order of birth and mean age at birth for selected populations. A linear association is found in almost every case with the lines of the low-fertility populations lying above those of high-fertility populations. This again proves that generally higher completed fertility is associated with younger mean ages at birth for given parities.

Table 2.8. Mean ages at births of order i for all women with seven or less and eight or more births.

| | Order of birth | | | | | |
| Country | Completed parity 7 or less | | | Completed parity 8 or more | | |
	1	3	5	1	3	5
AFRICA						
Benin	21.6	27.4	32.4	19.3	24.2	28.0
Cameroon	22.5	28.1	33.0	18.9	23.7	28.5
Egypt	21.2	25.7	30.1	17.8	21.8	25.9
Ghana	21.9	28.3	33.6	19.0	23.9	28.9
Ivory Coast	21.6	27.6	33.2	18.6	23.4	28.1
Kenya	22.5	28.2	33.4	19.0	23.6	28.2
Lesotho	22.1	28.7	34.3	19.2	24.4	29.4
Mauritania	22.2	28.4	32.7	17.9	22.6	27.2
Morocco	21.1	26.1	31.0	18.3	22.3	26.5
Nigeria	23.1	28.9	33.6	18.7	23.2	27.6
Senegal	20.0	26.5	32.4	17.8	22.9	27.8
Sudan	22.5	27.9	32.6	18.4	23.0	27.3
Tunisia	23.4	28.2	33.1	19.7	23.6	27.8
AMERICAS						
Colombia	23.0	27.8	31.8	19.7	23.4	27.1
Costa Rica	22.5	26.4	30.3	19.5	23.0	26.5
Dominican Republic	21.7	27.0	31.4	18.7	22.7	26.8
Ecuador	22.8	27.8	32.3	18.9	22.9	27.0
Guyana	21.6	26.4	31.0	18.4	22.5	26.2
Haiti	23.3	28.9	33.6	20.9	25.3	29.5
Jamaica	22.1	27.9	32.6	19.5	23.9	27.9
Mexico	22.5	27.3	31.8	18.9	23.0	27.1
Panama	20.7	25.3	29.4	17.9	21.9	25.9
Paraguay	22.5	28.1	32.4	19.2	23.4	27.7
Peru	22.7	28.1	32.7	19.3	23.5	27.6
Trinidad and Tobago	21.5	26.1	30.1	18.1	21.9	25.7
Venezuela	22.2	26.7	30.6	18.4	22.4	26.5
ASIA and PACIFIC						
Bangladesh	18.8	25.3	31.0	16.8	21.7	26.6
Fiji	21.4	26.6	30.9	18.2	22.3	26.4
Indonesia	20.9	27.2	32.1	17.9	22.6	27.2
Jordan	22.2	26.8	31.7	18.4	22.1	26.2
Korea, Republic of	21.3	27.2	32.3	19.0	24.2	29.4
Malaysia	21.0	26.3	31.0	18.6	22.8	27.1
Nepal	22.2	28.4	33.4	19.6	24.3	28.8
Pakistan	20.3	26.3	31.9	18.0	22.6	27.3
Philippines	24.2	28.6	33.1	19.7	23.7	28.1
Sri Lanka	22.1	27.0	31.7	18.5	22.6	27.1
Syria	23.9	28.4	33.0	19.8	23.8	27.9
Thailand	23.1	28.0	32.7	20.1	24.4	28.7
Turkey	20.8	25.7	30.6	18.9	23.1	26.6
Yemen	25.5	30.6	35.7	20.5	24.9	29.0
EUROPE						
Portugal	24.4	30.2	33.6	22.1	25.7	30.0

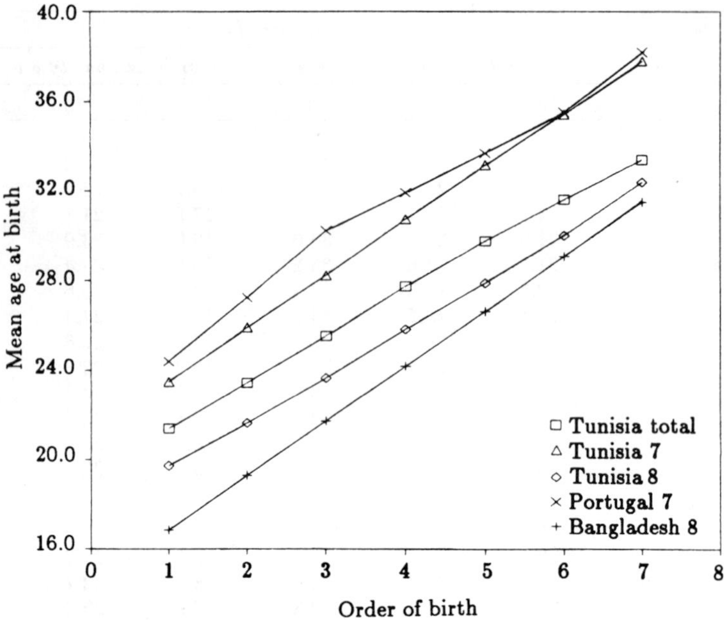

Figure 2.10. Mean ages of births of different orders for selected subpopulations of women with completed parities up to 7 or above in Tunisia, Portugal, and Bangladesh.

So far mean ages at births of various orders for complete cohorts and two sub-cohorts according to the level of fertility have been considered. Turning to the mean ages at births of various orders for all sub-cohorts broken down by individual completed parities, *Figures 2.11* through *2.14* illustrate this information in three-dimensional plots for four countries. Generally, the shape of the surfaces is very similar for all countries. Usually the shallowest point is that for the first births of women with highest completed parity. In the four countries studied, this lowest mean age is 15.9 in Morocco, 17.4 in Mexico, 18.0 in Yemen, and 18.8 in Portugal. The lowest mean age at first birth for women of completed parity 15 or above is again found in Bangladesh with only 14.6 years.

From this minimum in the center of the graphs the surface increases along both axes: to the right they must increase for directly mathematical reasons because for a given cohort the mean age at birth of order $i+1$ is always higher than that for births of order i; to the left the increase is of empirical nature. Theoretically, mean ages at births of certain orders could be invariant with respect to completed parity or could even be lower for lower-fertility women. Empirically, however, women tend to be heterogeneous in a way that sub-cohorts with higher completed fertility have their first child at younger ages than others. Or, put the other way round women who start later – for whatever reason – tend to have fewer children.

Generally, a smooth pattern of increase occurs along both axes with the level of the minimum and the speed of increase varying from country to country. Some of the irregularities in the graphs are most probably owing to small survey sample for each cell: the higher the sample size, the smoother the pattern. Smaller sample sizes yield a more ragged pattern, Yemen deviates from the expected monotonically increasing triangle because the number of women between the ages 40 and 49 is only 429. Even here, however, there is generally an increase along both axes.

There is also variation of mean ages at births within each group of completed parities. Appendix B shows not only the mean ages broken down by completed family size but also the standard deviations from those means. Generally, the standard deviation is significantly higher for women with low completed parities than for high-fertility women. In almost every country the highest standard deviations are for the group of women who had only one or two births. The variable is lowest for low-order births of high-fertility women. This is very plausible because there is much more potential for variation when placing only one or two births into the 30-year reproductive period, than for placing first births of a series of 12 or 15 births.

Another aspect of the tempo of fertility is the mean ages at last birth. The age at which women stop reproducing, either because of secondary sterility or because of parity dependent family limitation, is relevant to the nature of the fertility regime and possibly indicates the prevalence of fertility limitation. The relatively crude descriptive analysis in this section suggests the absence of such behavior for most cohorts considered. The next section on birth intervals also supports this.

Table 2.9 gives the mean ages at last birth for selected completed parities as well as the weighted average over all parities, i.e., the crude mean age at last birth. As expected, the mean age at last birth is lowest for women with only one child and increases as the woman's completed fertility increases. The mean age of first and only births ranges from 33.0 in Yemen to 21.3 years in Pakistan. It is also very low in the Caribbean, in some countries in Africa, and in Bangladesh. Women with completed parity nine have the highest mean ages at their last births in Yemen, Portugal, Haiti, and Lesotho and the lowest ones in Trinidad and Tobago, Egypt, Nigeria, Columbia, and Jordan. The picture of these mean ages at last birth does not follow any clear geographical pattern. Neither does it seem to depend on the country's level of fertility: we see that Portugal fits well into the pattern of LDCs. This implies that, across many cultures and fertility regimes, women who had the same number of children behaved similarly with respect to the timing of their births.

For the crude mean ages at last birth (last column in *Table 2.9*) the picture is quite different. The apparent ranking of countries combines the ranking according to fertility levels and the one according to parity standardized mean ages at last birth. This weighted average is lowest in Panama (32.5), Portugal (33.2), and Trinidad and Tobago (both 32.5), and highest in Yemen (38.9), Kenya (38.8), and Syria (38.2). Because in low-fertility countries the mean ages at births of lower order tend to be higher than in high-fertility countries, the inclusion of the quantum aspect results in a smaller reduction of the crude mean

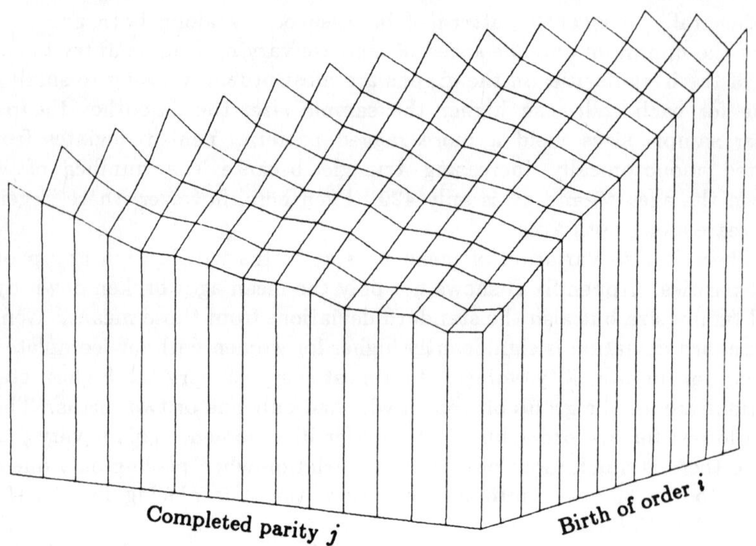

Figure 2.11. 3–D plot of mean ages and birth of order i at completed parity j for Mexico.

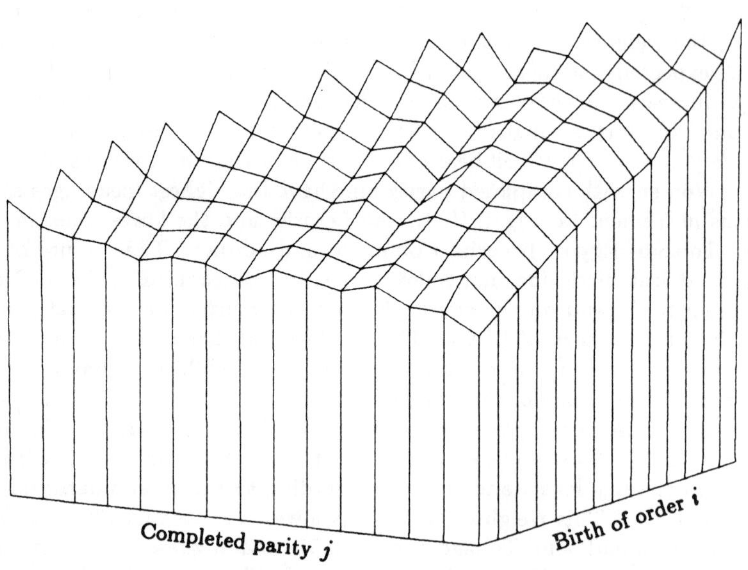

Figure 2.12. 3–D plot of mean ages and birth of order i at completed parity j for Portugal.

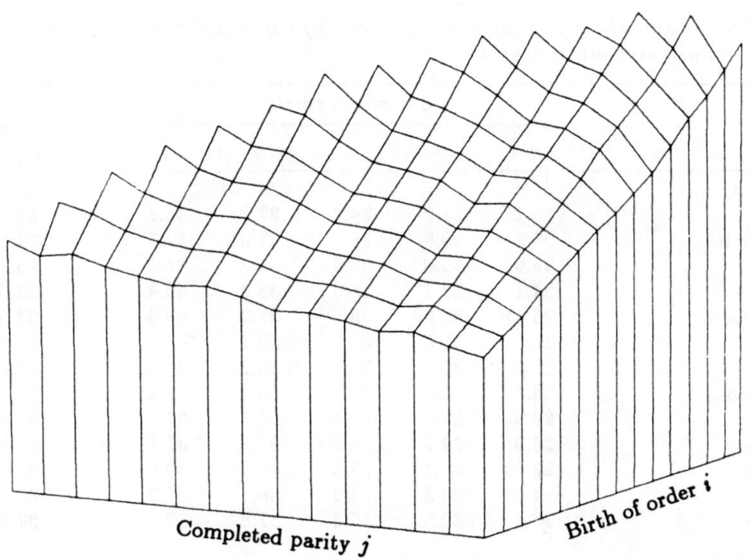

Figure 2.13. 3–D plot of mean ages and birth of order *i* at completed parity *j* for Morocco.

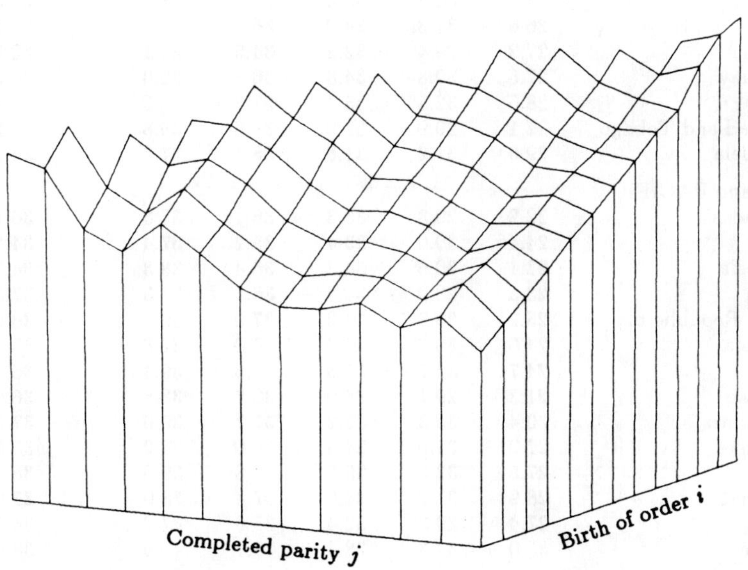

Figure 2.14. 3–D plot of mean ages and birth of order *i* at completed parity *j* for Yemen.

Table 2.9. Mean ages at last birth broken down by completed parity for cohort of ever-married women aged 40 through 49.

Country	Completed parity					Over all parities (weighted)
	1	3	5	7	9	
AFRICA						
Benin	25.1	31.9	34.3	37.3	40.1	37.0
Cameroon	23.8	29.8	35.1	37.3	39.5	34.2
Egypt	25.9	30.9	32.9	34.8	37.0	35.1
Ghana	24.1	32.3	35.8	38.3	40.4	38.0
Ivory Coast	23.5	30.6	35.9	37.7	39.8	37.5
Kenya	25.5	31.5	35.8	39.1	40.0	38.8
Lesotho	22.5	30.8	36.2	39.2	40.4	36.3
Mauritania	28.3	31.0	36.0	36.6	38.4	36.2
Morocco	22.9	28.6	32.4	36.7	37.8	35.9
Nigeria	25.9	32.7	35.7	37.5	37.1	35.6
Senegal	22.1	28.6	33.5	37.7	39.6	37.3
Sudan	24.4	30.3	35.2	36.7	37.7	35.1
Tunisia	26.2	32.5	35.8	37.8	39.0	37.3
AMERICAS						
Colombia	27.5	31.0	34.7	35.5	37.3	36.0
Costa Rica	29.4	32.6	34.3	37.0	37.8	33.6
Dominican Republic	23.8	30.5	31.0	37.6	37.9	34.9
Ecuador	28.6	32.3	34.7	36.3	38.9	36.8
Guyana	23.5	30.3	33.6	35.3	—	35.5
Haiti	24.3	32.5	35.6	37.9	40.4	37.2
Jamaica	23.5	30.2	33.4	37.1	38.2	34.5
Mexico	26.6	31.3	34.0	36.7	39.2	36.7
Panama	27.2	29.4	32.8	34.5	38.1	32.5
Paraguay	27.6	30.8	34.8	36.5	39.8	36.3
Peru	28.6	32.5	35.4	37.2	38.9	37.2
Trinidad and Tobago	22.1	29.9	31.9	34.6	36.8	33.2
Venezuela	29.6	31.2	31.8	35.1	37.3	34.8
ASIA and PACIFIC						
Bangladesh	22.2	29.3	33.3	36.1	37.8	36.1
Fiji	24.4	30.0	33.4	35.2	37.4	34.8
Indonesia	23.1	30.6	34.3	36.4	38.3	34.3
Jordan	23.5	28.9	34.2	36.5	37.3	37.5
Korea, Republic of	25.2	30.7	34.2	37.0	39.7	36.0
Malaysia	24.6	30.0	32.9	36.0	37.8	35.3
Nepal	24.7	32.7	35.5	37.6	39.4	36.6
Pakistan	21.3	29.1	35.0	36.7	38.6	36.6
Philippines	30.4	33.3	35.2	37.7	39.6	37.9
Sri Lanka	27.9	31.0	34.4	36.0	38.2	35.5
Syria	27.5	32.3	35.3	37.8	39.6	38.2
Thailand	28.9	31.3	34.5	37.4	38.9	37.0
Turkey	27.4	29.3	32.4	35.6	37.3	34.5
Yemen	33.0	34.3	38.4	39.1	40.9	38.9
EUROPE						
Portugal	27.3	32.4	34.8	38.2	40.7	33.2

age at last birth than might be expected intuitively. It is worth noting that despite the great variation in completed family sizes among populations the mean ages at last birth all fall within the range of six to seven years.

Unfortunately, the standardized WFS files do not include nearly as detailed information on the timing of fertility for industrialized countries. Mean ages at birth are only given for births up to order three. *Table 2.10* gives these means for cohorts of women aged 40 through 44 at the time of the survey. Because of a lack of data, the means correspond not to the one broken down by completed parity but rather to the crude means calculated as weighted averages in the above analysis of LDCs [see formula (2.8)].

Table 2.10. Mean ages at birth of orders one to three for ever-married women aged 40 through 44 in 12 European WFS countries and the USA.

Country	First birth		Second birth		Third birth	
	Mean age	*n*	*Mean age*	*n*	*Mean age*	*n*
Belgium	25.23	722	27.74	553	29.66	323
Czechoslovakia	22.99	520	25.93	422	28.15	183
Denmark	23.80	488	26.69	419	29.23	231
Finland	24.13	951	26.69	798	28.80	464
France	23.76	363	26.55	302	28.80	183
Great Britain	24.96	673	27.51	573	—	—
Italy	25.67	1069	28.76	866	30.98	427
Norway	24.13	423	26.72	378	30.05	246
Poland	23.53	1653	26.20	1411	28.49	794
Spain	25.75	1243	28.69	1140	31.27	745
United States	22.34	766	24.74	707	26.58	520
Yugoslavia	22.86	1284	25.67	1209	27.43	645

Among the 12 countries in *Table 2.10* mean ages at first birth were highest in Spain (25.8) and Italy (25.7) and lowest in the USA (22.3) and Yugoslavia (22.9). The United States has the lowest mean ages at births of all three orders, and the difference with the European countries becomes greater as birth orders increase. In all cases Yugoslavia is closest to the USA, and Spain and Italy are furthest away. It is interesting to notice that this ranking also seems to correspond grossly to patterns of ethnic, cultural, or political proximity.

2.3.3. Birth intervals

As pointed out in Section 2.1, the calculation of birth intervals from mean ages at birth of certain order requires some caution. To calculate differences the number of women included in the calculation of both means must be identical. Differences between the crude means may result in substantial errors. This is especially true for birth intervals in which the parity-progression ratios are low. For example, the application of formula (2.9) to the cohort fertility of Austrian women at the fourth and fifth intervals results in intervals of 2.00 and 1.61 years, whereas the wrong calculation using means that are based on different groups of women yields intervals of 3.93 and 3.47 years, respectively. The "wrong" intervals are almost twice as long as the "correct" intervals. This discrepancy increases for higher-order births in Austria (see Lutz and Feichtinger, 1985).

Table 2.11 presents the mean intervals between births of subsequent orders for LDCs and Portugal. What is striking about the table is the extreme uniformity. There are no significant changes across countries or within countries from one interval to the next: almost every interval seems to be between two and three years long. A closer look at the figures shows that generally the earlier birth intervals are somewhat longer than the later ones. The reason for this is a selection process. The lower-order births include low- and high-fertility women. The low-fertility women, who have controlled fertility or lower fecundability, tend to have longer birth intervals, and so the average length of birth intervals increases at lower-birth orders. High-fertility women with no birth control for either spacing or limiting family size dominate the picture after a certain parity.

This selection process becomes more apparent when the intervals for a group of low-fertility women and a group of high-fertility women are studied separately. In *Table 2.12*, the cohort is broken down into a group of women with seven or less births and a group with eight or more births. For each birth interval, the intervals are longer for low-fertility women. In some countries this difference is quite substantial: for first intervals it is highest in Indonesia (1.36 years of difference) followed by Mauritania, Nigeria, Senegal, and Portugal; in ten other countries it is more than one. As indicated, there are two possible explanations for this association between longer birth intervals and lower fertility. The first is biological and is based on the assumption that the low-fertility women had low fecundability and thus, longer waiting periods between births, which because of the limited reproductive period resulted in lower completed fertility. The second is behavioral and is founded on the argument that women who control their fertility limit the number of children and stretch the intervals between births.

This is better understood by looking at the mean intervals from first to last birth. *Table 2.13* provides the mean age span from first to last births for selected categories of completed parity and the weighted average over all parities. The figures for different completed parities come from the triangle matrices in Appendix B of mean ages at births of order *i* by completed parity *j* and are simply the differences between ages at first and last births. The average interval over all women was calculated according to formula (2.12).

Again the uniformity of the pattern is surprising. For instance, two countries as different in the state of their socioeconomic and demographic development as the Ivory Coast and Portugal have an identical age span of 4.8 years from first to last birth for women ending up with two children. For women with a completed parity of eight, the values only range from 15.4 years in Costa Rica to 19.8 years in Senegal. This geographic pattern did not become apparent in the study of individual birth intervals. It generally took a greater number of years to have a certain fixed completed family size in Africa than it did in Latin America. Asia has an intermediate position with intervals for women with eight children ranging from 16.5 in Turkey to 19.5 in Bangladesh. These differentials in the speed of reproduction may be due to marriages occurring at very young ages in

Table 2.11. Mean intervals between births of stated orders for completed cohort fertility, according to formula (2.9).

Country	1-2	2-3	3-4	4-5	5-6	6-7	7-8	8-9	9-10
AFRICA									
Benin	2.87	2.75	2.77	2.69	2.61	2.73	2.68	2.50	2.19
Cameroon	2.89	2.78	2.72	2.62	2.55	2.62	2.55	2.45	2.46
Egypt	2.31	2.30	2.30	2.37	2.37	2.45	2.78	2.77	2.48
Ghana	2.80	2.93	2.91	2.79	2.79	2.71	2.64	2.64	2.40
Ivory Coast	2.77	2.67	2.66	2.69	2.56	2.53	2.50	2.47	2.53
Kenya	2.46	2.45	2.49	2.48	2.41	2.42	2.36	2.41	2.39
Lesotho	3.16	3.10	3.06	2.88	2.72	2.81	2.72	2.52	2.55
Mauritania	3.16	2.73	2.68	2.54	2.44	2.61	2.51	2.30	2.72
Morocco	2.35	2.25	2.27	2.32	2.33	2.39	2.40	2.51	2.34
Nigeria	3.07	2.35	2.86	2.62	2.52	2.47	2.45	2.27	2.25
Senegal	3.04	2.83	2.72	2.72	2.59	2.53	2.57	2.53	2.37
Sudan	2.61	2.72	2.58	2.35	2.12	2.24	2.66	2.32	2.38
Tunisia	2.23	2.30	2.43	2.39	2.41	2.57	2.50	2.34	2.28
AMERICAS									
Colombia	2.27	2.20	2.22	2.21	2.22	2.02	2.21	2.16	2.10
Costa Rica	2.02	1.92	2.05	2.03	1.91	1.86	1.83	1.80	1.94
Dominican Republic	2.49	2.45	2.40	2.30	2.23	2.16	2.32	1.92	2.06
Ecuador	2.30	2.37	2.42	2.38	2.27	2.30	2.34	2.28	2.33
Guyana	2.44	2.30	2.26	2.25	3.82	2.23	2.19	2.18	2.16
Haiti	2.73	2.67	2.54	2.45	2.64	2.48	2.54	2.56	2.50
Jamaica	3.03	2.50	2.54	2.27	2.38	2.37	2.07	2.06	2.06
Mexico	2.36	2.34	2.40	2.36	2.46	2.35	2.40	2.30	2.26
Panama	2.28	2.33	2.35	2.24	2.25	2.30	2.28	2.04	1.93
Paraguay	2.59	2.80	2.70	2.39	2.49	2.36	2.27	2.24	2.15
Peru	2.51	2.49	2.45	2.49	2.39	2.39	2.41	2.42	2.34
Trinidad and Tobago	2.42	2.29	2.27	2.40	2.28	2.50	2.64	2.30	2.16
Venezuela	2.29	2.43	2.48	2.44	2.28	2.10	2.29	2.06	1.85
ASIA and PACIFIC									
Bangladesh	2.81	2.81	2.75	2.73	2.69	2.56	2.53	2.38	2.40
Fiji	2.50	2.44	2.39	2.31	2.34	2.44	2.40	2.54	2.23
Indonesia	3.09	2.97	2.81	2.71	2.68	2.53	2.57	2.55	2.30
Jordan	1.93	2.05	2.27	2.13	2.10	2.13	2.23	2.09	2.16
Korea, Republic of	2.99	2.90	2.83	2.81	2.76	2.82	2.82	2.65	2.55
Malaysia	2.59	2.63	2.57	2.57	2.51	2.45	2.42	2.34	2.39
Nepal	2.91	2.92	2.81	2.72	2.65	2.52	2.54	2.61	2.53
Pakistan	2.66	2.60	2.61	2.68	2.57	2.50	2.51	2.49	2.42
Philippines	2.18	2.36	2.49	2.38	2.42	2.42	2.34	2.43	2.36
Sri Lanka	2.50	2.63	2.65	2.72	2.65	2.57	2.53	2.58	2.20
Syria	2.09	2.26	2.21	2.29	2.39	2.21	2.24	2.31	2.26
Thailand	2.49	2.44	2.41	2.50	2.43	2.36	2.43	2.27	2.42
Turkey	2.35	2.53	2.26	2.56	2.47	2.47	2.39	2.35	2.45
Yemen	2.49	2.52	2.41	2.46	2.36	2.47	2.39	2.56	2.15
EUROPE									
Portugal	2.95	3.51	3.28	3.00	2.48	2.80	2.68	2.36	1.81

Table 2.12. Mean intervals between births of stated orders for women with completed cohort fertility of seven or less and eight or more, according to formula (2.9).

| | Interval between births of order | | | | | |
| | Women with 7 or less births | | | Women with 8 or more births | | |
Country	1–2	3–4	4–5	1–2	3–4	5–6
AFRICA						
Benin	3.18	3.17	3.16	2.57	2.45	2.38
Cameroon	3.28	3.13	3.10	2.39	2.38	2.30
Egypt	2.69	2.70	3.02	2.00	2.04	2.09
Ghana	3.15	3.45	3.30	2.47	2.48	2.55
Ivory Coast	3.39	3.35	3.20	2.37	2.33	2.37
Kenya	2.98	2.98	3.14	2.28	2.35	2.26
Lesotho	3.54	3.53	3.12	2.54	2.49	2.47
Mauritania	3.78	3.20	2.95	2.48	2.24	2.21
Morocco	2.29	2.82	3.05	2.05	2.05	2.15
Nigeria	3.56	3.07	3.10	2.34	2.15	2.18
Senegal	3.81	3.49	3.36	2.59	2.38	2.40
Sudan	3.09	3.12	2.61	2.20	2.23	1.95
Tunisia	2.66	2.87	3.07	1.92	2.14	2.13
AMERICAS						
Colombia	2.67	2.82	3.28	1.92	1.81	1.86
Costa Rica	2.22	2.44	2.32	1.82	1.74	1.76
Dominican Republic	2.94	2.82	2.88	2.02	2.06	1.97
Ecuador	2.61	2.95	2.70	2.03	2.05	2.10
Guyana	2.78	2.87	2.91	2.14	1.86	4.16
Haiti	3.19	2.99	3.29	2.15	2.10	2.30
Jamaica	3.64	3.12	3.07	2.26	2.05	2.11
Mexico	2.87	3.07	3.43	1.97	2.02	2.14
Panama	2.45	2.70	2.48	2.01	1.93	2.10
Paraguay	3.07	3.33	3.31	2.04	2.18	2.18
Peru	2.93	2.96	3.03	2.14	2.09	2.14
Trinidad and Tobago	2.70	2.61	2.88	1.98	1.87	1.92
Venezuela	2.48	2.97	3.03	2.07	2.07	1.95
ASIA and PACIFIC						
Bangladesh	3.40	3.35	3.32	2.45	2.45	2.48
Fiji	3.00	2.84	3.14	2.05	2.07	2.00
Indonesia	3.58	3.25	3.02	2.32	2.32	2.47
Jordan	2.15	2.87	2.60	1.87	2.12	2.01
Korea, Republic of	3.15	2.97	3.02	2.64	2.57	2.47
Malaysia	3.05	3.15	3.25	2.08	2.07	2.17
Nepal	3.30	3.31	3.16	2.36	2.26	2.34
Pakistan	3.24	3.21	3.38	2.32	2.31	2.33
Philippines	2.50	2.94	3.11	1.94	2.21	2.16
Sri Lanka	2.83	3.08	3.37	2.03	2.19	2.21
Syria	2.47	2.68	3.10	1.90	2.01	2.19
Thailand	2.84	2.73	3.17	2.13	2.15	2.09
Turkey	2.62	2.90	3.42	2.00	1.57	1.94
Yemen	2.72	2.96	2.65	2.30	2.00	2.23
EUROPE						
Portugal	3.05	3.53	3.02	1.91	2.11	2.04

Table 2.13. Mean interval (in years) between first and last birth by selected completed parities for cohort of ever-married women aged 40 through 49.

Country	2	4	6	8	10	Over all parities (weighted)
AFRICA						
Benin	4.6	10.9	16.2	19.0	21.2	17.0
Cameroon	4.1	9.9	15.6	19.1	21.1	15.3
Egypt	4.9	9.6	13.5	17.9	19.7	16.3
Ghana	4.9	12.1	16.5	19.2	22.2	18.0
Ivory Coast	4.8	12.3	15.6	19.4	22.2	18.3
Kenya	3.5	10.5	14.9	18.7	21.2	19.4
Lesotho	4.7	11.1	16.5	19.2	22.8	16.0
Mauritania	5.5	10.4	15.5	18.1	21.9	16.8
Morocco	4.4	9.6	14.1	17.8	21.0	17.7
Nigeria	4.9	11.6	14.7	18.0	19.7	15.2
Senegal	6.4	13.2	17.3	19.8	22.8	19.3
Sudan	4.0	10.9	14.3	17.8	20.3	15.9
Tunisia	3.7	10.0	14.1	17.1	20.2	16.6
AMERICAS						
Colombia	4.1	9.9	13.3	16.0	18.5	15.4
Costa Rica	4.5	9.5	12.8	15.4	17.8	12.9
Dominican Republic	3.4	10.6	13.3	16.9	19.3	15.3
Ecuador	4.0	9.7	13.1	17.6	19.6	16.2
Guyana	4.0	9.5	13.4	16.0	18.6	16.4
Haiti	5.4	9.8	14.7	17.6	20.7	15.4
Jamaica	5.4	10.7	14.4	16.7	19.3	14.5
Mexico	4.7	10.2	14.0	17.6	20.1	16.7
Panama	3.1	8.6	13.8	15.9	19.8	13.3
Paraguay	5.6	11.3	14.9	17.5	20.1	15.7
Peru	4.3	11.0	14.3	17.9	20.2	16.6
Trinidad and Tobago	3.8	8.7	12.9	17.5	18.3	13.7
Venezuela	4.4	9.9	14.0	17.1	18.7	14.6
ASIA and PACIFIC						
Bangladesh	4.9	11.7	16.5	19.5	22.6	18.9
Fiji	5.3	10.2	14.1	16.9	19.7	15.8
Indonesia	5.1	11.6	15.3	19.2	20.6	15.5
Jordan	3.2	8.9	12.3	16.9	19.4	18.5
Korea, Republic of	4.4	10.7	14.7	19.3	22.8	15.6
Malaysia	5.8	11.2	14.7	17.6	20.1	15.8
Nepal	5.4	12.0	15.3	18.5	20.6	16.1
Pakistan	4.7	11.2	16.3	19.1	21.3	18.3
Philippines	4.0	9.8	14.0	17.0	20.4	16.5
Sri Lanka	4.4	10.8	14.8	17.4	19.8	15.4
Syria	3.0	8.6	14.0	17.0	19.4	17.6
Thailand	4.7	9.0	13.9	18.1	20.0	15.7
Turkey	4.2	10.0	14.2	16.5	19.4	15.0
Yemen	3.5	10.8	13.5	17.6	19.2	16.3
EUROPE						
Portugal	4.8	9.8	13.1	17.2	18.8	9.6

Table 2.14. Mean duration from ith to last birth, $e(i)$, according to formula (2.12).

Country	2	4	6	8	10	12
AFRICA						
Benin	16.53	12.34	8.45	6.03	4.66	3.59
Cameroon	14.07	11.05	7.95	5.62	4.35	3.54
Egypt	14.43	11.07	8.31	8.49	4.42	3.31
Ghana	15.47	11.19	7.74	5.20	3.34	1.89
Ivory Coast	16.45	12.42	8.88	6.01	4.29	2.98
Kenya	17.32	13.20	9.34	6.48	4.66	3.23
Lesotho	13.90	10.38	7.46	5.17	4.05	2.09
Mauritania	14.33	11.01	8.50	6.47	4.67	3.74
Morocco	15.99	12.72	9.44	6.88	5.07	3.51
Nigeria	12.92	9.69	7.28	5.26	3.87	1.90
Senegal	16.92	12.72	9.15	6.17	4.24	2.63
Sudan	14.01	10.53	7.81	5.29	3.43	.90
Tunisia	14.64	10.90	7.97	5.49	4.07	2.96
AMERICAS						
Colombia	13.40	10.79	8.56	6.64	4.85	3.88
Costa Rica	11.27	9.36	7.35	5.71	4.02	2.56
Dominican Republic	13.64	10.58	8.54	6.28	4.52	3.21
Ecuador	14.33	11.29	9.07	7.00	5.44	3.77
Guyana	14.96	12.20	8.06	5.99	4.32	2.97
Haiti	13.55	10.20	7.62	5.36	3.49	1.79
Jamaica	12.63	9.82	7.73	5.72	4.71	3.85
Mexico	14.94	11.88	9.15	6.81	5.08	3.56
Panama	11.47	8.97	7.16	5.27	3.68	2.52
Paraguay	13.93	11.46	9.04	6.64	4.89	3.38
Peru	14.61	11.46	8.83	6.78	5.04	3.08
Trinidad and Tobago	12.16	9.88	7.99	6.17	4.75	3.01
Venezuela	12.85	10.26	8.04	6.27	4.65	3.41
ASIA and PACIFIC						
Bangladesh	16.53	12.34	8.45	6.03	4.66	3.59
Fiji	13.84	10.63	7.94	5.81	4.01	2.79
Indonesia	13.69	10.32	7.46	5.50	4.03	2.69
Jordan	16.73	13.13	9.96	7.29	5.17	3.51
Korea, Republic of	13.16	8.73	6.20	4.48	3.84	2.20
Malaysia	13.93	10.78	8.17	6.07	4.44	3.27
Nepal	13.66	9.74	7.14	5.17	3.83	2.60
Pakistan	16.11	12.12	8.49	5.92	4.16	2.93
Philippines	14.78	11.38	8.58	6.32	4.54	3.23
Sri Lanka	13.61	10.46	7.49	5.89	4.64	3.25
Syria	15.71	12.13	8.74	6.43	4.61	3.23
Thailand	13.79	10.51	7.88	5.88	4.44	3.10
Turkey	12.85	10.16	8.13	6.32	4.65	3.68
Yemen	14.13	10.53	7.95	5.70	4.25	1.19
EUROPE						
Portugal	8.23	7.50	6.54	5.18	4.14	2.44

The column group header is *ith birth* spanning columns 2, 4, 6, 8, 10, 12.

some countries—such as in Bangladesh where the longer interval might be caused by reduced fecundability at young ages—or probably more often to cross-cultural differences in birth spacing. Under this assumption *Table 2.13* indicates that even under natural fertility conditions (here assumed to be prevalent for women with 10 births), there are visible differences in birth spacing with the longest average birth intervals in tropical Africa and the shortest in Central America and the Caribbean.

The crude mean interval between first and last birth calculated over all parities shows a much wider range from 9.6 in Portugal to 19.4 in Kenya. The majority of less-developed countries lies between 13 and 18 years. *Figure 2.15* indicates clearly that this crude mean age is strongly associated with the mean completed parity in each country as measured by $F(0)$. A lower level of fertility implies a shorter average period from first to last birth, because there are more women with low completed family sizes who have their last birth generally at a younger age than high-fertility women. The slope of the regression line almost corresponds to the mean birth interval between subsequent births calculated over all 41 countries. This means that on the level of national averages lower fertility generally does not result in significantly longer birth intervals as indicated for national subpopulations.

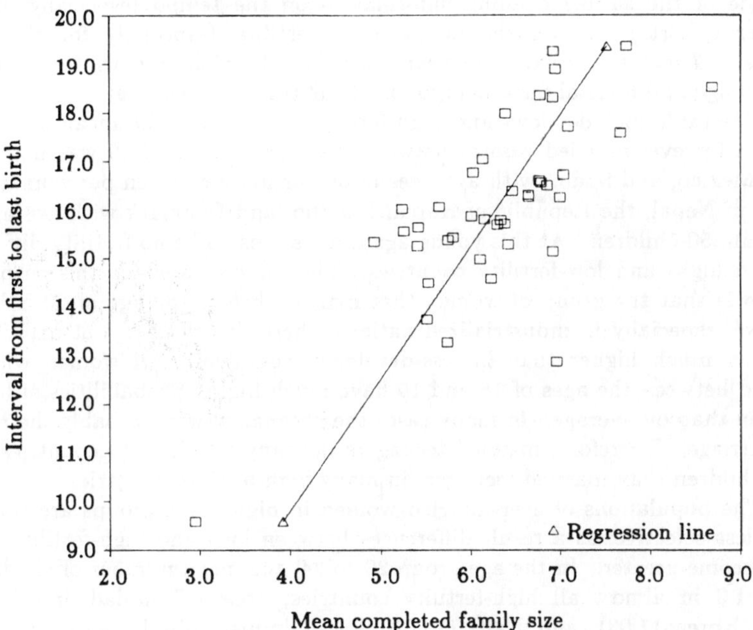

Figure 2.15. Cross-national association (for the 41 WFS LDCs, including Portugal) between the mean interval from first to last birth and the country's average fertility level, $F(0)$.

Table 2.14 finally gives the more general life cycle measure of $e(i)$, i.e., the mean interval from the birth of order i to the completion of childbearing. These again are weighted averages in which only women with more than i births were taken into consideration, and their distribution over the remaining parities provided the weights. Generally, for low i's the ranking is very similar to that of the intervals from first to last birth with Kenya at the top and Portugal at the bottom. The differentials clearly diminish for higher i's, and interestingly enough beyond parity six, Portugal no longer shows the shortest interval. Korea, Lesotho, and Nepal quickly pass Portugal with shorter intervals from births of orders six and above to the last birth. Hence, Portugese women with at least six children make up a population with a fertility regime quite comparable with that of corresponding populations in less-developed countries.

2.4. Current Parity Distributions

Until this point various aspects of completed fertility throughout the world have been described and analyzed. This section treats the analysis of women in the survey who are still within childbearing ages. Hence, their reproductive career is truncated by the interview, and the figures on the mean number of children at the date of the survey combine information on the tempo (especially for the younger cohorts) and on the quantum of fertility (especially for the older cohorts). *Table 2.15* gives the mean numbers of children born to women of selected age and marital duration groups at the time of the survey.

The table includes low- and high-fertility countries. The mean number of children for ever-married women between the ages of 15 and 19 was highest in Peru, Mexico, and Spain, with averages of one or more children per woman, and lowest in Nepal, the Republic of Korea, Lesotho, and Denmark with averages of less than .50 children. At this young age there seems to be no fertility difference between high- and low-fertility countries. The main reason for this surprising pattern is that the group of women that married before the age of 20 is highly selective, especially in industrialized nations where the mean age at marriage is generally much higher than in less-developed countries. All women who are married between the ages of 15 and 19 have much higher probabilities of having children than on average. In many cases the pregnancy was probably the reason for marriage. Therefore, married teenagers in many low-fertility countries have more children than married teenagers in many high-fertility countries.

The populations of ever-married women in higher age groups are progressively less selective; as a result differences between low- and high-fertility countries become greater. In the age group 20 to 24, the mean number of children is above 1.3 in almost all high-fertility countries, except Trinidad and Tobago (1.26), Korea (1.03), and Haiti (1.30). In all industrialized countries, except Spain and Czechoslovakia, it is lower. In the age group 30 through 34 the international average fertility ranking is already similar to that of completed cohort fertility with the highest means in Jordan and Kenya and the lowest in Europe. It is interesting to note that in high-fertility countries the ranking is very similar to that of completed fertility, whereas in Europe fertility beyond age 35 still appears to matter in terms of the final ranking. This may be because of the different structure of the reproductive pattern in natural and controlled fertility societies or it may be due to the fact that the means of two different age groups are being compared even though they belong to different cohorts that might have quite distinct reproductive patterns.

Analyzed with respect to marital duration, current mean parities are not necessarily reflective of the average age at marriage prevalent in a society. Chapter 1 showed that marriage and childbearing are very closely related; in most LDCs the highest birth intensities are during the years following marriage. The age at marriage may only have an indirect effect. Aside from declining fecundability, age only matters in cases where the mean age at marriage is extremely low; fecundability might be reduced during the first years of marriage. The average number of children for women married 0 to 4 years (which means an average marital duration of 2.5 years in the case of an even distribution) was highest in Kenya (1.39), Costa Rica, and Spain (both 1.31). Nepal (.47) and Bangladesh (.51) registered the lowest mean number of children for women married 0 to 4 years. Within the limits of these extremes, there is no clear differential between high- and low-fertility countries in the first duration category; whereas for higher durations, the less-developed countries clearly have higher mean numbers of children. This implies that for the cohorts considered

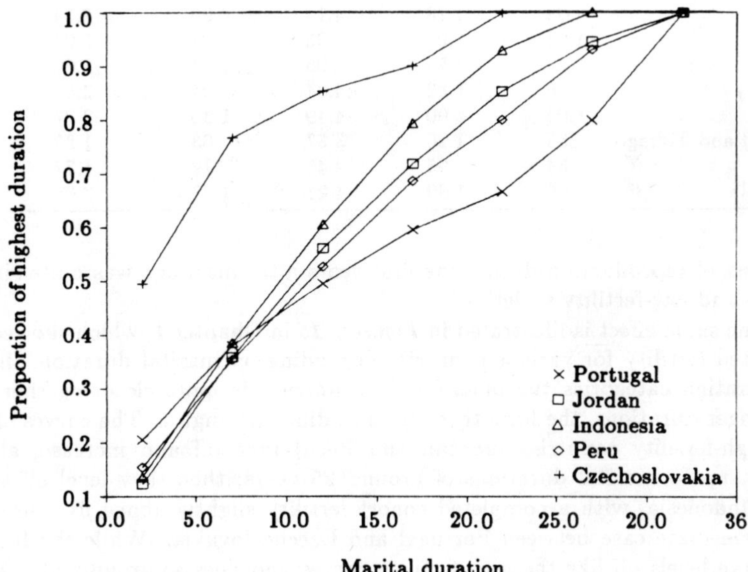

Figure 2.16. Proportion of fertility of highest marital duration category by current duration for five selected countries.

Table 2.15. Mean numbers of children ever born at time of survey for selected marital duration and age groups of ever-married women.

Country	Age group			Marital duration (in years)		
	15–19	*20–24*	*30–34*	*0–4*	*5–9*	*15–19*
AFRICA						
Benin	.63	1.68	4.73	1.17	2.68	5.65
Cameroon	.71	1.73	4.19	1.04	2.46	4.76
Egypt	.63	1.81	4.61	.91	2.64	5.46
Ghana	.71	1.59	4.06	.96	2.33	5.02
Ivory Coast	.76	2.01	4.78	1.09	2.69	5.45
Kenya	.94	2.16	5.62	1.39	3.31	6.36
Lesotho	.49	1.43	3.95	.82	2.31	4.63
Mauritania	.99	2.17	5.00	.89	2.29	5.03
Morocco	.77	1.92	4.91	.99	2.71	5.59
Nigeria	.83	2.10	4.36	1.02	2.50	4.85
Senegal	.71	1.95	5.26	.90	2.43	5.53
Sudan	.70	2.19	4.99	.86	2.67	5.60
Tunisia	.63	1.52	4.53	1.09	2.95	5.67
AMERICAS						
Colombia	.98	1.84	4.49	1.19	2.78	5.75
Costa Rica	—	1.61	3.90	1.31	2.48	5.48
Dominican Republic	.76	1.82	4.84	.91	2.58	5.82
Ecuador	.86	1.91	4.48	1.21	2.78	5.88
Guyana	.80	1.77	4.89	.93	2.54	5.43
Haiti	.66	1.30	3.54	.89	2.19	4.80
Jamaica	.88	1.78	4.14	.96	2.34	4.79
Mexico	1.03	1.99	4.95	1.21	3.04	6.14
Panama	—	1.74	4.05	1.21	2.66	5.07
Paraguay	.76	1.82	4.84	.91	2.58	5.82
Peru	1.04	2.00	4.49	1.30	2.97	5.78
Trinidad and Tobago	.55	1.26	3.37	.63	1.83	4.17
USA	.54	.95	2.45	.79	1.77	3.15
Venezuela	.86	1.89	4.21	1.07	2.68	5.31

the speed of reproduction during the first years after marriage was quite similar in high- and low-fertility societies.

The same effect is illustrated in *Figure 1.15* in Chapter 1, which showed the cumulated fertility for various countries depending on marital duration. In the first duration categories the plots for all countries lie quite close together, but with longer durations, the lines then curve at different angles. The curves of two very high-fertility countries (Jordan and Peru) take off and increase, almost linearly, up to marital durations of around 25 years; then they level off somewhat. Indonesia, with a completed cohort fertility slightly above five, presents an intermediate case between Portugal and Czechoslovakia. While the Indonesian curve levels off like the high-fertility curves and does so around 20 years of marital duration, the increase in the Portugese curve accelerates. This is probably a result of the selectivity of women who marry very young and tend to have significantly high fertility. The case of Czechoslovakia is interesting because it starts out faster than many other countries – even faster than Indonesia – and

Table 2.15. Continued.

Country	Age group			Marital duration (in years)		
	15–19	*20–24*	*30–34*	*0–4*	*5–9*	*15–19*
ASIA and PACIFIC						
Bangladesh	.71	2.40	5.67	.51	1.96	5.02
Fiji	.51	1.46	4.22	.96	2.56	5.01
Indonesia	.59	1.66	4.03	.73	2.07	4.27
Jordan	.89	2.45	5.89	1.18	3.44	6.90
Korea, Republic of	.47	1.03	3.37	1.10	2.71	4.42
Malaysia	.82	1.66	4.28	1.07	2.83	5.32
Nepal	.32	1.43	4.10	.47	1.72	4.42
Pakistan	.58	1.91	4.97	.63	2.46	5.46
Philippines	.85	1.89	4.27	1.24	2.95	5.77
Sri Lanka	.67	1.54	3.80	.92	2.44	4.84
Syria	.88	2.16	5.21	1.09	3.20	6.45
Thailand	.69	1.50	3.91	.95	2.53	5.02
Turkey	.67	1.81	4.28	.95	2.58	5.06
Yemen	.60	1.81	5.05	.68	2.31	5.79
EUROPE						
Belgium	.66	.66	1.95	.68	1.63	2.50
Czechoslovakia	.79	1.30	2.10	1.26	1.95	2.29
Denmark	.45	.90	2.10	1.01	1.86	2.57
Finland	.91	.94	1.79	.89	1.59	2.46
France	—	.92	2.25	.88	1.81	2.70
Great Britain	.60	.82	2.05	.64	1.69	2.54
Hungary	.78	1.13	1.86	1.03	1.77	2.01
Italy	.97	1.03	2.03	.95	1.75	2.60
Netherlands	.67	.82	1.94	.83	1.82	—
Norway	.74	.91	2.16	.91	1.87	2.73
Poland	.66	1.06	2.15	1.06	1.89	2.67
Portugal	.57	1.06	2.08	.95	1.75	2.75
Spain	1.00	1.46	2.38	1.31	2.13	3.04
Yugoslavia	.67	1.28	2.59	1.11	2.09	2.95

remains at an almost constant level after duration 10.

Standardizing these curves with respect to the quantum aspect as measured by the mean number of children for women in the highest duration category provides another interesting comparison. Because women in different duration categories come from different cohorts, the curves need not necessarily increase monotonically, but they do so empirically for most of the countries. *Figure 2.16* graphically displays cumulated fertility of various duration categories as a proportion of fertility of the highest duration category. The graph shows clearly what was already observed in *Figure 1.15*. Czechoslovakian women initially demonstrate a very high relative speed of fertility. Already after ten years of marriage, women had born more than 80% of the children that had been born by women married for more than 20 years. Conversely, the graph illustrates that in Portugal, the other low-fertility country in the graph, less than half of the children of the highest duration category were born after ten years of marriage.

This might be not only because of selectivity due to young marriage but also because of the result of a declining trend in fertility; in Portugal shorter duration cohorts may have quite a different fertility pattern from the longer ones.

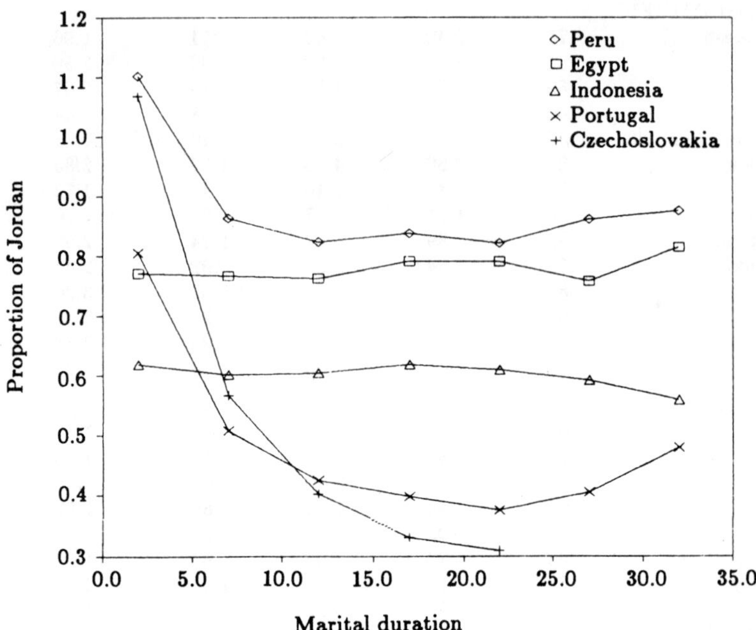

Figure 2.17. Current mean fertility by marital duration of five selected countries as a proportion of mean fertility in Jordan in respective categories.

As with mean parities in *Figure 1.15*, the high-fertility countries show a relatively stable increase toward high fertility in the high-duration categories. This indicates that in less-developed countries even young women who were newly married before the survey generally started out their reproductive career with the same speed as women in an essentially natural fertility regime.

Figure 2.17 compares the mean numbers of children for different duration categories in five selected countries with the fertility in Jordan, the country with the highest fertility in our study. Women in Czechoslovakia and in Peru began bearing children faster than women in Jordan but after 5 to 10 years of marriage fell way behind the Jordanians. While the curves for Czechoslovakia and Portugal decline to levels less than 40% of that of Jordanian women, the decline of the Peruvian curves stops around duration ten. In Indonesia and in Egypt the increase in mean family size from duration to duration is almost parallel to that in Jordan but at a lower level. In Peru it is parallel at a lower level after 5 to 10 years. In other words, the high-fertility countries show a similar tempo at different quantum levels.

So far the analysis has focused on the mean numbers of children at different ages and marital durations. The study will now consider the parity distributions. *Figures 2.18* through *2.23* depict comparisons of parity distributions for different countries, ages, and duration. *Figures 2.18* and *2.19* plot the current parity distributions for two European and three high-fertility countries for a selected age group (25 through 29 years) and a selected duration group (10 through 14 years). The two pictures look quite similar. In less-developed countries the distributions are spread out much more evenly over the parities than in Europe. All cases seem to be centered around the mode. Czechoslovakia has in both cases a very pronounced peak at parity two, whereas in France the prevalence of one-child families in the age group 25 through 29 is greater than that of two-children families. In *Figure 2.19* the curve representing French women refers to somewhat older cohorts than those referred to in *Figure 2.18*. This curve has the same shape as the Czechoslovakian curve. Thus, the initially different shape in *Figure 2.18* is a consequence of the differential tempo and hardly has implications on the eventual parity distribution.

Figures 2.20 and *2.23* compare the parity distributions across different age and duration categories for Jordan and Belgium. For Jordan the distributions according to duration are more centered around the mode than those with respect to age. This indicates that age at marriage is less homogeneous than fertility after marriage, which looks to be very homogeneous. At duration 0 through 4 years, 35% of the women have one child, at duration 5 through 9 years 56% of the women have three or four children, and at duration 15 through 19 more than half of all women are concentrated in the small parity range of six to eight children. Although *Figure 2.20* refers to the same sample of women as *Figure 2.21*, the different pattern of distributions is caused by the fact that women are grouped differently. Obviously age at marriage in Jordan is much less homogeneous than the tempo of fertility after marriage. This is the only explanation for the fact that the distributions of current parities are less centered around the mode for age cohorts than for marital duration cohorts.

In Belgium – an example of a low-fertility country – the differences between age and duration cohorts are less pronounced, *Figures 2.22* and *2.23*. This is probably due to the fact that few women have more than two births rather than to variation in the age at marriage. After the first five years of marriage or after age 25, the distributions of all age and marriage cohorts are clearly centered around two children with only an insignificant tail to the right representing a small number of high-fertility women.

2.5. Need for More Studies

This chapter discussed only a few aspects of cohort fertility. The data in Appendix A and Appendix B could be used for many more detailed studies on the quantum and tempo of fertility in individual countries. Because the primary focus of this study is the complete distribution of reproduction and its variation

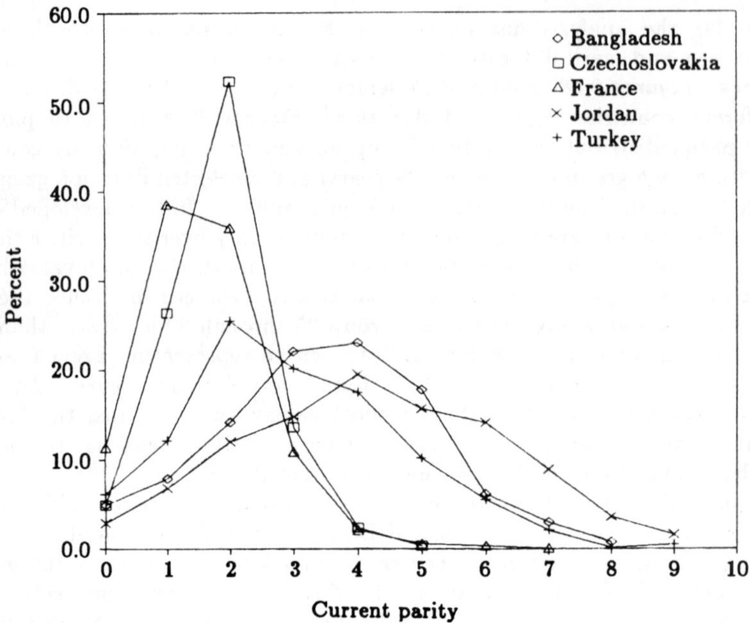

Figure 2.18. Current parity distributions in five selected countries for age group 25 through 29.

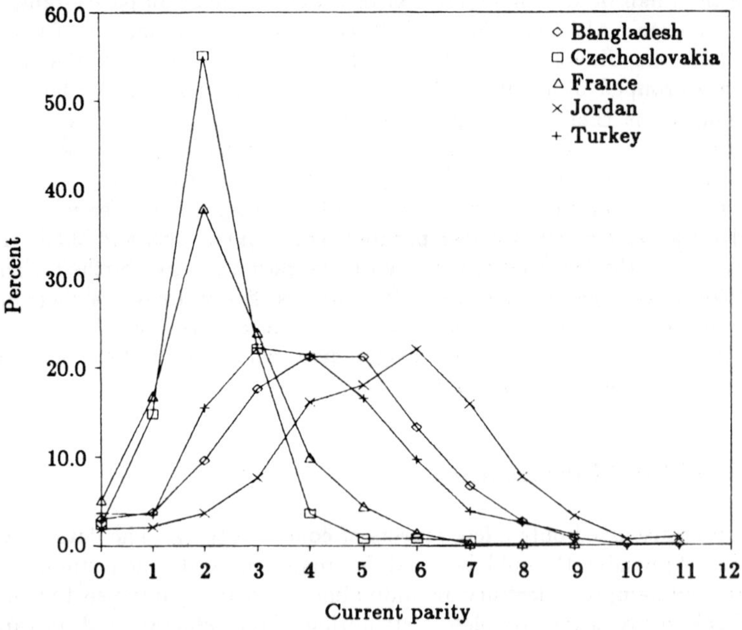

Figure 2.19. Current parity distributions in five selected countries for duration group 10 through 14.

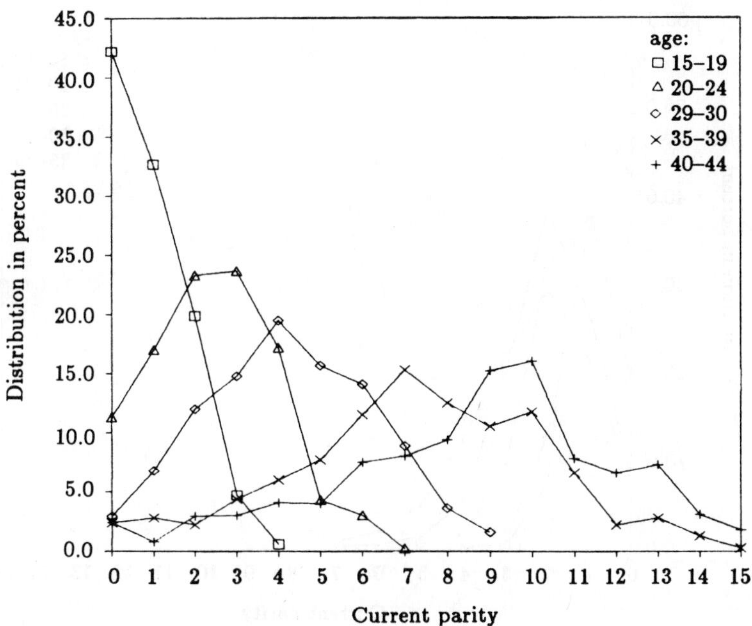

Figure 2.20. Current parity distributions in Jordan by age.

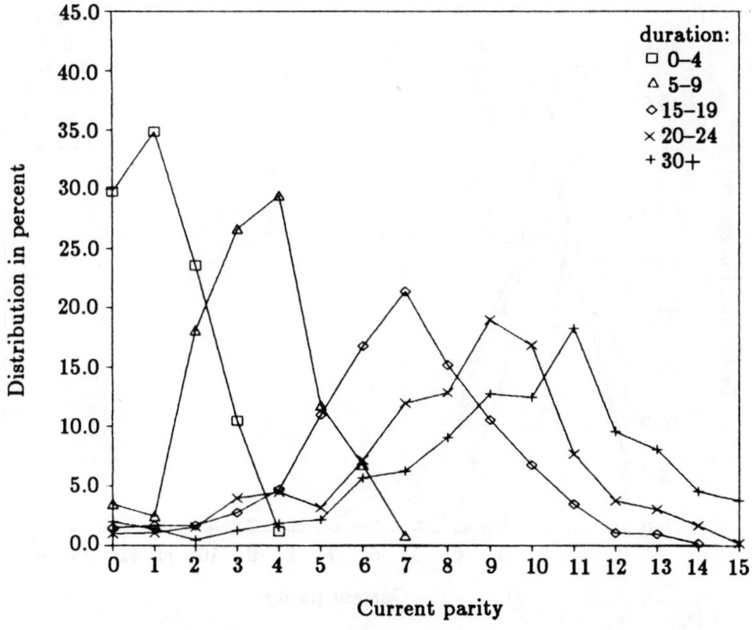

Figure 2.21. Current parity distributions in Jordan by marital duration.

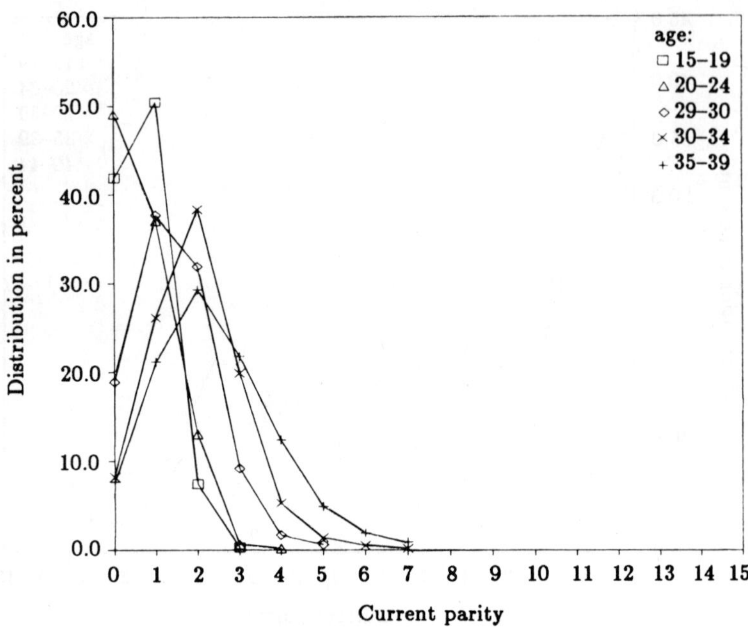

Figure 2.22. Current parity distributions in Belgium by age.

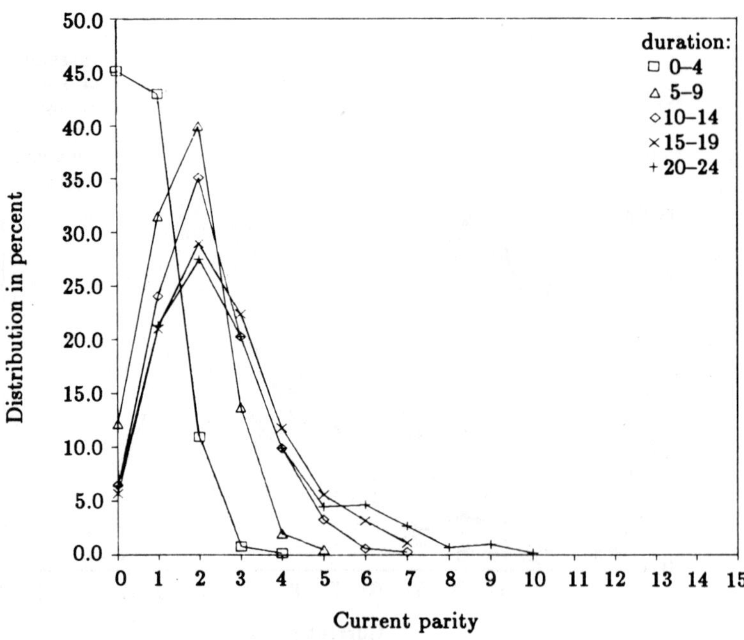

Figure 2.23. Current parity distributions in Belgium by marital duration.

across countries and socioeconomic groups, models that try to reduce the information into a few parameters, such as the relational logits models (see Pullum *et al.*, 1987), were intentionally disregarded.

Notes

[1]   If one of the subgroups in LDCs contains fewer than 120 cases, however, the table is not given. Also, categories including more than 80% of the total of the cohorts considered in a country are omitted because in such a category the pattern of fertility becomes almost indistinguishable from the total. Therefore, the table that was omitted can be seen from the n given in the other tables of the country.

[2]   In this context the Dutch data are not strictly compatible to the other countries because they are restricted to the marriage cohorts of 1963–1973.

CHAPTER 3

The Parity-Specific Analysis of Period Fertility

3.1. Parity-Specific Rates

3.1.1. Conceptual issues

This chapter examines the use of the period mode of temporal aggregation that cuts across several cohorts at one point (or period) in time. When these cross-sectional observations are arranged in a way that builds a *synthetic cohort*, meaningful life-cycle indicators can be derived that pertain to a period instead of a cohort. The great advantage of the period analysis of fertility is its greater contemporaneity.

A consideration of the demographic dimension parity in the study of period fertility has several important advantages. First, we know that parity empirically influences fertility, especially in low-fertility, developed countries. Second, a distinction between women of different parities at a given point in time introduces important information about very recent reproductive experience of the population into the measurement of current fertility. Furthermore, fluctuations and discontinuities in period fertility affect the parity composition of the population and for this reason measures that take explicit account of parity allow the construction of synthetic cohorts that come closer to that of real cohorts than the synthetic cohorts based on age-specific period rates only. This will be discussed in more detail in the following sections.

Generally, demographic rates are the appropriate *styles of measurement* of the intensities of demographic processes such as mortality, fertility, nuptiality in a certain period. Period probabilities in most cases cannot be observed directly. Under the conventional definition, demographic rates are calculated by dividing the number of observed events during the period by the number of person years of exposure lived during that period. The latter is mostly approximated by the *midyear population*. Because there is some confusion about the measurement of parity-specific fertility rates in the literature, it is necessary to clarify some terms that refer to the notion of demographic dimensions introduced in Chapter 1.

Every age-specific rate measures the events at a given age interval in relation to the exposure to the event in that age interval. When the continuous demographic dimension age – that in practice is mostly transformed to discrete age groups – is replaced by the discrete demographic dimension parity, one gets parity-specific fertility rates following the same logic: births of order $i+1$ should be divided by the number of women exposed to births of this order, i.e., women being at parity i. In other words, the one-dimensional parity-specific fertility rate is that of all births to women at parity i divided by the number of all women of parity i in a given period. This direct parity-specific rate, however, is hardly ever found in demographic literature. Usually parity is only considered in two-dimensional perspectives in addition to age or birth interval. The following sections discuss the way in which the simple one-dimensional rate is quite useful for the analysis of fertility behavior especially if some additional information on the mean ages of births of certain orders is taken into account.

When, in a two-dimensional perspective, parity and age (or any other dimension of individual time) are considered simultaneously, one must differentiate between two possible rates that may be computed: the two dimensions may be considered in the numerators only while using a one-dimensional denominator, or both numerator and denominator are specific for both dimensions. As has been briefly mentioned in Chapter 1, the latter possibility may be called real-specific rates; they are the real occurrence-exposure rates to be used, e.g., in every life-table model. For the other rates (often called reduced rates), there are theoretically two possibilities: a denominator that is parity-specific and one that is age-specific. While the first has almost never been used, the second is very common especially in descriptive studies. The reduced rates are smoother than the specific rates and may be summed up with respect to both age (to calculate synthetic cohorts for certain orders of birth) and parity (to get age-specific rates for a certain range of orders), but they are also bad statistics in the sense that they do not properly match numerator and demoninator. A more detailed analysis of this problem is given by Feeney and Yu (1987).

Figure 3.1 presents reduced parity-specific fertility rates for the birth cohort of 1936 in the Federal Republic of Germany, and *Figure 3.2* gives the real parity- and age-specific period rates for Finland in 1984. The patterns of first-order births are very similar in both cases because the denominators of the specific rates include almost the same numbers of women as that in the case of the reduced rates. For second-order births the picture becomes very different: while the rates in *Figure 3.1* are clearly lower than for first births (because of fewer second births than first births), the rates in *Figure 3.2* for second-order births are much higher, especially at younger ages (because the denominators include only women who already had a first birth). Third and fourth births are rare enough that even the age- and parity-specific rates diminish with order at all ages below age 30. Above age 30 in Finland the rate of having a fourth birth given that the woman already has three children is higher than the corresponding rates for lower-order births. The increase of the modal age at birth with the order of birth is more clearly visible in the case of reduced rates in *Figure 3.1*.

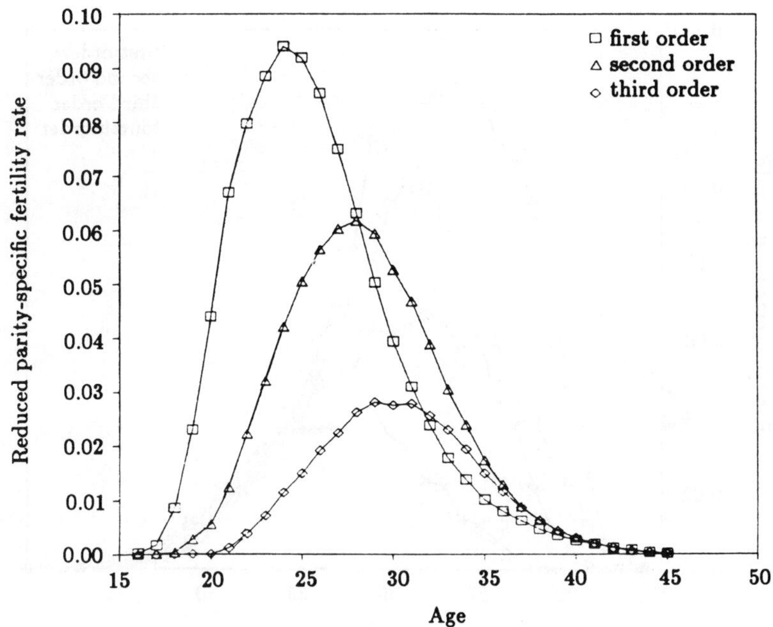

Figure 3.1. Reduced parity-specific fertility rates $\left(\dfrac{B(i,a)}{W(a)}\right)$ for birth cohort of 1936 in the FRG.

Is there any possibility to infer information on the parity-specific probabilities of birth from given period information? Luis Henry (1953) first approached this question in a systematic manner. He defined period parity-progression ratios (*probabilités d'agrandissement*) as the conditional probabilities of a birth of order $i+1$ given that the woman already had i births. However, the empirical measurement of period parity-progression ratios has always been a problem mostly because of lack of data. Henry suggested two methods for the indirect estimation of period parity-progression ratios. One uses tabulations of births by order and year of previous birth, whereas the second only needs a time-series of births by order. Similar methods have been applied more recently (e.g., by Marchal and Rabout, 1972; Feeney, 1983; and Bhrolchain, 1985). Several other studies tried to get more direct estimates by using fertility survey data (e.g., Brass and Juarez, 1983; Feeney and Wijeyesekera, 1983).

The crucial question in measuring the quantum aspect of period fertility lies in the conversion of observed parity-specific rates into probabilities, i.e., parity-progression ratios, that cannot be directly observed for period fertility. All attempts to estimate period parity-progression ratios are based on the concept of synthetic cohorts. The construction of some cohorts requires parity-

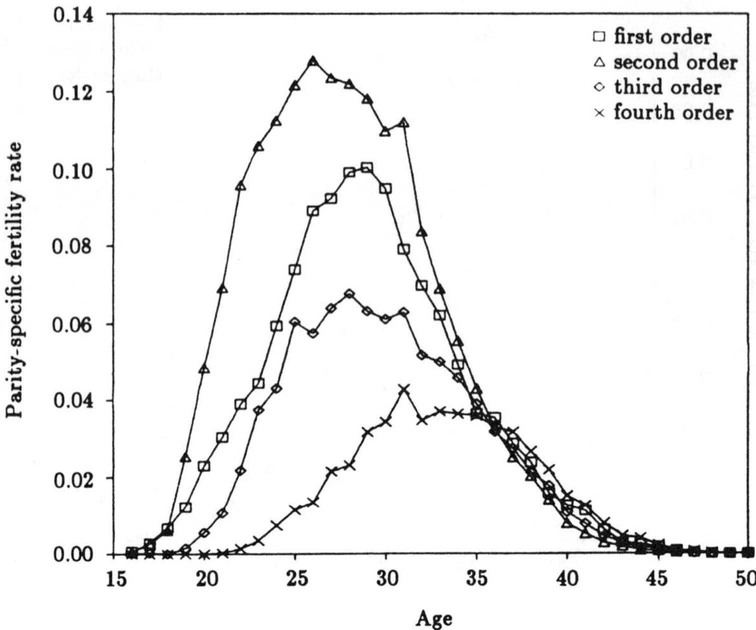

Figure 3.2. Age- and parity-specific period fertility rates in Finland, 1984.

specific data with respect to one time telling how long women remain in certain parities. Usually, the time dimension used is one of the following: women's age, birth interval, or marital duration. This first method leads to a two-dimensional approach, which will be described below. A second method uses only parity-specific fertility rates and mean ages at nth birth. Here, the empirical input is less complex and less specific than above, which reduces the risk of errors and makes data easier to obtain. The exact mathematics of transforming this input into parity-progression ratios is given in Section 3.2.

The basic idea of the first approach is that if a dimension of individual time is measured in addition to parity then standard life-tables techniques can be applied to estimate the progression probability from one parity to another by multiplicatively chaining the probabilities that are specific for parity and the units of the selected dimension of individual time. This dimension might be age, time since last birth, or marital duration. Most of the recent work in this area, especially the innovative work done by Feeney (e.g., 1983), concentrates on time since last birth. But it would be also justified to have age as the second dimension.

To illustrate this approach, *Table 3.1* gives a fertility table based on age- and parity-specific rates for the FRG and the birth cohort of 1936. A real cohort

Table 3.1. "Life table" of parity progression based on age, for birth cohort in the FRG, 1936.

| | Parity | | | |
	0	1	2	3+
Age				
15	100,000	0	0	0
16	99,970	30	0	0
17	99,790	209	1	0
18	98,912	1,078	10	0
19	96,547	3,345	108	0
20	91,929	7,692	377	2
21	84,714	14,137	1,125	25
22	75,992	21,119	2,752	136
23	66,189	28,063	5,299	449
24	55,683	34,485	8,735	1,097
25	45,459	39,447	12,983	2,111
26	36,105	42,622	17,660	3,614
27	28,133	43,732	22,570	5,564
28	21,708	42,970	27,285	8,037
29	16,886	40,834	31,413	10,867
30	13,332	38,311	34,561	13,796
31	10,678	35,658	36,811	16,854
32	8,742	33,314	38,205	19,739
33	7,372	31,413	38,846	22,369
34	6,352	29,924	31,935	24,590
35	5,634	28,865	39,196	26,305
36	5,079	28,117	39,170	27,634
37	4,660	27,657	39,061	28,622
38	4,356	27,324	38,984	29,336
39	4,128	27,123	38,919	29,829
40	3,964	26,994	38,863	30,180
41	3,843	26,920	38,823	30,414
42	3,765	26,874	38,809	30,552
43	3,716	26,848	38,805	30,631
44	3,694	26,827	38,804	30,675
45	3,680	26,821	38,795	30,704

perspective was taken here because the results can easily be verified (Birg *et al.*, 1984). We start from a radix of 100,000 childless females at age 15. The group of zero-parity women is gradually reduced at each age. These are derived from the rates by the usual transformation. Decreases in the childless category will result in increases in the one-child category, which at the same time shrinks due to second births. This table disregards the decreases due to death. It may be regarded as a hierarchical model with four states. The survivors at each parity at age 45 give the completed parity distribution of the cohort. The results nearly reproduce the distribution of the cohort in 1981 with slight differences owing to mortality and migration.

If period fertility rates were taken instead of cohort rates, the table could correspond to a synthetic life table. In further analogy to the conventional life table, one could also calculate life expectancies indicating the mean durations of sojourn in each parity status. An isomorphic table for marital fertility may be

Table 3.2. Annual parity-specific fertility rates (per 100) for all ever-married women in 55 WFS countries, three years before the survey.

	Parity												
	0	*1*	*2*	*3*	*4*	*5*	*6*	*7*	*8*	*9*	*10*	*11*	*12*
AFRICA													
Benin	19.2	28.0	28.1	27.3	24.6	24.6	22.2	17.2	17.1	13.0	18.8		
Cameroon	13.9	19.6	25.1	25.4	28.3	23.9	20.9	16.2	18.0	12.7	13.1		
Egypt	17.3	34.1	25.7	24.2	23.0	21.5	18.4	17.9	12.7	12.8	11.2	10.9	8.9
Ghana	19.6	24.3	24.7	22.9	18.3	23.7	23.7	17.0	18.1	12.6			
Ivory Coast	16.8	23.4	27.9	26.0	24.6	31.2	21.8	27.9	18.8	19.9	17.7		
Kenya	23.3	30.7	32.1	32.4	29.1	31.2	24.5	24.7	19.3	16.4	20.1	13.6	
Lesotho	16.9	23.7	22.7	21.1	19.6	20.7	18.2	22.3	17.5	16.6			
Mauritania	16.4	27.5	23.4	20.1	25.1	19.9	26.7	18.6	18.9	17.8			
Morocco	17.3	30.3	28.7	23.4	25.3	21.8	23.2	18.8	19.2	18.0	15.0	13.3	9.4
Nigeria	16.6	28.8	27.4	25.7	25.8	21.9	25.0	17.6					
Senegal	18.5	28.0	29.9	28.2	25.6	31.0	24.9	22.9	19.9	16.8	26.4		
Sudan (North)	14.0	28.8	25.7	27.5	29.0	22.7	23.3	21.1	20.7	19.9	10.8		
Tunisia	20.1	38.3	35.5	28.6	24.4	19.7	17.7	23.3	20.9	17.4	14.1		
ASIA & PACIFIC													
Bangladesh	13.2	28.5	27.8	26.2	25.3	19.2	16.5	19.3	11.9	12.0	10.2	10.8	
Fiji	15.4	28.3	23.3	21.2	16.8	12.0	10.1	8.6	9.2	8.6	6.1	12.3	
Indonesia	14.1	16.6	17.1	18.3	18.0	16.2	14.2	11.7	11.3	12.0	14.4		
Jordan	19.6	43.1	42.8	41.5	35.1	36.5	30.5	25.8	28.2	26.1	13.2	20.0	21.8
Korea, Rep. of	21.5	33.6	26.7	17.5	11.2	9.0	7.7	7.0	6.0	8.6			
Malaysia	18.2	31.3	23.4	17.5	21.5	13.5	17.4	8.8	14.4	9.2	10.5		
Nepal	12.3	30.0	26.9	25.4	18.9	21.1	20.3	18.0	12.8	17.3	12.0		
Pakistan	13.6	28.6	27.8	26.3	23.8	24.2	22.9	15.5	15.7	10.9	10.7	13.8	
Philippines	23.5	33.4	30.7	25.4	20.1	19.9	19.0	19.5	15.1	16.6	14.6	18.1	18.2
Sri Lanka	16.1	29.0	10.2	19.6	16.1	11.6	13.5	14.5	10.7	14.1	8.6		
Syria	20.8	44.4	39.8	32.1	28.8	31.5	31.0	22.9	21.7	17.2	12.3	14.8	19.2
Thailand	21.1	27.0	22.2	19.1	12.3	11.5	12.6	13.8	15.6	11.0			
Turkey	16.1	30.3	18.5	14.2	16.6	11.0	17.7	16.8	13.4	10.5	16.5		
Yemen	16.9	32.9	26.7	33.1	31.1	26.7	31.5	23.7	16.9	27.1	15.0		

constructed with marital duration replacing age as the indexing variable. If duration since last birth is selected as the basic time dimension, then the table should have a slightly different structure because each parity will be entered at duration zero. But the principal approach remains the same.

In the case of a one-dimensional approach, using only parity and not time, we could make a parity-progression table as we did in Chapter 2. The composition of such a table, using period parity-specific rates and mean ages at birth as input, is more complex than using completed fertility data. The data requirements, however, are much less demanding than in the two-dimensional case. For this reason more attention will be given to the one-dimensional period fertility table based on parity in Section 3.2.

Table 3.2. Continued.

	Parity												
	0	1	2	3	4	5	6	7	8	9	10	11	12
AMERICAS													
Colombia	19.9	28.0	19.6	16.1	17.8	14.7	19.7	14.3	15.3	18.1	15.7	17.1	
Costa Rica	25.3	21.9	13.4	13.0	11.6	16.7	12.3	9.6	13.9	16.4	8.6		
Dominican Rep.	16.3	30.6	27.8	21.3	21.3	21.4	16.8	25.9	31.3	27.9	1.61	17.1	19.4
Ecuador	20.6	30.4	20.1	21.1	20.4	17.8	19.6	18.2	19.6	18.3	20.0	19.5	15.9
Guyana	15.3	32.1	25.3	22.3	18.2	18.4	12.1	14.0	10.2	18.7	11.3	12.0	
Haiti	14.4	21.9	18.1	20.2	20.5	27.9	19.0	16.7	19.5	11.7			
Jamaica	13.3	19.6	17.2	21.8	18.0	19.9	18.5	14.8	16.7	13.8	26.8	26.9	
Mexico	21.3	35.1	30.3	23.6	25.3	23.8	21.3	20.6	24.2	20.9	13.8	26.7	21.2
Panama	21.8	22.3	19.8	11.8	16.2	11.7	14.5	15.7	13.0	19.2	13.8		
Paraguay	17.1	21.4	20.9	16.5	20.9	18.0	21.5	22.1	11.3	21.3	11.5	11.3	
Peru	23.5	31.1	26.0	24.5	22.5	21.1	19.0	18.5	18.2	17.8	18.4	18.8	
Trinidad & Tobago	11.5	21.4	12.8	16.0	11.9	10.3	1..8	8.6	7.3	13.5			
USA	33.7	16.8	5.8										
Venezuela	18.9	24.9	20.3	19.8	19.4	16.6	21.8	23.9	21.3	29.5			
EUROPE													
Belgium	20.2	9.6	3.8										
Czechoslovakia	37.8	18.6	3.9										
Denmark	27.3	21.0	4.5										
Finland	24.4	12.0	3.1										
France	21.4	12.9	4.9										
Great Britain	16.3	16.0	—										
Hungary	35.8	16.2	4.4										
Italy	28.6	12.9	3.8										
Netherlands	25.4	25.5	4.6										
Norway	23.5	19.2	6.0										
Poland	37.2	17.2	6.2										
Portugal	17.4	11.7	3.9	4.3	4.5	9.3	7.3						
Spain	34.2	19.5	6.5										
Yugoslavia	15.8	18.0	5.9										

3.1.2. Empirical period data

Empirical figures for period parity-specific fertility rates are given in *Table 3.2*
for the WFS countries discussed so far. The data pertain to the third year
before the survey was conducted. This year is frequently used in WFS studies
because more recent data on fertility tend to be biased by too many reports in
the first year and too few reports in the second year before the interview. The
denominators of the parity-specific rates have been calculated by using the
breakdown of current parity at the date of the interview and dividing it by the
number of births in the last three years before the interview. Rates based on less
than five women in the numerator are not shown in the table. For some countries only data on ever-married women are available. Therefore, to compare the
data across all countries, the rates pertain to ever-married women only.

Table 3.3. Mean ages at birth of order i for all ever-married women in 55 WFS countries, three years before the survey.

	Order of birth												
	1	*2*	*3*	*4*	*5*	*6*	*7*	*8*	*9*	*10*	*11*	*12*	*13*
AFRICA													
Benin	20.8	23.4	25.5	27.8	29.8	31.5	34.2	35.7	38.7	39.1	39.0		
Cameroon	19.8	22.2	24.9	28.3	29.7	32.8	34.6	35.2	37.8	40.0	38.5		
Egypt	21.1	22.9	24.8	26.7	28.5	29.6	32.2	34.2	34.8	36.7	36.1	38.2	39.0
Ghana	20.6	23.2	26.4	29.4	31.0	34.3	35.2	36.8	40.0	42.4			
Ivory Coast	18.8	21.5	24.1	26.5	28.7	30.9	32.9	36.7	38.0	40.3	39.6		
Kenya	19.5	21.7	24.0	25.7	27.8	30.8	33.5	34.5	38.2	37.7	38.9	39.4	41.7
Lesotho	20.7	23.9	27.0	28.5	32.6	35.2	34.6	38.5	39.2	39.2			
Mauritania	18.6	21.6	24.0	25.5	28.2	30.0	30.3	34.6	32.7	36.9			
Morocco	20.9	23.4	24.0	26.0	28.8	30.9	33.5	33.8	36.6	38.3	37.6	39.4	41.8
Nigeria	19.8	22.3	24.3	26.7	28.0	30.3	31.6	34.4					
Senegal	19.0	21.6	24.1	26.4	28.7	31.0	32.2	34.9	36.8	38.6	40.8		
Sudan (North)	20.7	22.1	24.1	26.1	27.9	28.9	32.9	33.0	35.2	36.0	37.0		
Tunisia	22.4	24.1	25.7	29.2	31.7	34.4	35.7	36.4	38.9	39.1	41.2		
ASIA & PACIFIC													
Bangladesh	17.0	19.7	22.5	24.3	26.7	28.9	31.0	33.5	34.9	36.1	36.3	37.3	
Fiji	21.0	24.1	25.5	28.0	29.8	31.1	32.8	33.4	38.7	37.8	35.6	38.7	
Indonesia	20.0	22.4	25.0	27.7	30.0	32.4	33.6	36.3	38.8	39.3			
Jordan	19.8	21.7	23.8	26.0	27.3	29.5	30.3	32.0	34.0	35.6	37.6	38.6	38.0
Korea, Rep. of	24.1	25.8	27.8	31.0	32.9	35.4	37.3	38.6	39.6	42.6			
Malaysia	22.2	23.5	26.6	28.0	29.8	32.0	33.2	34.7	36.1	37.8	37.6		
Nepal	20.8	23.0	25.8	28.0	30.2	32.8	34.5	37.0	37.0	38.9	41.3		
Pakistan	20.3	22.1	24.6	26.7	29.3	29.8	33.2	34.9	35.6	37.0	38.9	40.7	
Philippines	22.4	24.0	26.4	28.0	30.6	32.3	34.3	34.8	37.3	38.8	39.2	41.1	40.9
Sri Lanka	23.5	25.1	26.4	28.5	30.2	32.1	33.3	35.3	37.0	37.7	41.1		
Syria	20.5	22.6	24.6	27.3	24.6	30.9	32.3	34.4	35.8	38.3	40.9	38.4	38.7
Thailand	22.0	23.6	25.9	29.2	32.0	36.4	36.5	37.9	39.5	41.0			
Turkey	20.5	22.6	26.1	26.4	28.7	31.8	32.0	33.4	36.6	36.2	40.1		
Yemen	20.5	22.6	26.1	26.4	28.7	31.8	32.0	33.4	36.6	36.2	40.1		

The parity-specific rates given in *Table 3.2* may be interpreted as the fractions of women that had an additional birth of a certain order during the year of observation. At parity zero, i.e., the occurrence of first births, the highest LDC fertility rates are found in Costa Rica (.253), the Philippines (.235), Peru (.235), and Kenya (.233), while the lowest are in Trinidad and Tobago (.115) and Nepal (.123). In low-fertility countries the span of variation is greater, ranging from highs in Czechoslovakia (.378) and Spain (.342) to lows in Portugal (.174) and Yugoslavia (.158). There seems to be no clear difference between high- and low-fertility countries with respect to the rate of first-order births, and the level in individual countries seems to depend largely on the marriage pattern and on the mean age at first birth.

In LDCs highest fertility rates are generally those for second births (i.e., for women at parity one). In low-fertility countries the rates of second-order births are generally much lower. This is not due to a lower incidence of second births

Table 3.3. Continued.

					Order of birth								
	1	*2*	*3*	*4*	*5*	*6*	*7*	*8*	*9*	*10*	*11*	*12*	*13*
AMERICAS													
Colombia	20.9	23.1	25.3	27.5	28.1	29.9	32.0	34.1	35.7	37.1	35.6	38.3	38.8
Costa Rica	22.1	23.9	24.9	26.7	28.0	31.4	32.4	33.9	34.8	34.7	40.3	39.4	
Dominican Rep.	19.6	22.2	23.4	26.0	27.4	30.7	33.2	33.7	33.9	35.8	34.9	38.6	39.0
Ecuador	21.1	23.0	25.1	27.9	29.3	31.0	32.4	34.1	36.0	36.2	37.9	38.6	39.0
Guyana	20.4	22.4	23.4	26.2	27.4	31.7	32.3	32.5	34.5	34.9	36.7	37.2	
Haiti	22.0	25.4	28.1	29.9	31.4	34.1	33.9	38.4	40.2	40.2			
Jamaica	20.1	21.6	24.0	25.9	30.1	29.9	33.2	33.9	35.4	37.3	38.1	40.7	
Mexico	20.4	22.9	24.9	26.8	27.7	30.4	32.0	34.7	35.4	34.7	37.7	28.5	39.6
Panama	22.3	23.7	25.1	26.0	29.0	30.2	31.4	34.0	35.6	34.9	37.1		
Paraguay	21.5	24.3	26.4	28.2	29.2	31.6	32.7	33.8	37.5	37.2	39.4	40.7	
Peru	21.4	23.2	25.7	27.9	29.7	31.8	33.1	35.2	36.5	37.7	39.7	40.3	
Trinidad & Tobago	22.2	23.6	25.6	26.6	28.7	32.4	32.2	35.5	36.5	36.6			
USA	22.2	24.6	25.7										
Venezuela	21.1	23.2	25.0	26.6	27.3	29.3	31.3	32.3	34.7	35.4			
EUROPE													
Belgium	21.4	26.9	28.9										
Czechoslovakia	22.2	25.3	27.7										
Denmark	24.1	27.3	28.9										
Finland	24.7	27.6	28.7										
France	23.8	26.0	27.2										
Great Britain	24.2	26.4	—										
Hungary	21.5	25.2	26.8										
Italy	24.4	27.1	30.0										
Netherlands	25.0	26.8	29.0										
Norway	23.8	26.2	29.6										
Poland	22.6	25.6	28.6										
Portugal	23.8	27.2	30.4	32.7	31.8	34.5	40.5						
Spain	24.8	27.5	30.6										
Yugoslavia	21.6	24.4	27.0										

in low-fertility countries, but is due to longer birth intervals. These longer birth intervals are indicated by high mean ages for second births, illustrated in *Table 3.3*. In LDCs fertility rates at parities two to five usually show a slow decline after the steep increase from parity zero to one. The rates tend to peak at parities two to four only in tropical Africa. Aside from this weak trend, the patterns of parity-specific rates show great diversity. In some very high-fertility countries, we can observe a slight increase in the rates at very high parities. This pattern might have the same selection origin as the increase in parity-progression ratios at very high parities, which was identified in Chapter 2.

The European countries and the USA show a steep decline of rates when parity increases, which is especially strong between parities one and two. There is no data on fertility at higher parities in these countries, except for Portugal. Fertility there remains low at higher parities. This may indicate a concentration around the two-child norm with only a small fraction of women proceeding to higher parities. One must be cautious, however, not to interpret the parity-specific rates as if they were parity-progression ratios. To derive progression ratios from these fertility rates, timing and birth intervals must be considered. These can be derived from the series of mean ages at *i*th birth.[1]

Table 3.3 provides mean ages at *i*th birth for the third year before the survey. The mean ages at first birth are lowest in Bangladesh (17.0 years), Mauritania (18.6 years), and the Ivory Coast (18.8), and are highest in the Netherlands (25.0), [2] Spain (24.8), and Finland (24.7). Despite the general pattern of lower mean ages in LDCs and higher means in more-developed countries (MDCs) there is substantial overlap: e.g., Republic of Korea (24.1) and Sri Lanka (23.5) are clearly higher than Belgium (21.4) and Hungary (21.5). We can assume that age at first birth is closely related to the marriage pattern. A comparison of the cohort measure for women between the age of 40 and 49 in Chapter 2 with the current period measures reveals significant changes in a number of countries.

Confirming *a priori* expectations, mean ages at birth increase fairly smoothly with birth order. There are only a few discontinuities. This is possible because of the period nature of the data where the figures for different birth orders are from different women. When these data are used to construct synthetic cohorts, such discontinuities cannot be tolerated – a point to be discussed in more detail below.

Cross-national differentials in the period mean ages of fertility are large and increase by birth order. Generally, higher mean ages at given birth orders imply a later start in childbearing and fairly widespread use of modern or traditional spacing methods. This is true in Europe, where mean ages for the first three births are higher than they are in most LDCs.

For higher-order births data were collected only on LDCs and Portugal. For seventh births the mean ages range from 31.0 in Bangladesh to 40.5 in Portugal. For tenth births the difference is again larger, ranging from 34.7 in Costa Rica and 34.9 in Panama to 42.4 in Ghana and 42.6 in the Republic of Korea.

3.2. A Period Fertility Table Based on Parity

3.2.1. Structure of the period fertility table

Chiang and van den Berg (1982) first suggested a life-table approach to the analysis of period fertility, which was slightly modified later by Chiang (1984). The principle of the table is identical to that described in the previous chapter for cohort fertility: parity replaces age as the indexing variable of the life table, and the usual survival probabilities become parity-progression ratios.

Chiang and van den Berg considered the fertility table from a stochastic viewpoint in which reproduction is seen as a staging process, and each stage is defined by the birth of a child. The process advances from one stage to the next until the woman reaches her completed parity, which may be any parity between zero and the maximum considered. This model can be used to derive the maximum likelihood estimators for several table functions. For the purpose of this study, however, it is sufficient to consider the deterministic trunk model.

The period fertility table is entered through the empirical period mean ages at births of different order, $x(i)$, and the set of parity-specific fertility rates, $r(i)$. The definitions are isomorphic to that of the cohort fertility table

$$x(i) = \sum_{a=15}^{45} \frac{B(i-1,a)(a+.5)}{\sum_{a=15}^{45} B(i-1,a)} \tag{3.1}$$

and

$$r(i) = \frac{\sum_{a=15}^{45} B(i,a)}{\sum_{a=15}^{45} W(i,a)}, \tag{3.2}$$

where $B(i,a)$ is the total number of births at parity i to women aged a in the population in a given year, and $W(i,a)$ is the number of women with parity i aged a.

In the life table the parity-specific fertility rate is defined by

$$r(i) = \frac{l(i+1)}{L(i)}, \tag{3.3}$$

where $l(i)$ is the number of persons still in the process of reproduction at parity i, and $L(i)$ is the number of years lived at parity i. $L(i)$ consists of two parts: the number of person years lived by those who proceed to a higher parity, $l(i+1)$, and the years lived by those with final parity i, $d(i)$:

$$L(i) = d(i)\,[xw - x(i)] + l(i+1)\,[x(i+1) - x(i)]. \tag{3.4}$$

The years lived by an individual for whom i is the final parity are the years between entering parity i – on the average $x(i)$ – and the end of the process, i.e., the assumed age at menopause, xw. The number of years lived by an individual who goes on to the next parity is the difference between the mean age upon entering parity i, $x(i)$, and the mean age upon leaving parity i, $x(i+1)$. As defined the current form of the fertility table disregards mortality; it gives the implications of pure fertility net of all other effect.

The crucial point in the calculation of a period fertility table is the transition from annual parity-specific fertility rates to parity-progression ratios. Intuitively, the parity-progression ratio (a pure measure of the quantum aspect) is derived by applying the annual parity-specific fertility rates (containing both quantum and timing aspects) for a certain time to the mean duration of exposure to the next birth (a measure of timing only). Since the time that women are exposed to possible additional births, $L(i)$, contains also years of those women who do not proceed to higher parities, the formula for parity-progression ratios is not simply the rate times the mean birth interval. The parity-progression ratio for women at parity i may be defined as the parity-specific fertility rate times the exposure conditioned by the probability of having reached parity i:

$$p(i) = \frac{l(i+1)}{l(i)} = \frac{L(i)r(i)}{l(i)}. \tag{3.5}$$

The following algebraic transformations lead to an expression that is only written in terms of $x(i)$ and $r(i)$, the two empirically given pieces of information. By applying (3.4) to (3.5) one can write

$$p(i) = \frac{r(i)d(i)[xw - x(i)]}{l(i)} + \frac{r(i)l(i+1)[x(i+1) - x(i)]}{l(i)}; \tag{3.6}$$

by dividing both sides by $d(i)/l(i)$ one gets

$$\frac{p(i)}{1 - p(i)} = r(i)[xw - x(i)] + \frac{p(i)}{1 - p(i)}r(i)[x(i+1) - x(i)] \tag{3.7}$$

because

$$\frac{l(i)}{d(i)} = \frac{1}{1 - p(i)} \quad \text{and} \quad \frac{l(i+1)}{d(i)} = \frac{p(i)}{1 - p(i)}. \tag{3.8}$$

By splitting $[x(i+1) - x(i)]$ into the two components $[xw - x(i)]$ minus $[xw - x(i+1)]$ the formula becomes

$$\frac{p(i)}{1 - p(i)} = r(i)[xw - x(i)] + \frac{p(i)r(i)}{1 - p(i)}[xw - x(i)]$$

$$\tag{3.9}$$

$$- \frac{p(i)r(i)}{1 - p(i)}[xw - x(i+1)].$$

Division by $r(i)[xw - x(i)]$ and $p(i)/1-p(i)$ on both sides further yields

$$\frac{1 - p(i)}{p(i)} = \frac{1 + r(i)[xw - x(i+1)]}{r(i)[xw - x(i)]} - 1, \tag{3.10}$$

and since the solution for $\dfrac{1 - p}{p} = x$ is $p = \dfrac{1}{x + 1}$, the final equation is

$$p(i) = \frac{r(i)\,[xw - x(i)]}{1 + r(i)\,[xw - x(i+1)]}. \tag{3.11}$$

This transition formula is identical to the maximum likelihood estimator Chiang and van den Berg derived for their stochastic model of reproduction. Once period parity-progression ratios are determined, the $l(i)$ and $d(i)$ columns follow as described above for the cohort fertility table or as detailed below in the summary of table functions.

The calculation of a life expectancy that summarizes the fertility table with respect to the timing aspect of fertility is less straightforward. Chiang and van den Berg (1982) suggest a measure, $e(i)$, which they call "expected length of waiting time from age at ith birth to completion of family." In the equation, $e(i)$ is defined by

$$e(i) = \frac{T(i)}{l(i)} \tag{3.12}$$

where

$$T(i) = \sum_{j=i}^{m} L(j), \tag{3.13}$$

m being the highest parity considered. Because, however, in contrast to the ordinary life table no one leaves the fertility table before the end of the process xw, $e(i)$ becomes simply

$$e(i) = xw - x(i), \tag{3.14}$$

which is part of the empirical input and does not require any further calculations. Formally equation (3.14) can be deducted from (3.12) and (3.13) with consideration of (3.4) by recursion (see Feichtinger and Lutz, 1983):

$$T(i) = L(i) + L(i+1) + \cdots \tag{3.15}$$

$$= d(i)[xw - x(i)] + l(i+1)[x(i+1) - x(i)]$$

$$+ d(i+1)[xw - x(i+1)] + l(i+2)[x(i+2) - x(i+1)] + \cdots$$

$$= l(i)[xw - x(i)] - l(i+1)[xw - x(i)] + l(i+1)[x(i+1) - x(i)]$$

$$+ l(i+1)[xw - x(i+1)] - l(i+2)[xw - x(i+1)]$$

$$+ l(i+2)[x(i+2) - x(i+1)] + \cdots = l(i)[xw - x(i)].$$

In his 1984 book Chiang includes a less trivial definition of $e(i)$ with the same verbal description as before,

$$e(i)^* = \frac{1}{l(i)} \sum_{j=i}^{m} d(j)[x(j) - x(i)]. \tag{3.16}$$

This measure may be considered a weighted average of the differences between age at current birth and the various possible ages at last birth, the $x(j)$'s. For women with completed parity i, this waiting period is zero. The empirical values of $e(i)^*$ estimated by Chiang (1984) are very small; they reach a maximum of 3.4 years at parity one. As stated above the reason for this is the fact that all women who do not proceed to higher parities, $d(i)$ women, have $e(i)^*$'s of zero. From a behavioral point of view this seems a somewhat artificial measure, because it is not known if women still have a nonzero waiting period to complete their family size when they are still exposed to the risk of an additional birth. For this reason Feichtinger and Lutz (1983) introduced another timing measure, $v(i)$, defined by

$$v(i) = \frac{L(i)}{l(i)}. \tag{3.17}$$

This measure may be called the "mean waiting time from birth of order i to the end of exposure to an additional birth" by either reaching age xw or proceeding to parity $i+1$.

A more serious question than the selection of a summary indicator for the timing of fertility is the age span covered in the fertility table. Chiang suggests that xw may be either 45.00 or 50.00. Sensitivity analysis shows that results are significantly different under these two assumptions.

Another important value is $x(0)$, the beginning of the risk period. Fertility results are even more sensitive to what $x(0)$ is selected than to what xw is chosen. Chiang took the mean age of women of parity zero during the study year for $x(0)$. As will be demonstrated below this is not correct; it should be the age when entering into the risk population. Chiang's implausible result of more than 40% of the US white female population remaining childless under 1978 fertility rates is a direct consequence of a value of $x(0)$ that is too high: with too little exposure to a first birth and a given parity-specific fertility rate, the parity-progression ratio will be underestimated.

Generally, the given model of a fertility table based on parity works only if the risk population covered in the empirical parity-specific fertility rates corresponds to the risk population in the life-table model. Let $_yB(i)_a$ be the number of births to women aged a to $a+y$ at parity i in a given year and $_yW(i)_a$ the number of person years lived in that year by women aged a to $a+y$ at parity i. Then, the empirical parity-specific fertility rate is defined in (3.2) by

$$_yr(i)_a = \frac{_yB(i)_a}{_yW(i)_a}. \tag{3.18}$$

The same rate is defined in terms of fertility table functions by

$$_y r(i)_a = \frac{l(i+1)}{L(i)}.$$

(3.19)

From (3.18) and (3.19) we can easily see that the life-table births, $l(i+1)$, and especially the person years of exposure, $L(i)$, should cover the same age span a to $a+y$ as the empirical measure. Clearly, if $_y W(i)_a$ includes women between the ages 15 and 45, then $L(i)$ should refer to the same age group so that $x(0)$ should be 15.00 and xw should be 45.00.

Consider two theoretical cases with identical age- and parity-specific fertility rates. In both cases, no woman has a birth before age 15 or after age 45. In the first case, $W(0)$ includes all childless women aged 15 to 45; in the second case women aged 10 to 15 are also included in $W(0)$. Obviously, $r(i)$ will be greater in the first case than in the second case. The results of the parity tables, however, should be identical because the fertility pattern is identical. Taking the same $x(0)$'s – say 15.00 – for the fertility tables in both cases would result in a lower progression ratio at parity zero and consequently in a higher proportion of childless women in the second case. If, however, $x(0)$ were set to 10.00 in the second case, then the longer exposure to a first birth would exactly compensate for the lower parity-specific fertility rate, and the results of the two tables would become identical. The same line of reasoning applies to xw. Therefore, xw must be selected to equal the maximum age considered by the input data.

The next step is to consider the age structure of the empirical population. What about the case of a sample survey where the number of women at the upper or lower end of the age span considered is significantly smaller than at other ages? They would contribute less than average exposure at certain ages, whereas in the fertility table every age is assumed to have equal weight in the calculation of exposure. This problem can arise in surveys and in cases of an uneven age structure in the total population. However, it does not pose serious difficulties because empirically age and parity correlate strongly. This issue is discussed at length in Section 3.2.2.

Summary of Table Functions

The period fertility table applied in this chapter has eight columns and one summary measure (see *Table 3.4*). The model uses the data from the complete Finnish population in 1984 and the WFS. Listed below is an explanation of each column in the table.

Column 1: Parity, *i*.
The first column gives the indexing variable of the table, parity. In the Finnish data parity is defined as the number of living children a woman has born. Hence, it is not only the number of births but also all multiple births. The parities considered range from zero to $m+$. The value of m is selected according to two criteria: the availability of data and the fertility pattern of the population.

In this study m ranges from 3 in some European surveys to 15 in many less-developed countries.

Column 2: Mean age at birth of ith child, $x(i)$.
This is one of the two empirical input variables. It pertains to all births of order i in a given year and is defined in formula (3.1). In this formula $x(0)$ is the age of entry into the table and equals the age of entry into the observed risk population. In the case of a marital-fertility table, $x(0)$ is the mean age at marriage.

Column 3: Parity-specific fertility rate, $r(i)$.
This is the second empirical input variable to the table. It was defined in formulas (3.2) and (3.18).

Column 4: Parity-progression ratio, $p(i)$.
The information provided in columns 2 and 3 can be used to calculate period parity-progression ratios according to formula (3.11).

Column 5: Number of women with parity i or more, $l(i)$.
A radix of 100,000 women is assumed at the start. The parity-progression ratios are then multiplied (like the survival probabilities in the usual mortality life table) to obtain the $l(i)$ column:

$$l(i+1) = p(i) \cdot l(i). \tag{3.20}$$

Column 6: Mean waiting time from birth of order i to the end of exposure to an additional birth, $v(i)$. This measure of timing has been defined in formula (3.17). It is one of several possible timing indicators of fertility under a family life-cycle perspective. A woman's duration at parity i extends from the time she enters parity i, $x(i)$, to the birth of her next child, $x(i+1)$, or to the end of the process xw. As already mentioned, no woman leaves the table between $x(0)$ and xw.

Column 7: Number of women who stop reproducing after ith birth, $d(i)$.
This column gives the number of women who remain at parity i until the end of the process xw. Like in the mortality life table, $d(i)$ is defined by

$$d(i) = l(i+1) - l(i). \tag{3.21}$$

Column 8: Percentage of women with completed parity i, $c(i)$.
This column gives the completed parity distribution implied by the given period pattern of parity-specific fertility. It is the most significant result of the table. The numerical values are obtained by a simple modification of the $d(i)$ column:

$$c(i) = \frac{d(i)}{l(0)} \times 100. \tag{3.22}$$

Summary Indicator: Mean completed parity, MCP.
A summary indicator of the complete distribution should be comparable in size to the total fertility rate. It is the mean completed parity (MCP) or mean family size for women that is implied by recent period fertility behavior. Although the mean parity is derived by a completely different approach, its numeric value should not be too far from that of the regular total fertility rate calculated from age-specific fertility rates because both indicators can be interpreted to be the mean family size for a synthetic cohort based on observed period rates. The difference between the two indicators lies in the fact that the mean parity from the fertility table considers parity-specific behavior, whereas the total fertility rate disregards parity. MCP summarizes the quantum information provided by the fertility table in one measure. It is calculated as a weighted average of i, the weights being the $c(i)$'s

$$MCP = \sum_{i=0}^{m+} i\, c(i)/100. \tag{3.23}$$

This definition considers only births of orders lower than or equal to m. This is an approach taken, for instance, by Feeney and Yu (1987). This measure is not strictly comparable with the total fertility rate (TFR), which considers births of all orders. An attempt was made to approximate the TFR equivalent by assuming that the mean parity in the category of women with m or more children is $m+1$.

The great advantage of the parity-specific approach lies in the fact that it results in the estimate of the complete distribution of children among mothers in a synthetic cohort, whereas the age-specific approach can only provide a mean. The mean completed parity has some interest as the first distribution and is appropriate for assessing the difference between a parity-specific and an age-specific approach.

3.2.2. Sensitivity of the period estimates to age-structure distortions

There are two empirically derived variables in a period parity table: the mean age at birth of order i $[x(i)]$ and the annual parity-specific fertility rate, $r(i)$. Both variables depend on the age distribution of the population. They are specific with respect to parity but crude with respect to age. Like the crude birthrates and death rates, they reflect the age profile of the population. They should be different for populations with different age structures even when the age-specific pattern is identical. Since, however, age and parity tend to be strongly correlated, parity-specific birthrates are in reality less age dependent than crude birthrates. The strong correlation between parity and age is simply because of the hierarchical nature of the process of parity progression and the fact that birth interval must have a certain minimal length. Nevertheless, some age-distributional effects remain that will be analyzed in the following section.

Let $B(i,a)$ represent the number of births to women at parity i and age a, and $W(i,a)$ the number of women in that group. Then the previously defined parity-specific birthrate would be written as

$$r(i) = \frac{\sum\limits_{a=15}^{44} B(i,a)}{\sum\limits_{a=15}^{44} W(i,a)}. \tag{3.24}$$

In contrast to this the age- and parity-specific fertility rate had been defined by

$$r(i,a) = \frac{B(i,a)}{W(i,a)}. \tag{3.25}$$

Assuming that the age- and parity-specific intensity of reproduction – given by $r(i,a)$ – remains constant and only the distribution of women over age changes, then the number of births to women of parity i

$$B(i) = \sum\limits_{a=15}^{44} r(i,a)\, W(i,a) \tag{3.26}$$

would depend on the age distribution if $r(i,a)$ were invariant over age. In reality, however, $r(i,a)$ is far from constant. The intensity of birth, especially of lower orders, is heavily concentrated in the prime childbearing ages. For example, if the number of women aged 20 through 25 was significantly smaller than that of women aged 30 through 35, then the number of first births would be significantly smaller than in the case of an even age distribution, and smaller still compared with a population of mostly women in younger age groups.

The objective of this study is to standardize the parity-specific birthrates and the mean ages at births of certain orders with respect to the age structure to make them comparable with a cohort perspective disregarding mortality. In other words, all age groups should get equal weight. One seemingly obvious way to do this would be to calculate the age-specific rates as it is done in computing the total fertility rate,

$$r^*(i) = \sum\limits_{a=15}^{44} r(i,a). \tag{3.27}$$

Such a "total parity-specific fertility rate," $r^*(i)$, is, however, meaningless because it assumes that the exposure to a birth of order $i+1$ is evenly distributed over all ages such as for the total fertility rate in which we assume that every woman lives through the ages 15 through 45. In the case of a parity-specific perspective it cannot be assumed that every woman lives through all ages at each parity because women proceed to higher parities. The mean age of women exposed to the risk of first birth is much lower than that of women exposed to the risk of fifth births. A rate such as $r^*(i)$ would give equal weight to the intensity of first births at age 18 as it would to that of third births at 18. Such conditional probabilities at young ages are often quite high because of extreme selectivity, but the proportions of women they refer to are very small. To yield a correct elimination of age structural effects, one must adjust for age differential in exposure by weighting the age- and parity-specific rate, $r(i,a)$, by the proportion of women at parity i and age a among all women aged a:

$$B^{ast}(i) = \sum_{a=15}^{44} r(i,a), \frac{W(i,a)\ WT}{30\ W(a)} \tag{3.28}$$

where the superscript *ast* stands for age standardized, WT indicates the total number of women at all parities between ages 15 and 44, and $W(a)$ represents the total number of women at age a. For the age-standardized parity-specific birthrate, a combination of (3.24) and (3.28) yields the following:

$$r^{ast}(i) = \sum_{a=15}^{44} \frac{B(i,a)}{W(a)} \Big/ \sum_{a=15}^{44} \frac{W(i,a)}{W(a)}, \tag{3.29}$$

where the numerator of the expression includes reduced fertility rates with respect to age. The sum of these rates over all parities would yield the total age-specific fertility rate at age a. These reduced rates show a much more even picture than the age- and parity-specific rates.

In a similar manner to the parity-specific rate, the mean age of women at the birth of order i depends on the age distribution. The mean age is defined as:

$$x(i) = \sum_{a=15}^{45} (a + .5)\ \frac{B(i,a)}{\sum\limits_{a=15}^{44} B(i,a)}. \tag{3.30}$$

We see that $x(i)$ depends on the female age structure because the number of births at parity i depends on the number of women at each age.

By using the same reduced parity-specific fertility rates as in (3.29), we can standardize the mean age at births of a certain order by relating it to an age distribution with the same number of women in each age group

$$x^{ast}(i) = \sum_{a=15}^{44} (a + .5)\ \frac{B(i,a)/W(a)}{\sum\limits_{a=15}^{44} B(i,a)/W(a)}. \tag{3.31}$$

Empirical Sensitivity Analysis

The study now turns to conducting some empirical test of age-standardization on the completed parity distribution implied in the model, more generally to study the sensitivity of the estimations to various kinds of age-distributional distortions. To achieve this, existing sets of age- and parity-specific fertility rates must be subjected to a number of empirical and hypothetical age distributions and the results of the model of uneven age distributions must be compared with the model assuming an even age distribution. The discrepancy between the two results will be a measure for the sensitivity of the fertility table to age distribution.

For the pattern of age- and parity-specific fertility, data based on complete national populations were preferred over small sample surveys to avoid the problem of irregularities because of small cell sizes. The following analysis uses two data sets that were used in Chapters 1 and 2: the 1984 period fertility rates from the Finnish population register and the 1936 cohort fertility experience from the Federal Republic of Germany. For the FRG cohort, which consisted of women in their prime childbearing ages at the peak of the German baby boom, some estimations had to be made concerning the parity distribution of illegitimacy and the distribution of the denominator (see Birg *et al.* 1984).

Figure 3.3 shows four extreme age distributions that are used in the sensitivity study.

(1)   The even distribution of women over all ages corresponds to the age distribution that is assumed by the model of the fertility table in which the number of person years between the ages 16 and 17 is equal to those between the ages 42 and 43. The age standardization given above is oriented on this distribution. Mortality is disregarded.

(2)   The population-age distribution of the FRG in 1984 is characterized by irregular ups and downs. Women between ages 16 and 27 have more weight than the average age groups; they are the strong cohorts from the baby boom. Above age 28 the groups are smaller with a minimum at age 39. Ages 44 and 45 are again above average. Such fluctuations, mainly caused by fertility fluctuations in the past, are typical for many industrialized societies.

(3)   Because of the extremely high fertility in Kenya the population is very young and age-group sizes decline monotonically from younger to older. Although somewhat less extreme, many less-developed countries have a similar age structure in reproductive age.

(4)   This hypothetical distribution illustrates extreme ups and downs and is based on the assumption that women are only in every fifth age group and all other age groups are empty. Less extreme empirical cases of such fluctuations might result from incorrect reporting or possibly from strong fertility fluctuations in the past.

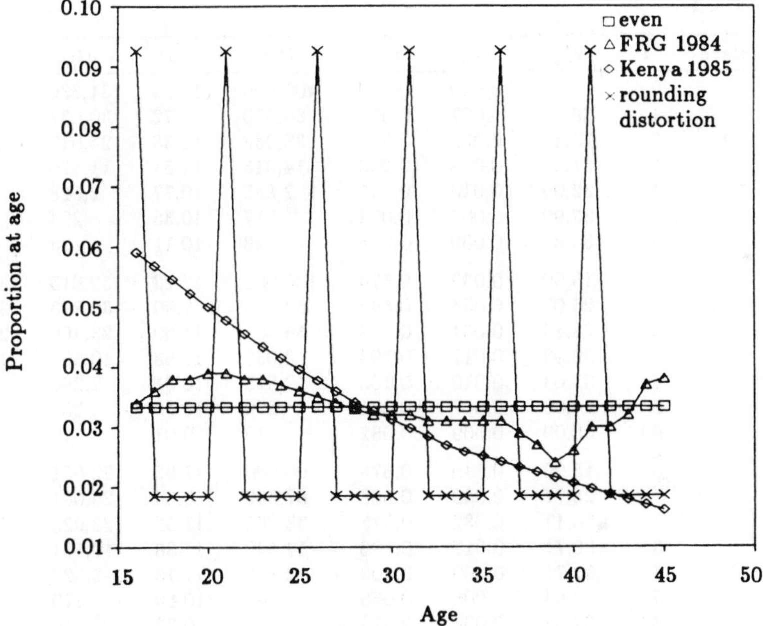

Figure 3.3. Four extreme examples of age distributions for sensitivity analysis.

Table 3.4 gives the result of this sensitivity study for the Finnish period data of 1984. The table gives the completely unweighted situation, i.e., the actual Finnish age distribution in 1984. The other four fertility tables result from weighting the given pattern of age- and parity-specific fertility rates by the four age distributions described above and then from reaggregating them as if they were crude parity-specific fertility rates and crude mean ages at marriage. *Table 3.5* is analogous to *Table 3.4*, but refers to the 1936 birth cohort in the FRG. Because of the cohort nature of the data it does not make sense to give a table for the crude data; they are essentially the same as in the case of weight A (even distribution), with slight adjustments for mortality and migration.

From *Tables 3.4* and *3.5* the following conclusions can be drawn:

(1)   For both the Finnish and the FRG data the crude fertility tables show little difference from the age-standardized data (weight A). The reproductive behavior of the 1936 birth cohort in the FRG resulted in a distribution in which only 5% of the women remained childless; however, the period fertility of Finnish women in 1984 implies that about 32% of the women remain childless. This difference between the childlessness in the cohort of 1936 in Germany and the recent situation in Finland (which is common in many

Table 3.4. Period fertility table for Finland, 1984, unweighted and weighted with age structures A–D.

Age structure	i	$x(i)$	$r(i)$	$p(i)$	$l(i)$	$v(i)$	$d(i)$	$c(i)$
Row	0	15.00	0.040	0.687	100,000	17.04	31,330	31.33
	1	26.13	0.057	0.554	68,670	9.72	30,637	30.64
	2	28.48	0.032	0.369	38,032	11.38	24,017	24.02
	3	31.05	0.018	0.203	14,015	11.51	11,170	11.17
	4	32.99	0.010	0.111	2,845	10.77	2,528	2.53
	5	33.90	0.007	0.074	317	10.35	294	0.29
	6+	34.89	0.009	0.086	23	10.11	23	0.02
A	0	15.00	0.039	0.674	100,000	17.23	32,615	32.62
	1	26.05	0.054	0.542	67,385	9.96	30,883	30.88
	2	28.40	0.031	0.357	36,501	11.60	23,466	23.47
	3	30.99	0.017	0.194	13,036	11.68	10,500	10.50
	4	33.03	0.010	0.106	2,535	10.81	2,266	2.27
	5	34.00	0.007	0.071	269	10.30	250	0.25
	6+	35.09	0.009	0.082	19	9.91	19	0.02
B	0	15.00	0.040	0.673	100,000	17.05	32,651	32.65
	1	25.77	0.059	0.568	67,349	9.64	29,081	29.08
	2	28.11	0.032	0.375	38,268	11.53	23,925	23.92
	3	30.71	0.017	0.196	14,343	11.88	11,531	11.53
	4	32.71	0.009	0.103	2,812	11.13	2,523	2.52
	5	33.64	0.006	0.066	289	10.68	270	0.27
	6+	34.68	0.008	0.078	19	10.32	19	0.02
C	0	15.00	0.036	0.629	100,000	17.55	37,102	37.10
	1	25.21	0.066	0.608	62,898	9.19	24,680	24.68
	2	27.55	0.034	0.398	38,218	11.54	23,020	23.02
	3	30.14	0.015	0.184	15,197	12.49	12,399	12.40
	4	32.12	0.007	0.088	2,799	11.83	2,552	2.55
	5	33.07	0.005	0.053	246	11.35	233	0.23
	6+	34.07	0.006	0.062	13	10.93	13	0.01
D	0	15.00	0.039	0.674	100,000	17.27	32,634	32.63
	1	26.11	0.059	0.565	67,366	9.54	29,289	29.29
	2	28.46	0.033	0.374	38,076	11.34	23,847	23.85
	3	31.06	0.018	0.202	14,229	11.51	11,351	11.35
	4	32.99	0.010	0.109	2,878	10.78	2,564	2.56
	5	33.78	0.007	0.071	314	10.50	292	0.29
	6+	34.87	0.009	0.085	22	10.13	22	0.02

industrialized countries), where almost one-third of all women are expected to remain childless, also illustrates the dramatic changes in reproductive behavior over the last 25 years.

(2) When a modern European fertility pattern is applied to an extremely young population (like Kenya), the proportion of childless women is overestimated by approximately 5% at the expense of the proportion with completed parity one. The rest of the distribution remains almost the same. The reason for this discrepancy is based on the fact that a very young age distribution biases downward in both the mean age at first birth and the rate of first-order birth, a combination that results in a lower parity-progression ratio.

Table 3.5. Cohort fertility table for birth cohort born in 1936 in the FRG, applying different weights A–D.

Age structure	i	$x(i)$	$r(i)$	$p(i)$	$l(i)$	$v(i)$	$d(i)$	$c(i)$
A	0	15.00	0.085	0.954	100,000	11.17	4,552	4.55
	1	25.27	0.088	0.694	95,448	7.93	29,170	29.17
	2	28.00	0.047	0.469	66,278	9.95	35,222	35.22
	3	29.96	0.048	0.440	31,056	15.04	31,056	31.06
B	0	15.00	0.086	0.950	100,000	11.04	4,978	4.98
	1	25.05	0.090	0.703	95,022	7.84	28,237	28.24
	2	27.77	0.048	0.478	66,785	9.94	34,883	34.88
	3+	29.73	0.048	0.446	31,903	15.27	31,903	31.90
C	0	15.00	0.076	0.892	100,000	11.77	10,772	10.77
	1	24.57	0.102	0.743	89,228	7.26	22,891	22.89
	2	27.29	0.057	0.533	66,337	9.32	31,007	31.01
	3+	29.23	0.058	0.504	35,330	15.77	35,330	35.33
D	0	15.00	0.083	0.947	100,000	11.37	5,343	5.34
	1	25.32	0.090	0.701	94,657	7.83	28,280	28.28
	2	28.11	0.049	0.477	66,376	9.76	34,722	34.72
	3+	30.05	0.050	0.453	31,654	14.95	31,654	31.65

This effect is especially strong if – such as in this case – the risk population at young age (denominator) is unproportionally great and the number of first births according to the European fertility pattern (numerator) is quite low and at higher ages. If, instead of the European age- and parity-specific fertility pattern, an African schedule were selected with young ages at first birth, the difference between the crude and the age-standardized model would be significantly less. The mean age at first birth was 19.5 in Kenya at the time of the WFS while it was above 25 in both the Finnish and the FRG fertility pattern. The deviation shown in this sensitivity analysis is a theoretical maximum distortion since, in reality, a European fertility pattern with high ages at first birth could never produce an age structure that is as young as the Kenyan one.

(3) A periodic distortion of the age structure, as could be produced by incorrect reporting of age or by extreme fertility fluctuations, has practically no effect on the estimation of period parity-progression ratios and the completed parity distribution in our model. The reason for the small effect of such distortions is based on the fact that numerators and denominators tend to increase and decrease proportionally and hence the level of the rate is not affected.

In summary, the fact that the fertility table based on parity disregards the age structure is reason for some caution but is not cause to prohibit the application of the model. If the fertility pattern and the age structure of the population stay empirically within a possible and plausible range, the errors caused by age structure are probably less significant than the instability of the estimated set of parity-progression ratios with respect to short-term fertility fluctuations.

Table 3.6. Fertility table for Mexico.

i	$x(i)$	$r(i)$	$p(i)$	$l(i)$	$v(i)$	$c(i)$
0	17.00	0.128	0.875	100,000	6.84	12.5
1	20.40	0.330	0.981	87,540	2.97	1.7
2	22.90	0.303	0.951	85,889	3.14	4.2
3	24.90	0.237	0.909	81,659	3.83	7.5
4	26.80	0.258	0.877	74,208	3.40	9.1
5	27.70	0.234	0.928	65,073	3.97	4.7
6	30.40	0.211	0.849	60,392	4.02	9.1
7	32.00	0.210	0.886	51,250	4.22	5.9
8	34.70	0.236	0.790	45,400	3.35	9.5
9	35.40	0.213	0.741	35,862	3.48	9.3
10	35.70	0.138	0.701	26,588	5.08	7.9
11	37.70	0.257	0.769	18,638	2.99	4.3
12	38.50	0.212	0.724	14,336	3.42	4.0
13+	39.60			10,383	8.40	10.4

Mean family size/woman: 6.68.

Table 3.7. Fertility table for Colombia.

i	$x(i)$	$r(i)$	$p(i)$	$l(i)$	$v(i)$	$c(i)$
0	13.00	0.059	0.795	100,000	13.47	20.5
1	20.90	0.244	0.935	79,457	3.83	5.2
2	23.10	0.195	0.895	74,255	4.59	7.8
3	25.30	0.155	0.842	66,442	5.43	10.5
4	27.50	0.178	0.803	55,961	4.51	11.0
5	28.10	0.144	0.795	44,956	5.52	9.2
6	29.90	0.196	0.858	35,722	4.38	5.1
7	32.00	0.149	0.776	30,640	5.21	6.9
8	34.10	0.153	0.738	23,785	4.82	6.2
9	35.70	0.134	0.670	17,552	5.00	5.8
10	37.10	0.193	0.700	11,757	3.62	3.5
11	37.60	0.143	0.623	8,225	4.36	3.1
12	38.30	0.171	0.645	5,124	3.77	1.8
13+	38.80			3,303	9.20	3.3

Mean family size/woman: 4.60.

3.2.3. Fertility tables for all women

If the age- and parity-specific fertility pattern is known, then the formulas given above may be used to adjust the age-distributional aspect. If only parity-specific rates are given (requires less than 3% of the information needed for age- and parity-specific analysis), then the model seems to be robust enough to give some reasonable information on the parity distribution implied by period fertility. This section looks at such tables in a selected number of countries.

Table 3.8. Fertility table for Cameroon.

i	$x(i)$	$r(i)$	$p(i)$	$l(i)$	$v(i)$	$c(i)$
0	13.00	0.107	0.936	100,000	8.74	6.4
1	19.80	0.199	0.920	93,562	4.62	7.5
2	22.20	0.246	0.953	86,080	3.87	4.0
3	24.90	0.257	0.981	82,051	3.82	1.6
4	28.30	0.277	0.908	80,477	3.28	7.4
5	29.70	0.238	0.949	73,038	3.99	3.8
6	32.80	0.210	0.853	69,278	4.06	10.2
7	34.60	0.162	0.734	59,101	4.53	15.7
8	35.20	0.170	0.818	43,397	4.81	7.9
9	37.80	0.124	0.675	35,519	5.45	11.5
10+	40.00			23,988	10.00	24.0

Mean family size/woman: 6.70.

Table 3.9. Fertility table for Kenya.

i	$x(i)$	$r(i)$	$p(i)$	$l(i)$	$v(i)$	$c(i)$
0	13.00	0.107	0.922	100,000	8.62	7.8
1	19.30	0.294	0.971	92,199	3.30	2.7
2	21.80	0.318	0.966	89,484	3.04	3.0
3	24.00	0.316	0.952	86,480	3.01	4.2
4	25.90	0.345	0.983	82,316	2.85	1.4
5	28.40	0.286	0.941	80,920	3.29	4.8
6	30.60	0.313	0.964	76,129	3.08	2.8
7	33.10	0.242	0.849	73,359	3.51	11.1
8	34.40	0.248	0.916	62,267	3.70	5.2
9	37.10	0.200	0.773	57,060	3.86	13.0
10	38.60	0.156	0.642	44,092	4.11	15.8
11	39.20	0.192	0.680	28,288	3.54	9.0
12	39.80	0.156	0.638	19,240	4.09	7.0
13+	41.00			12,284	8.00	12.3

Mean family size/woman: 8.16.

In parts of Africa and Latin America the WFS interviewed samples of all women; in Asia and Europe the interviews were restricted to ever-married women. The fertility table that is only based on the reproductive behavior of ever-married women raises some specific questions about the exposure to birth, which will be discussed in the next section. Here examples from countries in which all women in the reproductive age were interviewed are provided.

Tables 3.6 through *3.9* give the fertility tables for two Latin American and two African countries, namely, Mexico, Colombia, Cameroon, and Kenya. In these tables the start of exposure and the end of the process, $x(0)$ and xw, were set according to the age span of the population considered in the denominators of the empirical rates: $x(0)$ was 17.0 in Mexico and 13.0 in the three other countries; xw ranged from 48 to 50.

The empirically derived cohort mean ages at birth (see Section 2.3) must increase monotonically with parity in all countries. For empirical period data, however, it could well happen that the mean age at births of order $i+1$ in a given year is somewhat lower than that for births of order i. In the less-developed WFS countries, this happens only in a few instances and mostly at higher parities in which the number of cases are relatively small. For these instances some adjustments must be made if a synthetic cohort should be constructed from such data, because the model requires monotonically increasing mean ages for all birth orders.

Less evident but also problematic is the case when the differences among the period mean ages are very irregular. Again, this tends to happen primarily at higher parities where the cell sizes are small. There are three possible sources of uneven intervals in the sequence of mean ages at birth. The first refers to real differences under a cohort perspective; it might well be that the difference between mean age at seventh and eighth birth is greater than that between the eighth and the ninth for a real cohort without measurement error. The second source of irregularity lies in period fluctuations; in a given year eighth births might well be later or earlier on the average than in the surrounding years and also under a cohort perspective. The final source of unevenness is measurement error due to small sample sizes, incorrect reporting of differential age, or coding errors. While the third source of irregularity is clearly undesirable, the first two should be part of the model and should be reflected in the estimated period parity-progression ratios.

In every country the sequence of estimated parity-progression ratios is more even than those of mean ages at birth and those of parity-specific fertility rates taken separately. The reason for this is based on the fact that period fluctuations concerning only the tempo and not the quantum of fertility are reflected in both the mean ages and the period parity-specific rates and compensate for each other in the calculation of the parity-progression ratio. If, for example, women in a given year for whatever reason delay their second births (tempo only), then in this model the difference between mean ages at first and second births would increase. If the probability of having a second birth remained constant, this delay would also result in a decrease of the annual parity-specific fertility rate because an identical number of births would be spread out over more years. This intuitively described relationship is illustrated in formula (3.11). In the Mexican fertility table, *Table 3.6*, parity-progression ratios do not change dramatically from parity nine to ten although the difference between the mean ages increases from .3 to 2.0 years. A parallel decrease in the parity-specific fertility rate counteracts the increased exposure to the risk of another birth.

Such balancing does not always take place, and some implausible irregularities in the series of parity-progression ratios and consequently in the completed parity distribution, $c(i)$, of the synthetic cohort remain. One such irregularity is, for instance, that in Kenya 5% of the women end up with eight children, whereas 11% and 13% of the women have seven and nine children, respectively. Generally, however, the resulting distributions are plausible.

Table 3.10. Period fertility table for Austria, 1977–1980, by woman's education.

	i	$x(i)$	$r(i)$	$p(i)$	$l(i)$	$d(i)/l(0)$
Austria	0	15.00	0.05040	0.72115	100,000	27.9%
total	1	23.24	0.10229	0.76846	72,115	16.7%
	2	26.46	0.03404	0.41219	55,418	32.6%
	3	29.40	0.03282	0.35154	22,842	14.8%
	4	31.11	0.02945	0.30886	8,030	5.5%
	5	33.97	0.03694	0.30896	2,480	1.7%
	6+	36.35			766	.8%

Average number of children 1.62

Education

	i	$x(i)$	$r(i)$	$p(i)$	$l(i)$	$d(i)/l(0)$
Elementary	0	15.00	0.04444	0.66448	100,000	33.6%
	1	22.36	0.12110	0.82797	66,448	11.4%
	2	25.91	0.04061	0.46938	55,017	29.2%
	3	28.95	0.03636	0.38247	25,824	15.9%
	4	30.54	0.03090	0.33074	9,877	6.6%
	5+	33.62			3,267	3.3%

Average number of children 1.62

	i	$x(i)$	$r(i)$	$p(i)$	$l(i)$	$d(i)/l(0)$
Vocational	0	15.00	0.06143	0.79414	100,000	20.6%
	1	23.50	0.08041	0.70216	79,414	23.7%
	2	26.82	0.02568	0.34032	55,761	36.8%
	3	30.53	0.02775	0.29848	18,977	13.3%
	4	32.55	0.02670	0.26346	5,664	4.2%
	5+	35.17			1,492	1.5%

Average number of children 1.62

	i	$x(i)$	$r(i)$	$p(i)$	$l(i)$	$d(i)/l(0)$
Completed	0	15.00	0.04519	0.71847	100,000	28.2%
secondary	1	25.37	0.12391	0.76699	71,847	16.7%
	2	27.48	0.03668	0.40686	55,106	32.7%
	3	29.20	0.02173	0.27955	22,421	16.2%
	4+	34.51			6,268	6.3%

Average number of children 1.56

	i	$x(i)$	$r(i)$	$p(i)$	$l(i)$	$d(i)/l(0)$
University	0	15.00	0.03946	0.66046	100,000	34.0%
	1	24.92	0.18275	0.91504	66,046	5.6%
	2	28.53	0.9121	0.61977	60,435	23.0%
	3	29.38	0.05878	0.55816	37,456	16.5%
	4+	34.04			20,906	20.9%

Average number of children 1.95

In the two Latin American countries recent parity-specific fertility patterns imply a relatively high proportion of women remaining childless. The expected distributions of mothers, $c(i)$, reaches a clear peak at parity four in Colombia, whereas in Mexico the distribution is stretched out further with the highest proportions of women in the range between parities four and nine. In Cameroon there is a concentration of completed parities in the range six to nine, yet in Kenya the range is seven to ten. This is reflected in the $c(i)$ function.

This pattern is also reflected in the $l(i)$ function. As for the analysis of completed cohort fertility discussed in the previous chapter, this function tells what proportion of all women will be expected to have i or more children. In Kenya the country with the highest level of period fertility in our study, more than half of the women are still expected to have nine or more children under current fertility conditions. However, in Colombia only 18% of the women are expected to have nine or more children. Mexico and Cameroon lie between these two cases.

The summary indicator of the complete distribution is the mean completed parity. It should be comparable with the total fertility rate. As a matter of fact, for the four countries studied, the period total fertility rate – as calculated by standard procedures from the WFS files – comes reasonably close to the mean parities: the TFRs are 6.18 for Mexico, 4.70 for Colombia, 6.40 for Cameroon, and 8.26 for Kenya.

For low-fertility countries the WFS provides only samples of ever-married women up to parity two. The Austrian 1% sample survey of the population conducted in 1981 will be used to illustrate the fertility table for all women in an industrialized country. The Austrian data is even broken down by woman's education, enabling a comparison within subpopulations.

The fertility table (*Table 3.10*) for the complete female population of Austria between ages 15 and 45 in 1977–1980 implies that the fertility pattern of these years would result in 28% of all women remaining childless and about one-third having two children. This is comparable with the expected 31.4% childless rate found in Finland (see *Table 3.4*). *Table 3.10* also provides fertility tables for four different subpopulations according to the woman's education. The results demonstrate nicely that even with almost identical average family sizes (around 1.6), completed parity distributions may vary greatly. For women with only elementary education, the proportion with three or more children is quite large. In contrast, women with additional vocational training have a very high proportion (23.7%) at completed parity one; for women with university degrees, the picture is most extreme. There is clear heterogeneity with a large proportion expected to remain childless and also with a large proportion with four or more children. Because of small cell sizes, however, this result must be analyzed with caution.

3.2.4. Marital fertility tables

If data on unmarried women are available, it is preferable to calculate the fertility for all women. However, sometimes only marital fertility data are available, or only information on the effect of marriage on fertility and parity may be needed to be assessed. There are two possible ways to achieve these calculations. The first is to include additional transitions in the model and to extend it to a multistate model with progressions possible not only from one partity to the next but also from the unmarried to the married state, and further from the divorced to the remarried state. Such a multistate model has extensive data requirements. The following section discusses this multistate model for Austria. A second solution is to make marital fertility tables in those situations in which there is only data on ever-married women. This section also gives a few examples of the latter tables using WFS data.

To construct fertility tables using survey data that include only ever-married women, two difficulties must be overcome. First, the beginning of exposure no longer has a clearly defined age limit. This problem can be solved by taking the mean age at marriage as $x(0)$. Second, the table will include only legitimate births; however, premarital births that are later legitimized do influence the actual completed parity distribution of ever-married women but cannot be covered by the marital parity table. This problem cannot be resolved and must be kept in mind when interpreting results. The extent to which this second problem affects the estimated completed parity distributions may vary greatly from country to country according to the extent of illegitimacy.

Tables 3.11 through *3.15* illustrate the marital fertility tables for Syria, Colombia, Republic of Korea, Portugal, and Czechoslovakia. Except for completed parity zero, the tables are expected to be very similar to fertility tables for all women. Both tables are compared for Colombia.

The mean age at marriage, the $x(0)$ for a marital fertility table, is not unequivocal. One possibility is to take the *singulate mean age at marriage*. However, the singulate mean age at marriage reflects largely the nuptiality behavior of past periods. An appropriate measure is the median age at first union for women in their twenties at the time of the survey. This age is given by Singh (1984). For the selected marital fertility tables discussed here, the mean ages at marriage were taken from comparative WFS studies (Singh, 1984; Smith, 1980).

In Syria the marital period parity-specific fertility rates and mean ages imply a plausible completed parity distribution. About 11% of the ever-married women are expected to remain childless. When unmarried women are included – only 2% of all women in Syria – the expected rate of women who remain childless increases only to 13%. One-third of the women in Syria is concentrated around parities eight to ten. The mean family size resulting from this distribution in Syria is 7.8. This is similar to the total fertility rate of 7.5 estimated by the UN (1986).

In Colombia and the Republic of Korea the estimated marital fertility levels are much lower than in Syria, but, as in Syria, about 11% of all ever-married women are expected to remain childless. In the Republic of Korea, where marriage is universal, the marital pattern corresponds to the pattern for all women. However, in Colombia, about 10% of all women remain unmarried, which is reflected in a high rate of overall childlessness – 20.5% (see *Table 3.7*). In the Republic of Korea more than half of all married women are expected to have their completed fertility within the narrow range of 4 to 6 children. The range of modal parities is somewhat lower in Colombia with one-third of the married women expected to have 3 to 5 children. Nevertheless, women with large families are expected to be more common in Colombia. In the Republic of Korea the fertility patterns imply that only about 2% of the married women will have 10 or more births, whereas in Colombia this percentage increases to 15%. The mean family size in the Republic of Korea resulting from the distribution of ever-married women is 4.4. This is very close to the UN estimate of TFR of 4.3. In

Table 3.11. Fertility table for Syria.

i	$x(i)$	$r(i)$	$p(i)$	$l(i)$	$v(i)$	$c(i)$
0	19.3	0.208	0.892	100,000	4.29	10.8
1	20.5	0.444	0.995	89,169	2.24	0.5
2	22.6	0.398	0.981	88,695	2.46	1.7
3	24.6	0.321	0.983	87,006	3.06	1.5
4	27.3	0.288	0.909	85,550	3.16	7.8
5	28.6	0.315	0.959	77,765	3.04	3.2
6	30.9	0.310	0.908	74,568	2.93	6.8
7	32.3	0.229	0.880	67,735	3.84	8.1
8	34.4	0.217	0.820	59,640	3.78	10.7
9	35.8	0.172	0.741	48,895	4.31	12.7
10	37.0	0.123	0.627	36,231	5.10	13.5
11	38.0	0.148	0.634	22,727	4.28	8.3
12	38.4	0.192	0.684	14,404	3.56	4.6
13	38.7	0.250	0.912	9,845	3.65	0.9
14+	41.7			8,974	7.30	9.0

Mean family size/woman: 7.80.

Table 3.12. Fertility table for Colombia.

i	$x(i)$	$r(i)$	$p(i)$	$l(i)$	$v(i)$	$c(i)$
0	19.60	0.199	0.888	100,000	4.46	11.2
1	20.90	0.280	0.953	88,754	3.41	4.1
2	23.10	0.196	0.899	84,624	4.59	8.5
3	25.30	0.161	0.855	76,098	5.31	11.0
4	27.50	0.178	0.811	65,083	4.55	12.3
5	28.10	0.147	0.807	52,767	5.49	10.2
6	29.90	0.197	0.865	42,576	4.39	5.7
7	32.00	0.143	0.777	36,836	5.43	8.2
8	34.10	0.146	0.739	28,603	5.06	7.5
9	35.70	0.153	0.721	21,152	4.72	5.9
10	37.10	0.181	0.703	15,259	3.88	4.5
11	37.60	0.157	0.668	10,729	4.25	3.6
12	38.30	0.171	0.667	7,165	3.90	2.4
13+	38.80			4,778	10.20	4.8

Mean family size/woman: 5.39.

Colombia the mean of marital fertility is 5.4. This is considerably higher than the UN TFR estimate of 4.7. The discrepancy can be explained by the sizable proportion of unmarried women in Colombia: when all women are considered, the mean parity is 4.6.

Although the marital fertility patterns for these three selected countries differ, they are all characterized by relatively high and similar rates of childlessness, and by modes at fairly high parities. Portugal and Czechoslovakia, two industrialized countries, are characterized differently by lower rates of childlessness and modes at parity two. The low expected proportions of childless, married women is probably due to a lower incidence of involuntary sterility. The parity distribution is strongly peaked: 46% of the married women in

Table 3.13. Fertility table for the Republic of Korea.

i	$x(i)$	$r(i)$	$p(i)$	$l(i)$	$v(i)$	$c(i)$
0	22.80	0.215	0.887	100,000	4.12	11.3
1	24.10	0.336	0.951	88,660	2.83	4.3
2	25.80	0.267	0.930	84,337	3.48	5.9
3	27.80	0.175	0.894	78,437	5.11	8.3
4	31.00	0.112	0.719	70,120	6.42	19.7
5	32.90	0.090	0.652	50,429	7.24	17.6
6	35.40	0.077	0.551	32,856	7.15	14.8
7	37.30	0.070	0.474	18,100	6.77	9.5
8	38.60	0.060	0.399	8,579	6.65	5.2
9	39.60	0.086	0.521	3,423	6.06	1.6
10+	42.60			1,785	6.40	1.8

Mean family size/woman: 4.39.

Table 3.14. Fertility table for Portugal.

i	$x(i)$	$r(i)$	$p(i)$	$l(i)$	$v(i)$	$c(i)$
0	19.90	0.174	0.938	100,000	5.39	6.2
1	23.80	0.117	0.825	93,832	7.05	16.5
2	27.20	0.039	0.481	77,375	12.33	40.2
3	30.40	0.043	0.456	37,219	10.62	20.2
4	32.70	0.045	0.418	16,990	9.28	9.9
5	33.60	0.093	0.594	7,098	6.38	2.9
6	34.50	0.073	0.637	4,214	8.72	1.5
7+	40.50			2,684	7.50	2.7

Mean family size/woman: 2.42.

Table 3.15. Fertility table for Czechoslovakia.

i	$x(i)$	$r(i)$	$p(i)$	$l(i)$	$v(i)$	$c(i)$
0	21.70	0.387	0.915	100,000	2.36	8.5
1	22.20	0.186	0.905	91,453	4.87	8.6
2	25.30	0.039	0.446	82,807	11.43	45.9
3+	27.70			36,921	16.30	36.9

Czechoslovakia and 40% of the Portugese women are expected to have two children. Of the married women 37% will have three or more children in both countries if recent parity-specific fertility patterns are accurate. For Czechoslovakia it is not possible to calculate the mean parity because the distribution beyond parity three is not known. In Portugal the mean parity for married women is slightly higher than the official TFR because a sizable proportion of Portugese women remains unmarried.

For most countries the parity tables presented here are the first attempts to calculate parity distributions implied by recent period fertility patterns. The distribution of fertility has considerable impact on many aspects of the society, the economy, and the psychology of people. Hence, the estimated distribution is an important addition to the knowledge of a country's future population and its potential problems. In addition, the resulting mean parities seem to be a better summary indicator of the average level of fertility under a cohort perspective than the conventional total fertility rates, because they partly compensate for strong period fluctuations.

For several reasons the fertility table for ever-married women seems more problematic than a table referring to all women. The question of premarital births remains unresolved. To shed more light on the interactions between parity progression and marital status transition, a more sophisticated multistate model will be applied to Austria, a country with one of the highest rates of illegitimacy, in the following section.

3.3. A Parity- and Marital-Status-Specific Multistate Model for Austria

Especially in modern industrialized societies with high proportions of out-of-wedlock births, the study of marital fertility alone does not give a representative picture of population reproduction. Trends, such as a lower proportion of the population marrying, postponement of marriage to a later age, increasing divorce rates, and the popularity of cohabitation, weaken the role of marriage as the sole place of reproduction.

In many European countries high rates of illegitimacy are not a new phenomenon. In some regions of Austria (Styria and Carinthia), for example, the proportion of illegitimate births was above 40% around 1870 (Kytir and Münz, 1986). This coincides with high proportions of women that never married, e.g., about 25% of the women were reported to be unmarried at age 50 in 1880 (see Lutz, 1985b). Reasons for this are related to rural inheritance, law, and legal marriage restrictions. Both illegitimacy and the high proportion of never-married women did not decline substantially until the baby boom after World War II. However, the prevalence of marriage after World War II reduced illegitimacy by almost 10%. Of these births most were legitimized later by marriage.

Presently, this trend seems reversed; out-of-wedlock births in Austria are again between 20% and 25%, probably because of alternative life-styles. However, even today most children are born and raised in wedlock, and marriage is still the most important demographic covariate of fertility. The model below shows that many single mothers eventually marry, and, under the fertility and marriage pattern of 1981–1986, only 4.4% of the women aged 45 will be expected to remain never-married mothers.

A comprehensive picture of the implications of parity-specific and marital-status-specific fertility and of the interactions between these two important demographic dimensions of fertility cannot be drawn from the traditional approach of the family life cycle (see Glick, 1977; Höhn, 1982; Feichtinger, 1987) nor by one-dimensional demographic decrement tables. The family life cycle approach developed during the 1920s assumes a standard sequence of demographic events (birth, marriage, birth of first child, ..., death of spouse, own death) and gives the mean ages at these events. However, this seemingly very illustrative approach has two serious disadvantages. First, it is increasingly unrepresentative for modern populations since only a minority of women follows this predefined sequence of events. Second, as shown in Section 2.1, it is not possible to derive exact estimates of mean durations in the family life-cycle states by just taking the differences of the mean ages $x(i)$ and $x(i+1)$ because not all women that experience event i also experience event $i+1$. Hence, a more comprehensive framework for the analysis of family processes is needed.

The most general model based on individuals and not groups of individuals (families) that allows transitions in all directions between states defined by marital status and parity status is the multistate life table. The mathematics for this table have been described extensively elsewhere (e.g., Keyfitz, 1980; Schoen, 1974; Rogers, 1975; Land and Rogers, 1982) and shall not be discussed here. Applications of the model to marital transition have been given, e.g., by Willekens *et al.* (1982), Espenshade (1986), Wijewickrema and Alli (1984), and Krishnamoorthy (1979). In fertility analysis a multistate approach had been taken by Suchindran *et al.* (1977) and Suchindran and Koo (1980). In this study the state space is defined as a combination of parity and marital status. Related models have been used by Kuijsten (1986) and Lutz (1985b).

One shortcoming of the multistate model is the fact that it can only account for a one-time variable (age) and cannot consider other important time dimensions like birth intervals or marital duration. An extension of the model encompassing duration dependence is theoretically possible (Wolf, 1987) but data demands seem to be too high for this particular data set. This data set is the 1% sample survey of the Austrian population in 1986. The survey asked all women aged 18 to 60 for their birth- and marital-status histories. All transitions for the period 1981 through 1986 were reconstructed, and appropriate transition rates were calculated.

Figure 3.4 gives the 12 states defined by cross-classifying parity and marital status. Because of limited space and cases, higher parity categories could not be considered. The obvious hierarchical nature of parity is reflected in one-way transitions to higher parity levels. Double transitions in one year are allowed in only a few cases (such as marriage and first birth). Mortality is, of course, possible for all states. Because of the lack of information on parity- and marital-status-specific mortality rates, identical age-specific death rates are assumed for all states. These rates are from the 1981–1982 Austrian life table. The model contains 35 single-year groups, from ages 15 through 49.

The possible results from this particular multistate model with 12 states and 35 single-year age groups (15–49) are extensive. They consist of conditional probabilities of being in status j at age y given that the person had been in status i at age x $(x < y)$. Probabilities such as 90720 $[=(12\,{}^{*}12\,{}^{*}35)$ + $(12\,{}^{*}12\,{}^{*}34) + ...]$ are given by the model. *Tables 3.16* through *3.20* illustrate just a few such probabilities. Another result of the model consists of conditional life expectancies in the various states. *Table 3.16* gives a few selected values from the 5040 $(= 12\,{}^{*}12\,{}^{*}35)$ possible life expectancies.

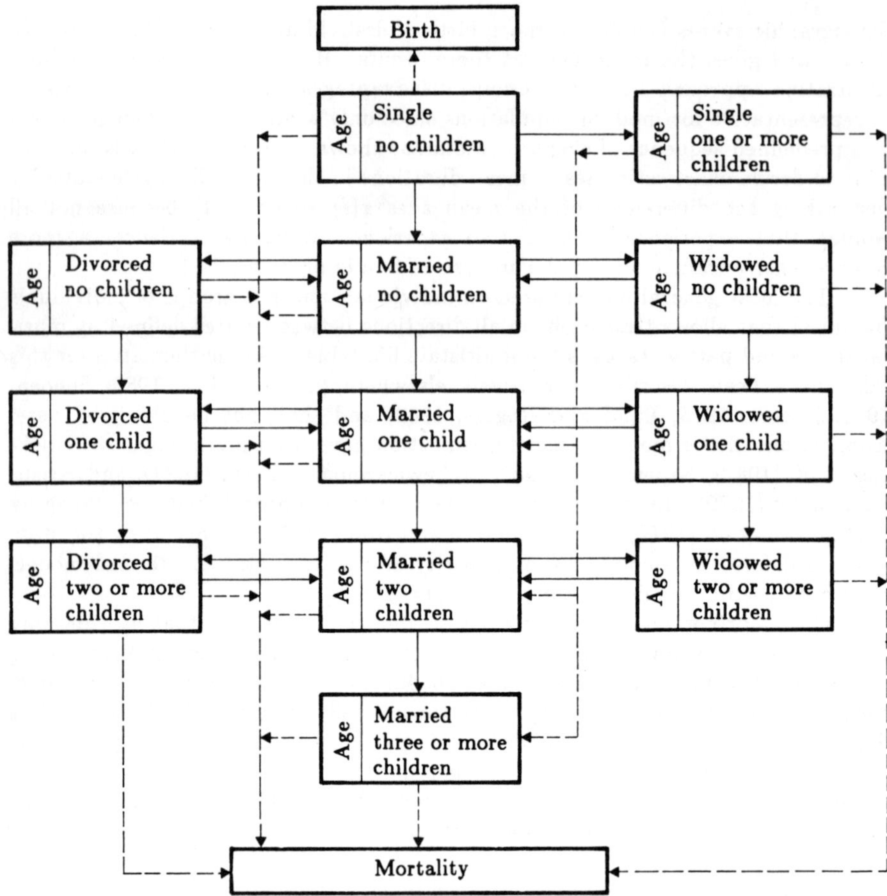

Figure 3.4. Illustration of potential transitions in the marital-status and parity-status life table.

Since the data are period rates for 1981 through 1986, the results on probabilities and distributions implied by the schedule can be interpreted in the same way as a synthetic cohort in other period life-table approaches. *Table 3.16* gives the distribution of 12 states at age 45 (= probability of being in status at age 45) for women who were unmarried and without children at age 15, i.e., for the complete synthetic cohort. The table shows that about 15% of the women will still be unmarried at age 45, 70% will be married, 9% divorced, and 3% widowed. With respect to fertility the pattern implies that 22% will remain childless over all marital states and 26% will have one child; about half of all women will have two or more children according to the period fertility pattern of 1981 through 1986.

Table 3.16. Expected durations (life expectancies) in the various states in years and distribution over states at age 45 for all women (= unmarried, no children at age 15).

	Mean duration up to age 50	%	Distribution of all women at age 45
Unmarried, no children	11.49	33.26	10.62
Unmarried, one or more children	1.86	5.40	4.37
Married, no children	3.31	9.58	9.61
Married, one child	5.50	15.92	17.69
Married, two children	6.99	20.23	26.96
Married, three or more children	3.29	9.52	16.16
Widowed, no children	0.07	0.21	0.64
Widowed, one child	0.13	0.38	0.67
Widowed, two or more children	0.23	0.67	1.51
Divorced, no children	0.32	0.92	1.24
Divorced, one child	0.63	1.82	3.36
Divorced, two or more children	0.73	2.10	4.57
Total	34.56	100.00	

Table 3.17. Percentage distributions of the effect of age at marriage on later fertility.

		Status married with no children at age			
	x	20	25	30	35
Married	0	2.12	11.99	44.18	75.02
with x	1	13.65	28.47	28.22	9.55
children at	2	38.68	30.68	9.19	.70
age 45	3+	28.34	11.85	1.27	.02

	No children			
	Age 20		Age 25	
Status at age 45	Married	Unmarried	Married	Unmarried
Unmarried, no children	—	13.06	—	27.33
Married, no children	2.12	11.62	11.99	19.93
Widowed, no children	.17	.77	1.02	1.25
Divorced, no children	.39	1.49	1.80	2.39
Total	2.68	26.94	14.81	50.90
Unmarried, one or more children	—	5.01	—	7.30
Married, one child	13.65	19.17	28.47	18.63
Widowed, one child	.80	.66	1.02	.54
Divorced, one child	3.49	3.53	5.31	2.97
Total	17.94	28.37	34.80	29.44
Married, two children	38.68	24.47	30.68	12.12
Married, three or more children	28.34	12.69	11.85	3.48

Table 3.18. **Effect of premarital births on later marital status and fertility.**

| | Unmarried at age 20 | | Unmarried at age 25 | |
Status at age 45	Without child	With child	Without child	With child
Unmarried, no children	13.06	—	27.33	—
Unmarried, one or more children	5.01	5.07	7.30	19.63
Married, no children	11.62	—	7.30	19.63
Married, one child	19.17	13.07	18.63	25.25
Married, two children	24.47	37.45	12.12	30.58
Married, three or more children	12.69	29.46	3.48	12.73
Divorced, no children	1.49	—	2.39	—
Divorced, one child	3.53	2.46	2.97	3.57
Divorced, two or more children	3.88	7.01	1.46	3.96

Table 3.19. **Effect of early marital births on subsequent marital fertility.**

| | Married | | | |
| | Age 20 | | Age 25 | |
Status at age 45	No children	One child	No children	One child
Married, no children	2.12	—	11.99	—
Married, one child	13.65	8.14	28.47	21.31
Married, two children	38.68	39.99	30.68	41.71
Married, three or more children	28.34	35.35	11.85	21.28
Mean 3–5	82.79	83.48	82.99	84.30
Mean	2.30	2.54	1.58	2.13

Table 3.20. **Effect of divorce on fertility.**

| | No children | | One child | | | |
| | Age 25 | | Age 25 | | Age 30 | |
At age 45	Divorced	Married	Divorced	Married	Divorced	Married
Married, no children	17.49	11.99	—	—	—	—
Married, one child	25.61	28.47	27.83	21.31	28.59	49.80
Married, two children	17.17	30.68	23.59	41.71	13.83	29.51
Married, three or more children	4.11	1..85	6.31	21.28	1.60	5.66
Divorced, no children	4.97	1.80	—	—	—	—
Divorced, one child	16.94	5.31	23.00	4.05	36.66	7.44
Divorced, two or more children	9.18	4.33	15.42	6.45	16.37	3.12
No children	22.46	13.79	—	—	—	—
One child	42.55	33.78	50.83	25.36	65.25	57.24
Two or more children	30.46	46.86	45.32	69.44	31.80	38.29

The given life expectancies in *Table 3.16* may by no means be interpreted as an average or standard sequence of a "typical" woman. There is probably not one woman in Austria who has gone through all the phases of a life cycle described here and certainly not within the given time frame. The figures for life expectancies rather reflect an expectation on the aggregate or, in other words – assuming that women are homogeneous at the beginning – the probability distribution of the expected person years to be lived over all states. When assuming an even age distribution, the given life expectancies (divided by the total life expectancy) may also be interpreted as the proportions of women in the given status in a stable population, assuming current transition patterns. This interpretation is of great importance for social policy questions. The life expectancies given in *Table 3.16* reflect a combination of both the quantum and the tempo of the transitions in the family life cycle. After accounting for mortality, women have 34.56 person years on average to live between ages 15 and 50. One-third (i.e., 11.5 years) is, on the average, spent in the status unmarried without children. This includes women who later married and might have had children and women who remained single and childless.

Table 3.16 also indicates that about 20% (i.e., 7 years) of an average woman's life can be expected to be in the state married with two children and almost 10% in the state married with three or more children. Mean durations in the widowed states are naturally very short because of the low incidence of widowhood below age 50. Also, the mean duration in a divorced state is only about 1.5 years despite sharply increased divorce rates (almost one-third of all marriages is expected to end in divorce). The reason for the small proportions of women in the divorced state is due to relatively high rates of remarriage and to the fact that divorces often occur at ages closer to 50. In fact, despite decreasing fertility, increasing mean ages at birth, decreasing nuptiality, and increasing divorce probabilities, all women still spend, on the average, more than half the years between ages 15 and 50 with at least one child.

Table 3.17 looks at the effect age has on later fertility in first marriages. The table predicts the expected family status for women currently between the ages of 20 and 25. The survey finds that of the childless women at age 20 less than 3% of those married can expect to remain childless, whereas for unmarried women the chance is about 27%. This differential with respect to childlessness becomes even greater when taking age 25 into consideration: about 15% of these married women will remain childless, while more than half of the unmarried women are expected to have no children.

As expected, young marriages also reduce the probability of ending up with just one child and conversely increases the probability of two or more children considerably (*Table 3.17*). This can be clearly seen from the difference between childless married and unmarried women at age 20. For childless married women at age 25, the average expected fertility is much lower than for the 20-year-old childless married women.

The proportion that will be married with two, three, or more children at age 45 confirms the pattern observed so far: young marriage is associated with significantly higher completed fertility. This pattern cannot be explained solely by the practice to marry at a very young age when a child is underway still common in Austria. This practice should only have impact on the degree of childlessness among women who marry very early. The much higher probability of ending up with two, three, or more children for women who marry at a young age is most probably due to the value system of such women, who simultaneously tend toward higher fertility and lower age at marriage. Longer exposure to marital births resulting from early marriage probably does not play a significant role in explaining the differences between one, two, and three births, because these few births could easily be spaced in much shorter intervals. Under a sociological perspective, however, a marriage with an early birth is likely to restrict the number of options a woman has and might make the high-fertility option more attractive.

Table 3.18 looks at the effect of an illegitimate birth on a woman's later marital status and fertility. Women unmarried at age 20 with one or more children have only a 5% chance of remaining unmarried by age 45, compared with about 18% for childless women. By age 25 the chances of remaining unmarried increase to 20% for single mothers. At ages 20 and 25 unmarried women with a child have a much higher probability of being married with two, three, or more children by age 45. Generally, *Table 3.18* indicates that a premarital birth at a young age has pretty much the same effects on completed fertility as an early marriage.

Table 3.19 focuses on the effects of an early marital birth on subsequent marital fertility. There is clearly a positive association between an earlier marital birth and completed marital fertility at age 45. Of the married women who are childless at age 20, 28% are expected to have three or more children, while 35% are expected to have at least one child by age 20. For 25-year-old married women the same association appears, although at a lower fertility level. In terms of the mean number of children born by married women by age 45 (assuming a mean of 3.5 for the category 3+), women who were already married and had a child by age 20 are expected to have the highest mean with 2.54 children. Childless married women aged 25 have only a mean completed family size of 1.58. Again this association is probably based on the value system of the woman and a certain predetermination of the woman on whether to have a child early in marriage.

Also, it is of interest to study the effects of divorce of fertility, *Table 3.20*. This model makes it possible to look at the number of children of those women aged 45 who were divorced at an earlier age. Generally, divorce is negatively associated with fertility. For instance, of the divorced women without children at age 25, 22% are expected to stay childless, whereas only 14% of married, childless women of the same age have no children. Almost half of the married, childless women at age 25 will have two or more children, whereas divorced women of the same age have only a 30% chance to end up with the same number of children. A similar pattern of lower fertility also holds when comparing married and divorced women with one child at ages 25 and 30. It is interesting to see that among divorced women with one child at age 30, the majority does not remarry by age 45, whereas 58% of the women five years younger will remarry.

Many more such questions could be addressed by this multistate model. Marital status, even in a modern industrialized society, is an extremely important factor in the determination of a woman's fertility. Compared with less-developed countries, however, completed parity remains within a rather narrow range of family sizes at a low level: even the highest-fertility women in our model – those married with one child at age 20 – will have less than three children on average at the end of their reproductive career.

3.4. Non-demographic Factors Associated with Progression to Parities Two and Three in Austria

The demographic analysis above indicates that in industrialized societies with widespread use of contraceptives, only the first few parity-progression ratios are crucial in determining the distribution of fertility and, consequently, the level of reproduction. Usually, the parity outcome is the result of conscious decision making. The reasons behind progressions in parity are beyond demographic analysis in a stricter sense because they concern sociological, economic, and psychological factors.

In previous chapters attention was given to amount of education and place of residence to explain differentials in the observed fertility patterns. Especially in less-developed countries, such differentials often reflect the partition of the society into more advanced and less advanced segments. This pattern is not as clear for parity progression in industrialized countries. To shed some light on the complex determination of parity progression in European populations, an example for a multivariate analysis of marital fertility is given for the progression to second and third births in Austria.

The data used in the following analysis stem from a survey of young married couples in Austria. A sampling of about 2,000 women of the marriage cohorts first questioned in 1974 and 1977 were interviewed again in 1978 and 1981–1982. The questionnaire covered many aspects that could be related to reproduction (see Münz, 1985). In the following multiple classification analysis nine aspects of a woman's life that could be relevant to her reproductive decision-making process were selected. These are her occupation, education, emancipation, degree of church attachments, age at first marriage, number of siblings, income, residence, and amount of help from the husband in the household (see Lutz, 1985c, for further explanations).

The first model, *Table 3.21*, focuses on the birth of a second child, given that the woman had a least one birth by the date of the first interview. The dependent variable is a dummy that is 0 if no second child had been born by the time of the second interview and 1 if a second child had been born. This is analogous to the parity-progression ratio except for the time constraint: only second births are considered that occurred within the first 4 to 7 years of marriage. The model, therefore, does not refer to the pure quantum of fertility but does include some tempo aspects.

Table 3.21. Multiple-classification analysis of progression to parity two in Austria. Dependent variable: was a second child born before 1981–1982? 0 = no, 1 = yes. Survey includes all women with at least one child in 1981–1982.

Independent Variable Main effects	n	Raw effects	η	Adjusted effects	β	Significant at 0.95 level
Occupational status			0.34		0.29	
Farmer	150	0.27		0.19		
High white-collar						
Independent	148	-0.12		-0.08		
White-collar	367	-0.22		-0.18		Yes
Blue-collar	209	-0.18		-0.18		
Housewife	857	0.11		0.10		
Education			0.12		0.04	
Elementary	533	0.08		0.00		
Vocational	986	-0.03		-0.01		
Completed college	213	-0.06		0.04		No
Emancipation index			0.07		0.02	
Often goes out						
without husband	804	-0.04		-0.01		No
Seldom goes out						
without husband	929	0.03		0.01		
Degree of attachment						
to church			0.14		0.06	
High	568	0.09		0.04		
Medium	952	-0.03		-0.02		Yes
None	211	-0.11		-0.03		

Covariates	Mean of variables	Multiple regression coefficients	Significant at 0.95 level
Age at first marriage	20.88	-0.004	No
Number of siblings	2.90	0.019	Yes
Monthly net household income (in AS 1000s)	12.48	-0.007	Yes
City-Country			
0 = City			
1 = Country	0.49	0.120	Yes
Help with the household			
0 = Seldom	0.45	-0.013	No
1 = Very often			

$R^2 = 0.106$ (without interactions).

The second model, *Table 3.22*, focuses on the progression to the birth or expected birth of a third child to women who planned to have at least two children. Because in the case of a third child the temporal constraint (marital duration 4 to 7 years) would be too restrictive, the expectation to have a third child is included in the dependent variable. It is 1 in the case that the woman had or expressed the expectation to have a third child. Again, the dependent variable is comparable with the parity-progression ratio, this time without a temporal constraint but with uncertain fertility expectations. The results of the two models show that the various aspects have differing effects on the birth of a second or third child.

Table 3.22. Multiple-classification analysis of progression to a third child born or desired. Dependent variable: was a third child born or desired in 1981–1982? 0 = no, 1 = yes. Survey includes all women who had or desired at least two children.

Independent Variable Main effects	n	Raw effects	η	Adjusted effects	β	Significant at 0.95 level
Occupational status			0.24		0.19	
Farmer	149	0.30		0.24		
High white-collar						
Independent	150	-0.06		-0.04		
White-collar	332	-0.11		-0.07		Yes
Blue-collar	193	-0.12		-0.12		
Housewife	811	0.03		0.02		
Education			0.06		0.06	
Elementary	502	0.05		-0.02		
Vocational	918	-0.02		-0.01		Yes
Completed college	216	-0.01		0.08		
Emancipation index			0.08		0.06	
Often goes out without husband	752	-0.04		-0.03		Yes
Seldom goes out without husband	883	0.04		0.03		
Degree of attachment to church			0.20		0.15	
High	564	0.13		0.10		
Medium	892	-0.06		-0.05		Yes
None	180	-0.12		-0.06		

Covariates	Mean of variables	Multiple regression coefficients	Significant at 0.95 level
Age at first marriage	20.86	-0.002	No
Number of siblings	2.92	0.025	Yes
Monthly net household income (in AS 1000s)	12.60	-0.006	Yes
City-Country 0 = City 1 = Country	0.52	0.040	No
Help with the household 0 = Seldom 1 = Very often	0.45	-0.015	No

$R^2 = 0.106$ (without interactions).

The tables show that the number of a woman's siblings exerts a significant positive influence on the probabilities of having a second or third child even after controlling for the eight other background variables. This finding also confirms the assumption, to be discussed in the epilogue, that mothers' and daughters' family sizes are correlated. The mechanisms of this transmission probably include attitudes adopted from the parents concerning large or small families as well as the experience of growing up in a family of a particular size. One could also think of psychological mechanisms inducing an inverse relationship between mothers' and daughters' family size, but the net effect seems to be positive in the Austrian case as well as in several other cases studied (see Anderton *et al.*, 1987).

A comparison of *Tables 3.21* and *3.22* also indicates that the effect of sibship size is more pronounced for a third child than for a second.

Education is generally considered to be negatively associated with fertility, both in less-developed and in developed countries. Cochrane *et al.* (1980) listed three mechanisms through which higher education may lead to lower fertility: higher education is mostly associated with an older age at marriage, which in turn is associated with lower fertility; more educated women use more efficient contraception; and education tends to influence the desired family size through changes in the value system. In our study this negative association is true from a bivariate perspective. Under a multivariate perspective, however, the pattern changes to the contrary. After accounting for age at marriage, some attitudinal, and all the other socioeconomic indicators, higher education seems to result in higher propensities of having a second or third child. In other words, from the Austrian data it can be concluded that more education would slightly increase womens' family sizes if this did not affect their professional career, their independence, etc. – a very hypothetical situation, indeed.

Among the attitudinal variables, a woman's degree of attachment to a church seems to play an important role with respect to her family size. It has been shown in several studies that the fertility differentials between Christian denominations have clearly diminished in modern European societies (e.g., the Netherlands). However, in our survey the *intensity* of attachment to the church (in Austria almost exclusively the Roman Catholic church) and its norms remains a significant factor. Particularly in regard to addition of a third child, this variable becomes very important. This indicates that the effect of traditional Roman Catholic norms on fertility in a multivariate setting is an especially important variable for explaining above average fertility.

The occupational status of women interacts with fertility in a complex manner: a woman might not work outside the home because she has children or she has children because she prefers domestic activity. Despite the uncertainty about the causal structure, a very strong negative association between economic activity and fertility appears empirically. It turns out that occupational status is the major explanation for the progression to a second birth within the first 4 to 7 years of a marriage. Among women who worked or said that they want to work in the future, only 52% had a second child; whereas among women who were not oriented toward work 78% had a second birth. The sector of female employment also plays an important role: even after accounting for urban-rural differentials and the other independent variables in the model, farmers show a 40% higher probability for a second birth than blue- or white-collar workers. Being a farmer *ceteris paribus* affects the probability of having a third child, whereas being a housewife does not.

Another aspect of a woman's orientation is the degree of her intra-familial emancipation. This is measured here by questioning a woman on whether she sometimes goes out without her husband.[3] It turns out that this indicator has a slight but clearly negative effect on third-birth probabilities but hardly any influence on second births. From this it could be inferred that intra-familial emancipation of women does not inhibit the birth of a second child, but that more emancipated women are clearly less likely to have a third. It seems to be a fallacy to assume that more independence within marriage generally leads to lower fertility; the analysis shows that this association is parity-specific.

Often, economic fertility emphasizes the positive effect of income on fertility. The analysis shows that under a bivariate perspective the relationship between income and fertility is U-shaped. In a multivariate setting a low but statistically significant negative multiple-regression coefficient results. This means higher income *ceteris paribus* seems to lower the probabilities of second and third births. The absence of a positive income effect on fertility in Austria is also confirmed by another survey question: 90% of the women stated that a hypothetical doubling of their income would not affect their desired family size.

Residency is the second most important variable after occupational status. The proportion of women with a second birth in rural areas is 22% higher than in urban areas. This socio-regional differential pertains also in the multivariate setting. For those women considering a third child, the residential variable is less important. It appears that even the residents of rural areas orient their family size (after controlling for the other important variables like farm versus non-farm) to the generally prevailing two-child norm.

Another aspect considered is the question of how much a woman's husband helps with the housework. This variable was dichotomized and includes five specific household activities. The multiple-regression coefficients for this variable are slightly negative – indicating lower birth probabilities for women with husbands who help – but statistically not significant. By itself help in the household does not lead couples to wish for more children. In fact it might be seen as an expression of the "modern partner" relationship that is generally associated with lower fertility or at least somewhat later second births and fewer third children.

In summary, of the variables determining the probability of the progression to second and third births during the first 4 to 7 years of marriage, the occupational status of women is the most critical one. This includes both quantum and tempo aspects. For the threshold to a third child (birth or expectation), occupational orientation becomes less important. Here, the degree of attachment to the Catholic tradition is most decisive. Also the sibship size, education, and intra-familial emancipation are more important influences in the decision to have a third child than to have a second child.

This analysis covers only the experience of two marriage cohorts in Austria. Without doubt the findings would be somewhat different for other cohorts and in other countries, but the general pattern can be expected to be similar in many other industrialized societies. It was also interesting to see that a parity-specific approach to the analysis of fertility determinants yields quite different results for different parities. Hence, the results also differ from the usual approach that takes the mean expected family size as the dependent variable. From this it is learned that the distributional aspect should not only be considered in the description of fertility but also in the analysis of its determinants.

3.5. Summary

The first two sections of this chapter on parity-specific period analysis are closely related. Section 3.1 discusses conceptual issues of parity-specific measurement under a period perspective. A principal distinction is made between one-dimensional approaches that consider births only in relation to the parity of the mother and two-dimensional approaches that consider a variable of individual time (age, marital duration, birth interval) in addition to parity. Section 3.1.2 also provides the empirical data that are needed for the one-dimensional approach of a period fertility table based on parity. The data requirements for this approach are much less than those for any two-dimensional approach.

Section 3.2 presents the period fertility table based on parity in a somewhat different form than that originally proposed by Chiang and van den Berg (1982). Since this one-dimensional approach disregards age distributional aspects, considerable effort is spent to assess the sensitivity of the model to age distributional distortions. Except for some extreme cases, the model is relatively insensitive to the age distribution. This is mainly due to the high correlation between age and parity. An application of the model to several more- and less-developed countries results in plausible estimates of the completed parity distribution implied by recent period fertility. If only information on marital fertility is available, the results become difficult to interpret especially in countries with high illegitimacy rates and a widespread practice of later legitimation of premarital children.

Section 3.3 attempts to solve this problem of interactions between marital-status changes and parity progression. For this the methodology of a multistate life table is used where the state space is defined by a cross-classification of marital statuses and parities. The model is applied to data from a recent Austrian survey. The results of the model provide information on a large number of questions relating to the family-related life cycle of individuals – e.g., what is the influence of early marriage on the completed parity distributions; how does a divorce affect a woman's further fertility; and how does the number of children influence remarriage after divorce?

The last section of this chapter leaves the strictly demographic field and looks at socioeconomic, psychological, and other factors that influence parity progression. Data again pertain to Austria. Multivariate models are used to study the influence of eight selected variables on the probability of having a second or third child. The results show that the pattern of determination is quite different for births of different orders. This also indicates that in the analysis of fertility determinants the study of means only tells part of the story and that a parity-specific approach reveals additional aspects that are necessary for understanding current and future fertility patterns.

Notes

[1]   It was shown in Section 1.2 that the difference between two subsequent mean ages may not be regarded as the correct birth interval because not all women who had an ith birth also have an $i+1$th. The formulas for calculating period parity-progression ratios in the following section will take this into account.

[2]   The Dutch survey is problematic in such comparisons because the sample was restricted to selected cohorts.

[3]   From the study of related variables it is clear that this is not an indicator of alienation from the partner but rather one of emancipation within stable relationships.

CHAPTER 4

The Concentration of Reproduction

4.1. The Measurement of Concentration in Demography

4.1.1. Static and dynamic concentration

Every real population is heterogeneous with respect to various aspects: individual survival, reproduction, migration, marriage, divorce, etc. There are always some subgroups of the population that have a higher risk of death, marriage, or divorce at certain ages. There is also no population where all women bear the same number of children. Furthermore, considerable diversity among the populations of the world is found when using a total (e.g., national) population as the unit of observation.

Dispersion and concentration are two notions that are closely related. Without dispersion in the distribution, there is no concentration and vice versa. The questions behind these two notions are, however, somewhat different: the indicators of dispersion tell how strongly the units of observation differ from each other with respect to their *output*, whereas indicators of concentration signify how the total *output* is attributed to individual units.

The concept of concentration usually covers two quite different aspects. We may refer to dynamic concentration, i.e., the *process* of a distribution becoming more concentrated, or to static concentration. Static concentration observes the *status* of the distribution at a given point in time. This second type seems to be used more frequently, at least in the economic literature (see Bruckmann, 1981). The dynamic process of concentration is usually studied by looking at a sequence of the distribution statuses, i.e., by taking a comparative statics approach. This implies the calculation of static concentration measures at different points in time and their comparative analysis.

For demographic applications the static understanding of the word concentration also seems to be more natural than the dynamic. Demographers may study the distribution at one point in time and then possibly compare its changes over time. The static meaning seems easier to define unambiguously than the dynamic meaning that, in the field of population analysis, would only make sense under a spatial perspective, e.g., concentrating troops in one place.

The question of clear definition is crucial to an application of concentration analysis in demography. In contrast to many economic questions, in population science the *output* and the producing units must first be defined. As mentioned above, the units may be all individuals, individuals with certain characteristics (e.g., women of a certain age group), or population groups. The *output* may be anything (e.g., birth, marriage, migration) that is measured in demography. Only events that cannot be repeated and that occur in everyone's lives, such as death, are not appropriate for concentration analysis. But *aspects* of mortality, such as the concentration of child mortality among families, might well be studied. This study, however, focuses on the concentration of fertility. The birth of a child is, on a global perspective, the most often-repeated demographic event (except perhaps for local migrations), and its distribution has important consequences for the mother, the child, and the population as a whole. Population reproduction seems to be the demographic field that fits best for concentration analysis.

Before discussing specific indicators of concentration, an important distinction must be made between absolute and relative terms. Absolute concentration focuses on the proportion of total output produced by a small absolute number of the highest producing units, whereas relative concentration looks at the proportion of units that produce certain proportions of the total *output*. The essential empirical difference is that if a great number of additional units with little *output* were added to the total, the measure of absolute concentration should remain essentially unchanged, whereas relative concentration should increase significantly. This will be discussed in greater detail below.

4.1.2. Absolute concentration of fertility

Because of the nature of demographic phenomena, the study of absolute concentration is only reasonable and informative for a very restricted number of questions. Generally, the analysis of relative concentration is more appropriate because demographic information is mostly related to the total of the population or certain subgroups (e.g., age groups). One great advantage of measures of absolute concentration is that they may be applied to distributions that are truncated at the lower end (e.g., in tax records or lists of companies of a certain size). In population fertility statistics, this kind of data problem usually does not exist because information on low-fertility women is mostly at least as good as that on high-fertility women. Furthermore, in demography there is a natural limit to concentration. The number of children women can bear during their lifetime is biologically limited, and it is very small in relation to the total number of children born in a society. Hence, a small absolute number of even extremely fertile women would never account for a sizable proportion of the total number of births in a society.

However, there are a few questions in demography where the study of absolute concentration is informative – for example, if the units of observation are aggregate populations instead of individuals. In this case the reservations mentioned above would not apply. For the most part it is accurate to say that in 1950–1955 more than one-quarter of all children in the world were born in the People's Republic of China (PRC), and that the People's Republic of China, India, and the Soviet Union accounted for almost half of all births (see *Table 4.1*). Similar calculations can be made for other periods, and the static statements on absolute concentration may then be compared over time.

Table 4.1. Absolute concentration of average annual numbers of births by countries in 1950–1955. (Herfindahl index: 0.1079.)

Rank order	Country	Number of births $a(i)$	Proportion of total births $p(i)$	Concentration ratio $\sum p(i) = c_m$	m
1	PRC	26,675	0.2647	0.2647	$m = 1$
2	India	17,024	0.1689	0.4336	$m = 2$
3	USSR	4,947	0.0491	0.4827	$m = 3$
4	USA	3,946	0.0392	0.5128	$m = 4$
5	Indonesia	3,573	0.0355	0.5573	$m = 5$
6	Brazil	2,569	0.0255	0.5828	$m = 6$
7	Pakistan	2,091	0.0207	0.6035	$m = 7$
8	Japan	2,052	0.0204	0.6239	$m = 8$
9	Nigeria	1,784	0.0177	0.6416	$m = 9$
10	Bangladesh	1,769	0.0176	0.6591	$m = 10$
11	Mexico	1,378	0.0137	0.6728	$m = 11$
12	Vietnam	1,206	0.0120	0.6848	$m = 12$
13	Korea, North & South	1,121	0.0111	0.6959	$m = 13$
14	Philippines	1,094	0.0109	0.7067	$m = 14$
15	Thailand	1,016	0.0101	0.7168	$m = 15$
16	Egypt	1,014	0.0101	0.7269	$m = 16$
17	Turkey	1,003	0.0100	0.7368	$m = 17$
18	Iran	920	0.0091	0.7460	$m = 18$
19	Ethiopia	885	0.0088	0.7547	$m = 19$
20	Italy	870	0.0086	0.7634	$m = 20$

How can absolute concentration be measured adequately? Bruckmann (1969) specified four conditions that every indicator of concentration should meet. The first two hold for both absolute and relative concentration, the third and fourth are differentiating criteria between absolute and relative concentration.

(1) Indicators of absolute and relative concentration must be insensitive to proportional changes in the *output* per unit; instead they should only depend on the proportion of the total *output* produced by each unit.

(2) Given $p(A) > p(B)$, an increase of the proportion $p(A)$ at the expense of $p(B)$ by a certain amount e should lead to an increase in the indicators of absolute and relative concentration (and vice versa). For maximum concentration the indicator should be equal to unity and otherwise be greater than or equal to zero.

(3) An increase in the number of producing units drawn from the same distribution should affect the indicator of absolute concentration but not that of relative concentration. In other words, only the indicator of absolute concentration should depend on the sample size if the distribution remains unchanged.

(4). The inclusion of a greater number of producing units with very little *output* should influence the indicator of absolute concentration only marginally, whereas the indicator of relative concentration should respond markedly to such a change.

These criteria will be used as guidelines for measuring absolute (this section) and relative (Section 4.3) concentrations.

The most frequently used indicator of absolute concentration, the concentration ratio, is defined as follows: let $a(i)$ be the absolute amount of *output* produced by unit i (i.e., birth), and let m equal a certain small integer. Then the concentration ratio c_m in a sample of size N, where cases are ordered by the size of $a(i)$, can be written as

$$c_m = \frac{\sum\limits_{i=N-m+1}^{N} a(i)}{\sum\limits_{i=1}^{N} a(i)} = \sum\limits_{1}^{m} p(i) \tag{4.1}$$

where $p(i)$ is the proportion of total output produced by unit i. For this ratio the producing units are ranked by *output* size, and the m greatest producers are compared with the rest of the units. The selection of m is arbitrary. The ratio gives the proportion of the total output produced by the greatest 3, 5, 10, 25, or more production units.

The concentration ratios of the global distribution of births for the top 20 countries, can be seen in *Table 4.1* for the period 1950–1955 and *Table 4.2* for the period 1975–1980. The projected concentration ratios for 1995–2000 are given in *Table 4.3*. In all three tables m ranges from 1 to 20. The top 20 countries accounted for more than 80% of all children born in the 156 countries considered by the UN population statistics for 1950–1955. This percentage declined to 77% in 1975–1980 and is projected to decline to 74% by the next survey in 1995, indicating a decrease in absolute concentration of births among all countries in the world. As indicated by the tables, this decline is mainly due to the success of the birth control program in the People's Republic of China, although it is offset partly by a number of other countries where the number of births increased considerably. The proportion of all births taking place in the People's Republic of China declined from 26.5% in 1950–1955 to 17.1% in 1975–1980; it is expected to decline further to 15.3% by 2000. This decrease is largely responsible for the lowering in the concentration ratio for $m = 5$ (the five countries with the highest number of births), which was 55.7% in 1950–1955, only 47.2% in 1975–1980, and which is expected to be 43% by 2000.

Table 4.2. Absolute concentration of average annual numbers of births by countries in 1975–1980. (Herfindahl index: 0.0758.)

Rank order	Country	Number of births $a(i)$	Proportion of total births $p(i)$	Concentration ratio $\sum p(i) = c_m$	m
1	India	23,583	0.1893	0.1893	$m = 1$
2	PRC	21,313	0.1711	0.3603	$m = 2$
3	Indonesia	5,220	0.0419	0.4022	$m = 3$
4	USSR	4,745	0.0381	0.4403	$m = 4$
5	Bangladesh	3,889	0.0312	0.4715	$m = 5$
6	Nigeria	3,751	0.0301	0.5016	$m = 6$
7	Brazil	3,671	0.0295	0.5311	$m = 7$
8	USA	3,621	0.0291	0.5601	$m = 8$
9	Pakistan	3,569	0.0286	0.5888	$m = 9$
10	Mexico	2,433	0.0195	0.6083	$m = 10$
11	Vietnam	1,995	0.0160	0.6243	$m = 11$
12	Japan	1,757	0.0141	0.6384	$m = 12$
13	Egypt	1,593	0.0128	0.6512	$m = 13$
14	Philippines	1,540	0.0124	0.6636	$m = 14$
15	Iran	1,526	0.0122	0.6758	$m = 15$
16	Ethiopia	1,507	0.0121	0.6879	$m = 16$
17	Korea	1,478	0.0119	0.6998	$m = 17$
18	Turkey	1,475	0.0118	0.7116	$m = 18$
19	Thailand	1,380	0.0111	0.7227	$m = 19$
20	Burma	1,264	0.0101	0.7328	$m = 20$

This decline in absolute concentration can also be described by giving the number of countries that account for about half of all births in the world. Such figures cannot be exact because countries may not be interpolated. In 1950–1955 three countries accounted for almost half of all births in the world, in 1975–1980 six countries produced half the children, and by 2000 seven to eight countries are expected to produce half the births in the world. Two-thirds of the births were in 11 countries in 1950–1955 and in 15 countries in 1975–1980. Eighteen countries are expected to produce two-thirds of the children by 2000.

Hence, in this case of the distribution of births during 1950 through 2000, any selection of m observed over time results in the same finding: absolute concentration of births among countries diminishes considerably during the second half of the twentieth century. But the selection of different m does not necessarily always yield equivalent results. In some cases and distributions a certain m indicates an increase in concentration, yet in other cases m may indicate a decrease. Even though all m's indicated the same direction of change, the *extent* of change measured still depended on the arbitrary selection of m. Such properties of the concentration ratio are clearly not desirable.

Another index that overcomes this deficiency in consistency by considering all information given by the distribution, not only that of those at the top of the list, was suggested by Herfindahl (1950). He first provided a consistent indicator for absolute concentration, the Herfindahl index, which is defined by

Table 4.3. Projected absolute concentration of average annual numbers of births by countries in 1995–2000. (Herfindahl index: 0.0603.)

Rank order	Country	Number of births $a(i)$	Proportion of total births $p(i)$	Concentration ratio $\sum p(i) = c_m$	m
1	PRC	22,786	0.1584	0.1584	$m = 1$
2	India	22,007	0.1530	0.3113	$m = 2$
3	Nigeria	7,208	0.0501	0.3614	$m = 3$
4	USSR	5,038	0.0350	0.3965	$m = 4$
5	Bangladesh	4,798	0.0333	0.4298	$m = 5$
6	Indonesia	4,436	0.0308	0.4606	$m = 6$
7	Pakistan	4,355	0.0303	0.4909	$m = 7$
8	Brazil	4,121	0.0286	0.5195	$m = 8$
9	USA	3,810	0.0265	0.5460	$m = 9$
10	Mexico	2,668	0.0185	0.5646	$m = 10$
11	Ethiopia	2,563	0.0178	0.5824	$m = 11$
12	Zaire	2,096	0.0146	0.5970	$m = 12$
13	Vietnam	1,868	0.0130	0.6099	$m = 13$
14	Iran	1,801	0.0125	0.6225	$m = 14$
15	Kenya	1,765	0.0123	0.6347	$m = 15$
16	Egypt	1,758	0.0122	0.6469	$m = 16$
17	Tanzania	1,731	0.0120	0.6590	$m = 17$
18	Philippines	1,682	0.0117	0.6707	$m = 18$
19	Turkey	1,637	0.0114	0.6820	$m = 19$
20	Japan	1,627	0.0113	0.6934	$m = 20$

$$H = \frac{\sum\limits_{i=1}^{N} a(i)^2}{[\sum\limits_{i=1}^{N} a(i)]^2} = \sum\limits_{i=1}^{N} p(i)^2 \tag{4.2}$$

where $p(i)$ again is the proportion of *output* produced by unit i. In the case of maximum concentration, i.e., all output being produced by one unit, this index reaches unity. In the case of no concentration, i.e., an even distribution, the Herfindahl index will be $1/N$. As a measure of concentration, the Herfindahl index meets the four conditions given by Bruckmann (1969) and described above. The minimum value of $1/N$ is necessary to meet condition 3, i.e., the sensitivity of the index to changes in the sample size. A further practical advantage of H lies in the fact that units i need not be ordered by output because all $a(i)$'s enter the calculation.

The Herfindahl index for the three periods is also given in *Tables 4.1* through *4.3*. It confirms the above finding that absolute concentration declines significantly from 1950 to 2000 and also shows that the decline was significantly stronger during the first 25 years than the expected decline in the coming decade. The main reason for the change of rates of decline is a shift in the major causes of the birthrate decrease. Chinese fertility decreased greatly between 1965 and 1980, and reached such low levels that it cannot decline much further.

Parallel to the Chinese decline, the number of births in a large fraction of less-developed countries, most prominently in India, increased substantially, a fact that also brought about more evenness among the countries with the highest numbers of births, i.e., less absolute concentration. For the period up to the end of the century, absolute numbers of births are expected to decline in several large Asian countries, whereas they are projected to increase in parts of Latin America and especially in Africa. This will further diminish the differentials between numbers of babies born in most populous countries of the world and therefore reduce the absolute concentration of births, though at somewhat slower speed.

4.1.3. Relative concentration of fertility

The major criterion that distinguishes relative concentration from absolute concentration is that measures of relative concentration should also be sensitive to the addition of units at the very end of the list, ranking units by output. Suppose two populations, A and B, had exactly the same numbers of fertile women and identical parity distributions but population B had – in addition to the fertile women – a sizable number of childless women, then the relative concentration of fertility in B should be higher than that in A although the absolute numbers of children born and their distribution are identical.

The Lorenz curve provides a natural tool to describe relative concentration. Introduced by Lorenz (1905), it depicts the relationship between cumulated producing units and cumulated output units as fractions of the total of producing units and the total output. This basic setup of the Lorenz curve makes it especially useful to the analysis of relative concentration. Almost all further generalizations in the measurement of relative concentration are based on the Lorenz curve and focus on specific features, e.g., the slope at different points (see Piesch, 1975).

The Lorenz curve clearly refers to relative concentration because on both axes there are cumulated proportions: the x axis shows the cumulated proportion of producing units; the y axis that of output units. If the ranking of producing units by output is done in a way that puts the most productive units to the left, then the curve comes to lie above the diagonal, otherwise below. Lorenz originally worked with curves that lie above the diagonal but especially in economic concentration analysis the setup is often so that the curves lie below the diagonal. Whether the ranking goes from lowest to highest or highest to lowest does not affect the mathematics or the general setup of the curve. It only reflects the focus of the specific research, whether one is more interested in the lower end (such as poverty analysis in economics) or in the upper end of the distribution. In the life sciences and animal ecology where questions of dominance play an important role (see Goodwin and Vaupel, 1985), researchers usually put the most productive at the beginning.

Figures 4.1 to *4.5* show ways in which the Lorenz curve may be built up by a graduation scheme (see Piesch, 1975). These steps from the density distribution of children ever born to the inverted distribution function and finally to the Lorenz curve shall be illustrated using fertility patterns from three countries.

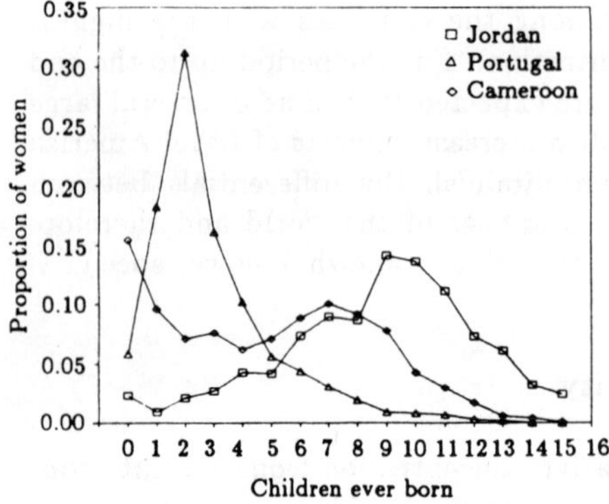

Figure 4.1. Distributions of children ever born in Jordan, Portugal, and Cameroon to ever-married women aged 40–49 (WFS).

Figure 4.2. Distribution functions for the three densities from *Figure 4.1.*

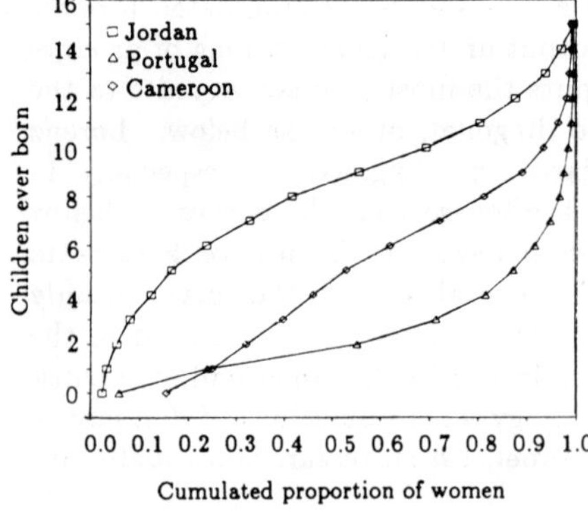

Figure 4.3. Inverted distribution function, based on *Figure 4.2.*

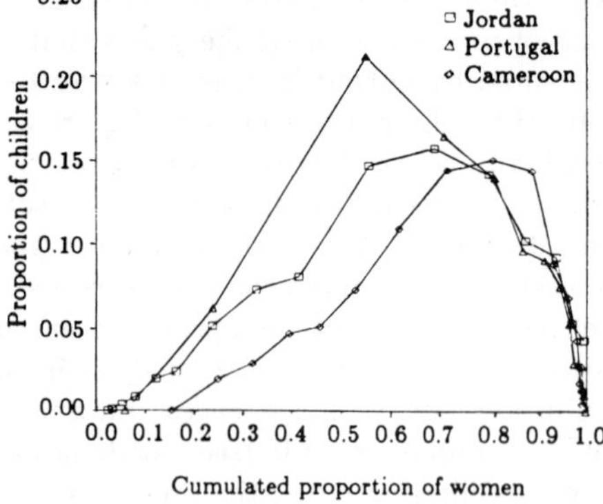

Figure 4.4. Adjusted inverted distribution function.

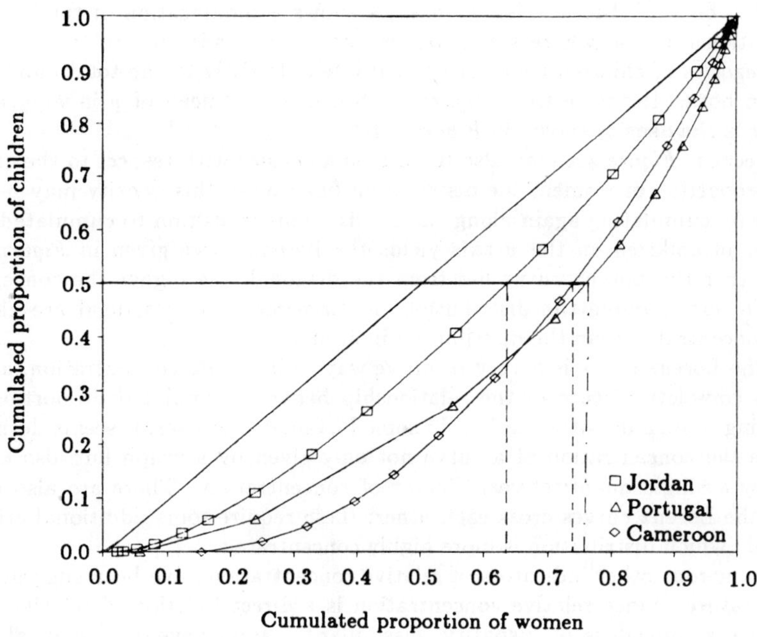

Figure 4.5. Lorenz curves resulting from cumulation of adjusted inverted distribution functions.

Figure 4.1 gives the three densities, indicating the way in which women are distributed over 16 possible completed parities (0 to 15 children) in three WFS countries with distinct reproductive patterns: Jordan, Cameroon, and Portugal. Women between the ages 40 and 49 in Jordan at the time of the survey had the highest fertility of all countries considered in WFS with the mode at parity nine. In Cameroon the pattern is quite different mainly because of a high proportion of childless women (15%). The distribution of women with more than one child peaks at parity seven in Cameroon. Portugal is an example of a country that has essentially completed the fertility transition. In Portugal marital fertility of women beyond reproductive age clearly peaks at parity two (31%), with more than 15% of the women each at parities one and three and around 10% at parity four.

Figure 4.2 gives the distribution functions of the three countries. This is simply the cumulated densities over all parities from lowest to highest. Because of the concentration of women at lower parities in Portugal, the distribution function there increases sharply. In Portugal women with 0 to 3 children already make up more than 70% of the adult female population. In Jordan the corresponding figure is under 10%.

The inverted distribution function depicted in *Figure 4.3* presents the cumulated proportion of women shown on the x axis and the distribution of children ever born on the y axis. *Figure 4.4* shows a modification of the inverted distribution function where the y axis is normed and adjusted to the fact that the categories of children ever born contribute differently to the total number of children born. Hence, y from *Figure 4.3* becomes $y \cdot c$/mean of y in *Figure 4.4*, where c is the density shown in *Figure 4.1*.

Because *Figure 4.4* may also be seen as a density with respect to the cumulated proportion of women, the distribution function of this density may be calculated by cumulating again along the x axis. This transition to cumulated proportions of children on the y axis yields the Lorenz curve given in *Figure 4.5*. The further the Lorenz curve lies from the diagonal, the higher the concentration. In our example the distributions in Cameroon and Portugal are clearly more concentrated than the distribution in Jordan.

The Lorenz curve is a very intuitive way to illustrate concentration, and it gives a complete picture of the relationship between cumulated proportions of producing units and output units. In some instances, however, it seems desirable to have the concentration of a curve not only given by a graph but also calculated by a single quantitative indicator of concentration. There are also cases where the Lorenz curves cross each other; these require some additional criteria to decide which distribution is more highly concentrated.

Numerous other indicators of relative concentration have been suggested in the literature. Since relative concentration is a direct function of relative variance, many indicators of disparity, dissimilarity, and unevenness may also be taken as indicators of the degree of concentration. Other concentration coefficients are based directly on the Lorenz curve. Perhaps the best-known indicator of this kind is the Gini coefficient. In terms of the Lorenz curve approach, the Gini coefficient is twice the area between the concentration curve and the diagonal (Foster, 1985). The Gini coefficient has the advantage of summarizing the complete information given by the Lorenz curve. It may be used to compare the degree of concentration of two different distributions; however, it is not easy to interpret it in terms of the original data.

What does a Gini coefficient of .7 in the distribution of births mean in terms of certain fractions of women having certain proportions of all children born? In this context it seems desirable to use an analogue to the concentration ratio, c_m, which was introduced for the study of absolute concentration. The concentration ratio shows what proportion of the total output was produced by a certain absolute number of producers. For relative concentration the proportion of children born by a certain *proportion* of women would be needed. These proportions may be called fractiles. If women are ordered by their family size the question of what proportion of women gave birth to 10% (.1 fractile), 50% (.5 fractile), or 90% (.9 fractile) of all children must be answered. These values may be readily seen from the Lorenz curve.

Being very intuitive and easy to interpret as quantitative indicators of concentration, the fractiles have the shortcoming of not reflecting all the information given in the curve. The .1 fractile gives the percentage of highest-fertility women that gave birth to 10% of all children. It mainly reflects the distribution among very high-fertility women and does not tell much about the degree of concentration at the lower end of the distribution. The .9 fractile suffers from the opposite shortcoming. The least amount of information is lost when using the .5 fractile because it is at the center of the distribution and reflects the shape of the curve both before and after the .5 fractile.

This may be illustrated with the help of *Figure 4.5*. When the horizontal line drawn at the level of 50% of all children crosses the Lorenz curves, the x axis values of these points indicate the proportions of all women that had 50% of the children. Since in this figure women were ranked from low fertility (at the left) to high fertility, the curve lies below the diagonal. This is a consequence of the graduation of the Lorenz curve described above. In the rest of the study, however, the fractiles will consistently be defined as percentages of a distribution ordered from highest to lowest. In *Figure 4.5*, the x fractiles should thus be read as $1-x$.

Although the Gini coefficients and other concentration indices are at similar magnitude for Portugal and Cameroon, the curves look quite different. In Cameroon the curve is steeper for high-parity women and less steep for low-parity women, mainly because of high proportions of childless women. This results in a crossover in the concentration curves, which means that the fractiles from highest fertility down to about the center of the curve indicate higher concentration for Portugal and thereafter higher concentration for Cameroon. In this specific case the .5 fractile indicates a still somewhat higher concentration for Portugal, since it is above the crossover of the two curves. But generally the correlation between the Gini coefficient and the .5 fractile should be higher than that for other fractiles (e.g., .1, .25, .4 fractiles). For most other countries in the world the Lorenz curves are of a similar, rather symmetric, shape without crossovers and vary only in their distance from the diagonal. Empirical studies (Goodwin, Lutz, and Vaupel, 1986) on 41 WFS countries result in correlation coefficients between the Gini index and the .5 fractile of above .9.

Vaupel and Goodwin (1986) call these fractiles *have-statistics* because they indicate what proportion of women *has* a certain proportion of children. Clearly the .5 is then the *havehalf*. Because of its easy interpretation and the fact that it is a consistent statistical measure (Goodwin and Vaupel, 1985) sensitive to nonproportional changes in any of the values of the underlying frequency distribution, the .5 fractile will be used (interchangeably called *havehalf*) as the basic measure of relative concentration in the following analysis.

4.2. Relative Concentration of Fertility along Various Demographic Dimensions

Concentration analysis always refers to the distribution of *output* units among *producing* units. In this study the output units are always births; the producing units may be individual women but also aggregates of women defined with respect to different demographic dimensions. Regarding the dimension of historical time, the definition given to time unit (year, month, day) is the producing unit, which allows for the study of the distribution of births over those time

units. With respect to subjective time (i.e., age or duration), certain years of age
are defined as the producing units, permitting the observation of the distribution
of births over ages. An equivalent approach can be taken of the study of the distribution of births over marital durations. Finally, not only temporal aggregates
but also spatial aggregates may be regarded as producing units, for instance, the
distribution and relative concentration of births over all countries in the world or
over all km^2 of land on the planet. Several of these dimensions are discussed
separately below.

4.2.1. Time

This section focuses on the distribution of births over historical time, starting
with very long time periods and progressing to shorter periods. The longer time
periods have much more concentrated Lorenz curves. *Table 4.4* and *Figure 4.6*
show the concentration of births over 10,000 years, from 8000 B.C. to A.D. 2000.
The estimates for the period before modern demographic records became available are based on population sizes and average annual increases suggested in
United Nations (1973), assuming a crude birthrate of 50 per thousand up to
1900. For the period after 1900 more empirical figures are available. For the
period A.D. 1950–2000, United Nations (1985) estimates and projections have
been used.

Table 4.4. Estimates of the distribution of total births (about 80 billion) from A.D. 2000
back to 8000 B.C.

Fractile	Birth	Time period	Proportion of time
.10	8 billion	A.D. 2000 back to A.D. 1931	.007
.25	20 billion	A.D. 2000 back to around A.D. 1760	.024
.5	40 billion	A.D. 2000 back to A.D. 1000	.100

The estimates suggest that half the children ever born within these 10,000
years were born within the last 1,000 years, i.e., in only one-tenth of the time
considered. World population growth has speeded up also within the last century, so that the most recent percentiles show an even greater discrepancy
between cumulated births and cumulated years: 10% of all births were and will
be during the 70 years from 1931 to 2000. This is only 0.7% of the total time
considered. Including estimates on the distribution of births over time and the
number of people alive at any point in time would increase the concentration
because of significant improvements in life expectancy.

More reliable records are available to analyze of shorter time periods.
Sweden and Finland, for example, have reliable annual figures on fertility since
the beginning of the eighteenth century. The concentration of births in Finnish
population history from 1722 to 1985 is plotted in *Figure 4.6*. Here, 32% of all
years considered (e.g., 85 years) produced half of the Finns born over the last
264 years. These 85 years do not include the most recent years since 1968; they
include years from the mid-nineteenth century to the postwar baby boom. Even

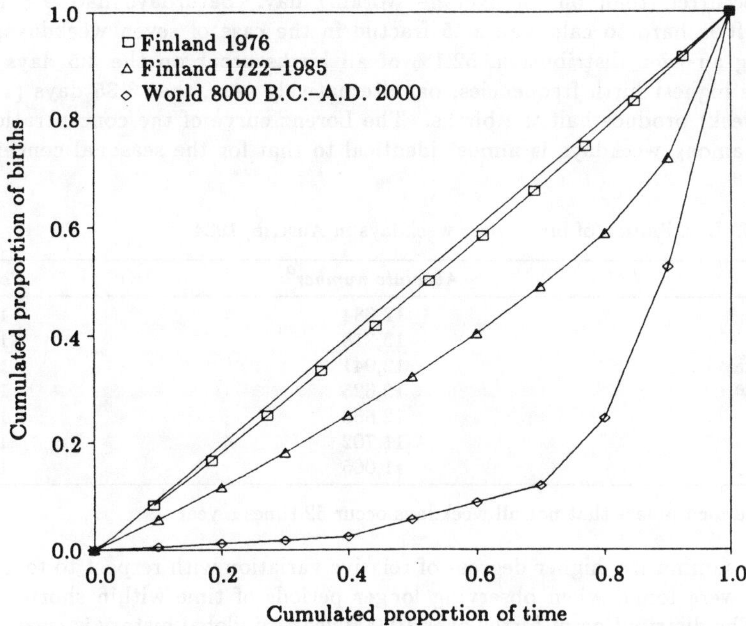

Figure 4.6. Lorenz curves for the temporal concentration of fertility over the period 8000 B.C. to A.D. 2000, for 1722–1985 in Finland and for monthly variations within the year 1976 in Finland.

though the total fertility rate was highest in the eighteenth century, these early periods contributed relatively little to the total number of births because the size of the population in 1750 was less than one-tenth of today's population size. But still the 264 years of Finnish fertility history are much less concentrated than the 10,000 years of world fertility history.

Temporal variations of births occur not only between years but also within a year. In most countries births show some distinctive seasonal pattern and also some variation between different days of the week. The seasonality of births seems to be especially strong in a northern climate (see Rantakallio, 1971) and in countries where the marriage pattern is strongly seasonal. For this reason Finland was again selected to demonstrate the concentration with respect to the month of birth. In 1976 – a year with higher seasonal variation than most recent years – 53% of all births occurred within 50% of all months. In other words, 47.2% of the months produced half the births. This calculation adjusted for the fact that months are of different length. By far the greatest numbers of children were born in the months of March and April, nine months after midsummer. A second smaller peak occurred in September, nine months after Christmas.

Very short-term variations in births, namely, variations by weekdays, are not likely to depend on the time of conception but rather on the working hours in hospitals around the time of birth. *Table 4.5* gives the adjusted distribution of births over weekdays in Austria. The pattern reveals that on Sundays 15% fewer births occurred than on an average working day. Saturdays had 9% fewer births. It is hard to calculate a .5 fractile in the case of seven weekdays; but assuming an even distribution, 52.1% of all births occur on the 3.5 days that have the highest birth frequencies, or, alternatively seen, that 3.35 days (47.8% of the week) produce half the births. The Lorenz curve of the concentration of fertility among weekdays is almost identical to that for the seasonal concentration.

Table 4.5. Distribution of births over weekdays in Austria, 1984.

	Absolute number[a]	*Percent*
Monday	12,684	14.5
Tuesday	13,318	15.3
Wednesday	12,941	14.8
Thursday	12,625	14.5
Friday	12,868	14.8
Saturday	11,702	13.4
Sunday	11,065	12.7

[a]Adjusted for the fact that not all weekdays occur 52 times a year.

To summarize, higher degrees of relative variation with respect to temporal changes were found when observing longer periods of time within shorter time units. The distribution of births over 10,000 years of global history is clearly one of the highest concentrated curves that can be found in the field of fertility analysis. Monthly and daily variations are minimal.

4.2.2. Age

The concentration of fertility with respect to the subjective time dimension of age is very different from that of historical time. Observing the distribution of births over the average life course of a real or synthetic cohort allows each distribution to be subjected to static concentration analysis. A comparative analysis might then be done by comparing the static concentration measures of cohorts varying in historical time or nationality.

To do such a concentration analysis of fertility, three factors must be studied: the distribution of births over the potentially fertile ages (15–49), the rank of single-year age groups according to fertility, and the calculation of what proportion of ages produces (single-year age groups being the producing unit) a certain fraction of all births. *Table 4.6* shows how many single-year age groups produce half the number of children born to all women in five selected LDCs participating in the WFS. The first three columns give the figures that reflect the actual age distribution of period fertility in the year before the survey. Column four gives results for age-standardized distributions, i.e., assuming the same

Table 4.6. Number of single-year age groups that produced 50% of all children in the year before the survey for five WFS countries.

Country	Rural women	Urban women	Total	Total Age-standardized
Costa Rica	9	5	7	8
Kenya	9	7	9	11
Pakistan	9	6	9	9
Peru	9	7	9	10
Sri Lanka	8	6	7	8

number of women are in each age group. If 6 years out of 35 produce half the births, the 0.5 fractile is 0.17. Eleven years indicate a value of .34 for the havehalf.

The table demonstrates that the age concentration of fertility is higher among urban women than among rural women. The value referring to all women is usually close to the rural value because of high rural percentages in the populations considered. In most cases age-standardization seems to make the distribution over all ages more even.

The difference between the age concentration of Finnish fertility in 1776 and 1983 plotted in *Figure 4.7* is similar to the urban-rural differential observed

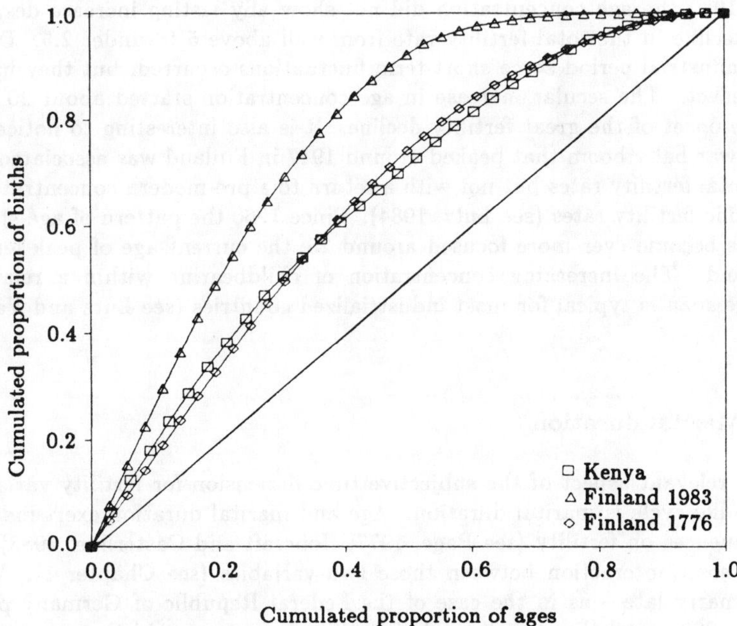

Figure 4.7. Lorenz curves for the age concentration of births (ages 15–49) in Kenya (WFS), Finland 1776, and Finland 1983.

in *Table 4.6*. Since *Table 4.6* shows that urban fertility levels are lower than rural ones and it is known that in Finland fertility was much higher in 1776 than in 1983, a lower level of fertility can be associated with higher age concentration. An explanation for this may be found in the concepts of natural fertility and controlled fertility. As discussed above natural fertility exists if the birth of a child does not depend on the number of children already born by the mother. The existence of natural fertility may be inferred from the age pattern of fertility. The natural fertility pattern is concave, e.g., shows a relatively slow decline after the age of peak fertility. In contrast to this, the pattern of controlled fertility produces a convex age pattern of fertility with a rather pronounced peak and fertility sharply declining after the peak ages. Therefore, a higher age concentration is expected in the controlled fertility pattern than in the natural fertility pattern as demonstrated in Finland in 1776 or in many rural, less-developed populations today.

In *Figure 4.7* the age concentration curves for the two high-fertility populations – Kenya in the 1970s and Finland in 1776 – are contrasted against the pattern of much higher concentration for the low fertility of Finland in 1983. For Finland, where data are available on the annual time-series of age-specific fertility rates for more than 200 years, the development can be followed and identified for the period during which the transition from low to high age concentration took place. *Figure 4.8* plots the total fertility rate against the .5 fractile of ages for 67 three-year periods in Finland for 1776–1976. (Since only five-year age groups are given, interpolations were made to single-year age groups.) Until around 1930 the age concentration did not show any lasting increase despite a strong decline in the total fertility rate from well above 5 to under 2.5. During the preindustrial period some short-term fluctuations occurred, but they had no lasting effect. The secular increase in age concentration started about 20 years after the onset of the great fertility decline. It is also interesting to notice that the postwar baby boom that peaked around 1947 in Finland was associated with higher total fertility rates but not with a return to a pre-modern concentration of age-specific fertility rates (see Lutz, 1984). Since 1960 the pattern of age-specific rates has become ever more focused around 25, the current age of peak fertility in Finland. The increasing concentration of childbearing within a relatively short age span is typical for most industrialized countries (see Lutz and Yashin, 1987).

4.2.3. Marital duration

Another relevant aspect of the subjective time dimension for fertility variations over the life cycle is marital duration. Age and marital duration exert independent influences on fertility (see Page, 1977; Hobcraft and Casterline, 1983), and there is some interaction between those two variables (see Chapter 1). When women marry late – as in the case of the Federal Republic of Germany period data for 1983 – and the overall level of fertility is low, most births occur within the first few years of marriage (see *Table 4.7*). The other extreme is Nepal, where women marry at a very young age (often before sexual maturity) and

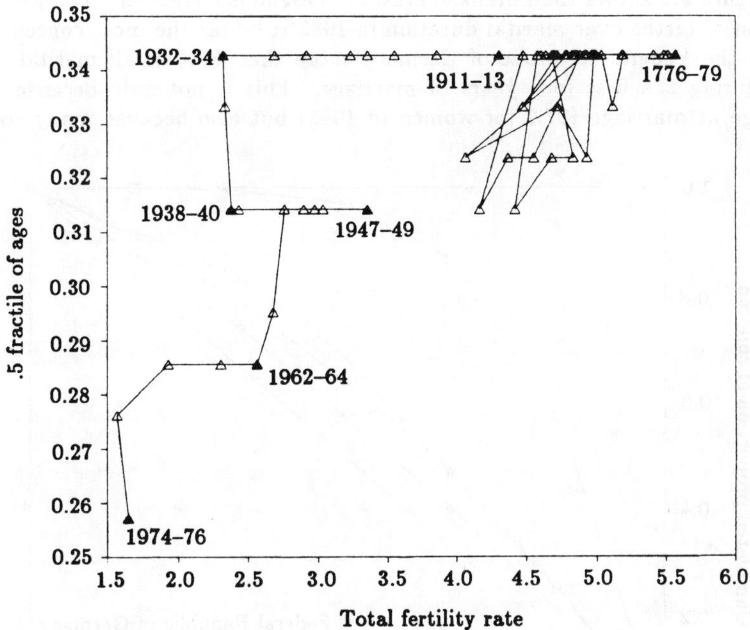

Figure 4.8. Changes in the relationship between the age concentration of fertility and the total fertility rate in Finland, 1776–1976, in three-year steps.

Table 4.7. Fraction of children born to certain marital durations of all children born up to duration 25–29.

Country	0–4	5–9	10–14	15–19	20–24	25–29
FRG	.573	.291	.106	.025	.004	.001
Nepal	.081	.216	.250	.216	.150	.086
Peru	.166	.213	.188	.171	.121	.140
Portugal	.257	.217	.146	.125	.089	.165

almost no voluntary family limitation takes place over the life course. In such a case childbearing is concentrated around some central marital duration of 10–14 years.

For Peru, the distribution over marital durations is somewhat less concentrated than in Nepal, mainly because of a higher age at marriage, which results in higher birth frequencies during the first 0–4 years of marriage. Marital fertility in Portugal shows the most even distribution of the four countries considered here, with a substantially lower age at marriage than in the FRG and some degree of voluntary spacing of births combined with a rather strong heterogeneity of the population with respect to the quantum and timing of births. Portugal has the Lorenz curve for duration that lies closest to the diagonal.

Figure 4.9 shows the Lorenz curves for these four countries. The FRG distribution of births over marital duration in 1983 is by far the most concentrated one: in the Federal Republic of Germany more than 57% of all marital births occur during the first four years of marriage. This is not only because of an older age at marriage (27.2 for women in 1983) but also because many couples

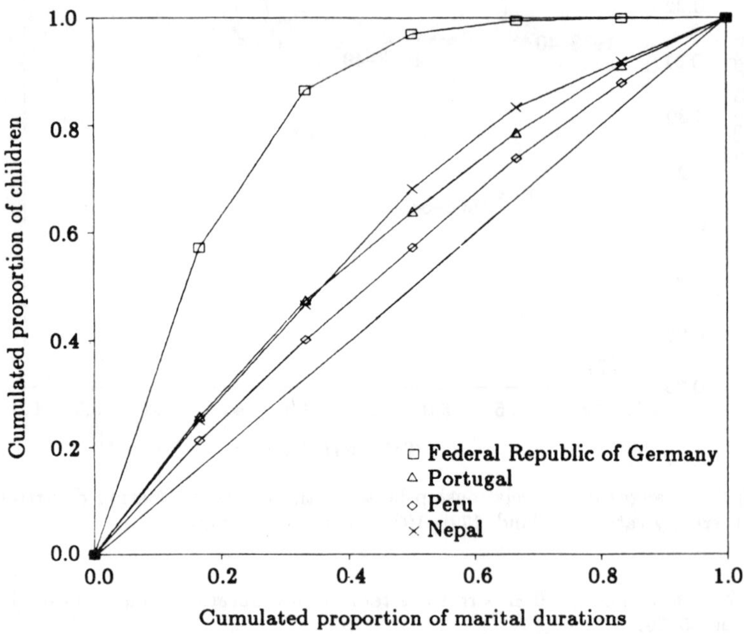

Figure 4.9. Lorenz curves for the concentration of births along six marital duration categories (see *Table 4.7*) for the Federal Republic of Germany in 1983 and the WFS data for Portugal, Peru, and Nepal.

have only one child, and if they have two they often try to space them close to each other. All in all, it can be said that marital duration concentrations of fertility vary within the same range as age concentration and both depend crucially on the fertility and nuptial pattern of the population concerned.

4.2.4. Space

Next to time aggregates, concentration can also be analyzed for spatial entities. The section on absolute concentration already considered nations as producing units, but it can also be applied to the analysis of relative concentration.

Figure 4.10 plots the Lorenz curves for the 100 countries that produce the most births. The figure shows curves for 1950–1955 and 1995–2000. The Lorenz curve for 1975–1980 lies between them. In 1950–1955 the People's Republic of China is to the very left and contributes by far the largest proportion of births. The People's Republic of China is expected to contribute a smaller fraction to the total number of children born in the world as a whole in 1995–2000 than it did in 1950–1955. This is a major reason for the fact that concentration in 1995–2000 is less, bringing the curve closer to the diagonal. The analysis of relative concentration here is very similar to that of absolute concentration above.

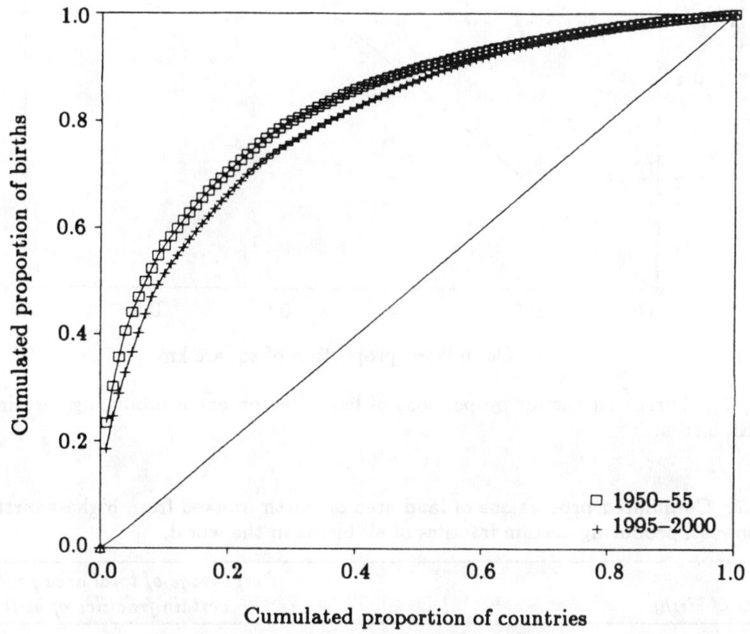

Figure 4.10. Lorenz curve for the 100 countries that produced the most births in 1950–1955 and that are expected to produce the most births in 1995–2000.

Countries are of very different size, and it is not at all surprising that large countries contribute a higher fraction of all births. A way to compensate for this bias is to take the area of a country into account. We then may ask what proportion of all km^2 of land on earth produces what proportion of children. This is done by calculating a birth density for each country (i.e., birth per km^2) and ranking the countries according to that density. The countries are then weighted again by the land area they cover to calculate fractiles. *Figure 4.11* shows the Lorenz curve for the proportions of land area on earth producing fractile of all births.

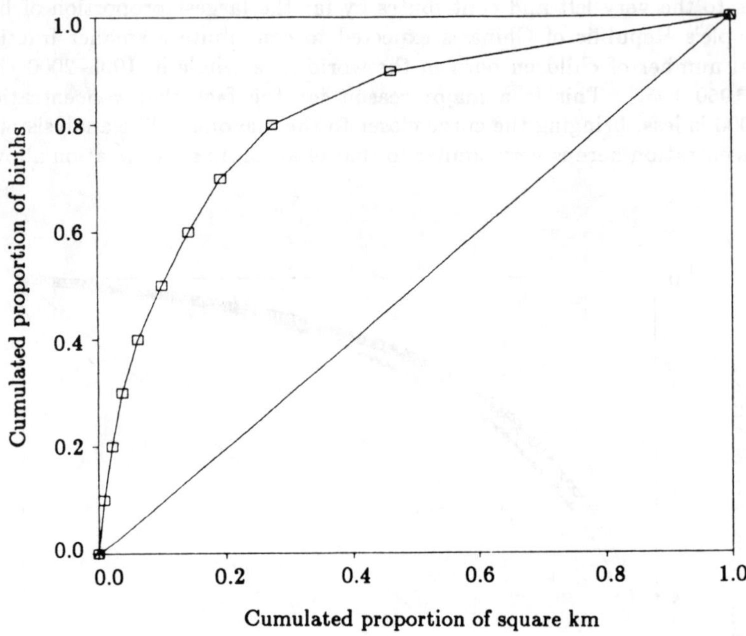

Figure 4.11. Lorenz curves for proportions of land area on earth producing certain fractiles of all births.

Table 4.8. Cumulated proportions of land area on earth, ranked from highest birth density to lowest, producing certain fractiles of all births in the world.

Fractiles of births	*Percentage of total area producing certain fractiles of births*
.10	0.9
.20	2.2
.30	3.7
.40	6.2
.50	10.0
.60	14.2
.70	19.3
.80	27.4
.90	46.2

Table 4.8 shows that less than 1% of land area produces 10% of all children, exactly 10% of all land produces half the children, and less than half of the

land produces 90% of all children. This already indicates a very high concentration of births with respect to spatial distribution. To calculate this, one very restrictive and unrealistic assumption must be made, namely, that within each nation births are evenly distributed over all km^2. Especially for countries like the Soviet Union or nations with high fractions of their territory being desert or rain forest, this is very misleading. In reality the spatial concentration of births is much higher, especially if considering the great urban agglomerations separately.

Without going into the vast geographical literature on spatial distribution, it shall be pointed out that the distribution of births in some respects is an important additional piece of information on the distribution of people. The spatial distribution of births is crucial for future food supply, industry, education, etc., all factors that affect the standard of living and the level of development.

4.2.5. Micro-level

So far the temporal and spatial aggregates that produced children have been studied. These were aggregates of women that gave birth to children at different times, at different ages, during different marital durations, and in different places. These aggregates all showed specific macro-aspects of the distribution of births. To study the concentration of reproduction within a specific group of women at a specific time and place, however, one must to go back to the micro-level and consider the original producing unit: the individual woman. All the remaining sections of this chapter will be a micro-level analysis of the concentration of fertility among individual women in certain countries or socioeconomically defined subpopulations in certain historical periods.

One important demographic aspect of the microanalysis is the difference in mean family size from the mothers' perspective and the mean family size from the children's perspective, originally discussed in the 1970s by Goodman, Keyfitz, and Pullum (1975) and Preston (1976). The difference in mean family size from women's and children's perspectives is intuitively obvious. Consider, for example, a family of eight. In the calculation of the mean family size for women, this family will count once. In the calculation of the mean family size for children, however, this family will count *eight* times – since each child perceives himself or herself in a family of eight. Thus, large families will receive considerably more weight in the calculation of the mean family size for children, which will also be denoted as mean sibship size.

Preston (1976) formalized this relationship in the following way: let $f(x)$ be the proportion of women with completed parity x. Then the mean family size for women is

$$\bar{x} = \sum_{x=1}^{n} f(x)x \tag{4.3}$$

where n is the maximum parity considered. The average family size for children is then

$$\bar{c} = \sum_{1}^{n} \frac{f(x)x}{\sum_{1}^{n} f(x)x}\, x = \frac{\sum f(x)x^2}{\bar{x}} \qquad (4.4)$$

where the weight in the summation represents the proportion of children from families of size x.

It can be shown (Preston, 1976) that the difference between women's mean family size ($\bar{x}$) and children's mean family size ($\bar{c}$) is a function of the variance of the distribution:

$$\bar{c} = \frac{\sigma_x^2}{\bar{x}} + \bar{x} \qquad (4.5)$$

where σ_x^2 is the variance of the distribution of family sizes among women.[1] This difference between the mean family sizes for women and children has several demographic and non-demographic consequences that will be considered in the concluding section of this study.

The following sections will give empirical studies of the concentration of fertility among individual women. The study of distributional aspects of fertility is a necessary complement to the usual study of average levels of fertility, and will lead, especially in the analysis of periods of demographic transformations, to surprising results.

4.3. Demographic Transition and Concentration

This section focuses on the relationship between changes in the average level of fertility and changes in the relative concentration of fertility during demographic transition. Wherever possible this relationship is observed separately for different socioeconomic strata. Germany and Austria from the late 1800s to 1939 are studied in one case. Then, a time-series of selected LDCs and a cross section of 41 LDCs are treated. It will become clear that during demographic transition, concentration increases as fertility decreases.

To do this analysis, data sets provided information on the number of children ever born at completion of childbearing for different cohorts, and on some socioeconomic variables. The data set that provides the historical information for Germany and Austria is the German census (Reichsfamilienstatistik) of 1939. For the LDCs, the data were provided by the WFS and figures were provided by the *UN Demographic Yearbooks*.

4.3.1. Marital fertility in Germany and Austria from the late 1800s to 1939

The German census of 1939 asked all women living in the German Reich (Germany and Austria at that time) their completed parity, first marriage date, and husband's occupation. Women over 40 participated in the census and provided family histories reaching back to the end of the last century. This is precisely the period when much of the fertility transition took place in Europe.

Using this census, Spree (1982, 1984) calculated parity distributions up to parity 5+ and mean numbers of children per women (calculated from a longer parity distribution). He classified the women according to husband's occupation using 64 job categories and three marriage cohorts: the cohort of women that married before 1905, between 1905 and 1910, and between 1920 and 1924. The mean age at marriage was above 25 for women in the 1920s, so even the youngest cohort should have almost completed its reproductive career by 1939.

Table 4.9 gives measures of fertility and reproductive concentration for the three marriage cohorts and 13 selected occupational groups. The mean number of children ever born declined significantly in all groups. Among the oldest cohort, those who had married before 1905, agricultural workers, miners, and independent farmers had the highest fertility with, on the average, more than 5.5 children. The lowest fertility was found among the families of self-employed physicians and university professors, social elites who had anticipated the fertility decline. Concentration in this cohort was lowest in the highest fertility groups: 31% of families of agricultural laborers bore half the children in that group. Only 4% of the agricultural families remained childless, while 64% had five or more children. The distribution was similar among independent farmers, miners, and construction workers. For the other occupational groups, the havehalf concentration coefficient ranges from 22% to 28%, generally being lower (i.e., concentration higher) when fertility levels are lower. The major exceptions to this pattern are the families of the self-employed physicians and university professors, who have the lowest fertility of the entire cohort, but also low concentration (havehalf = .28).

The couples who married between 1905 and 1909 had, on average, more than one child less than those who married before 1905. Simultaneously, concentration of reproduction increased in most occupational groups. This implies that some members of the groups moved toward the new fertility regime more quickly than others, thus increasing the relative variance. Among those employed in the selected 13 occupational groups, only for church officials and ministers did the completed parity distributions become more even.

This trend continued between 1905–1909 and 1920–1924. For several occupational categories the mean number of children per couple had fallen to 2.0 or below. With 1.4 children per couple, independent artists and actors were even well below the fertility rate of physicians and professors and showed extremely high concentration; this was mainly due to childlessness among 35% of the couples. At the upper end of the spectrum agricultural laborers still averaged 3.5 children. Concentration also continued to increase in most occupational groups. It is interesting to notice that the concentration within the aggregate of all 64

Table 4.9. Concentration of fertility among marriage cohorts by occupational groups for Germany and Austria according to the German census of 1939. (Source: Spree, 1984.)

Occupation of husband	Year of marriage	Mean number of children		.5 fractile
		Point of view		
		Mother	Children	
Laborers in	before 1905	6.0	7.6	0.31
agriculture	1905–1910	5.2	6.7	0.30
	1920–1924	3.5	4.9	0.26
Independent	before 1905	5.6	7.5	0.29
farmers	1905–1910	4.7	6.7	0.27
	1920–1924	3.1	4.6	0.25
Miners	before 1905	5.7	7.7	0.29
	1905–1910	4.9	6.8	0.28
	1920–1924	2.9	4.4	0.25
Construction	before 1905	5.2	6.7	0.30
workers	1905–1910	4.4	5.8	0.28
	1920–1924	2.9	4.5	0.24
Self-employed	before 1905	4.4	5.7	0.28
craftsmen	1905–1910	3.5	5.3	0.24
	1920–1924	2.2	4.0	0.22
Self-employed in	before 1905	4.4	6.4	0.26
transportation	1905–1910	3.3	5.1	0.23
	1920–1924	2.0	3.5	0.22
Workers in	before 1905	4.3	5.8	0.28
iron and metal	1905–1910	3.4	5.3	0.24
industry	1920–1924	2.1	3.4	0.23
Self-employed	before 1905	4.0	6.3	0.24
innkeepers	1905–1910	3.0	4.5	0.25
	1920–1924	1.8	3.1	0.23
Church	before 1905	3.9	5.8	0.26
officials,	1905–1910	3.4	4.5	0.29
ministers	1920–1924	2.7	3.8	0.27
Civil servants	before 1905	3.5	5.2	0.25
with railroad	1905–1910	2.9	4.4	0.25
and postal service	1920–1924	1.9	3.5	0.22
Independent	before 1905	3.1	5.1	0.22
artists,	1905–1910	2.3	4.3	0.20
actors, etc.	1920–1924	1.4	3.7	0.15
University	before 1905	2.7	3.8	0.28
professors	1905–1910	2.6	3.7	0.28
and deans	1920–1924	1.9	3.1	0.24
Self-employed	before 1905	2.6	3.6	0.28
physicians	1905–1910	2.5	3.9	0.26
	1920–1924	2.0	2.3	0.30
All	before 1905	4.7	6.5	0.27
	1905–1910	3.6	5.3	0.24
	1920–1924	2.3	4.0	0.21

occupations in the pre-1905 marriage cohort was about the mean of the values of the .5 fractile of the individual groups. For the marriage cohort of 1920–1924,

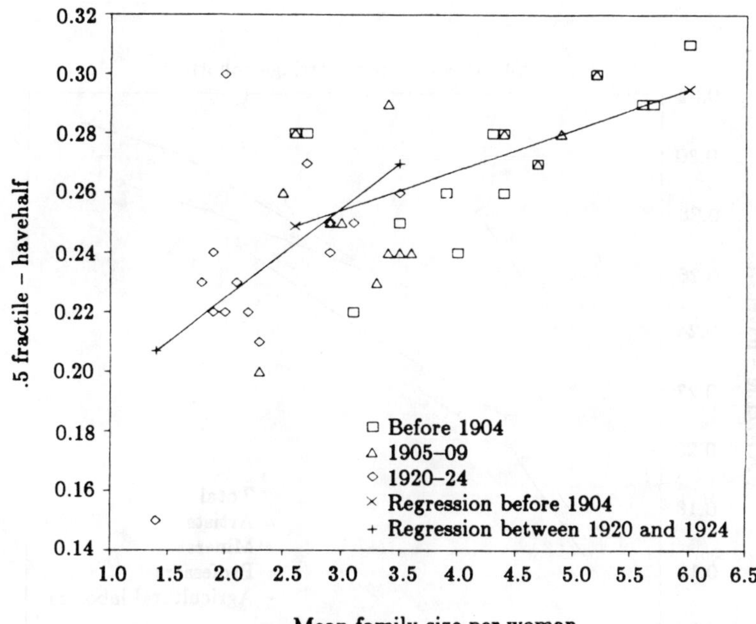

Figure 4.12. Relationship between mean family size per woman and the .5 fractile for different occupational groups in Germany and Austria and marriage cohorts from before 1904 to 1920–1924.

however, the aggregate is clearly more concentrated than the majority of the occupational groups taken separately. This indicates that variation between the occupational groups had increased even more strongly than the variation within the occupational groups.

Figure 4.12 plots the average level of fertility per couple against the concentration coefficient for the 13 selected groups and the total of all occupational groups for the three different marriage cohorts. The figure also shows the regression lines of this association for the oldest and the youngest cohorts, calculated by giving equal weight to all groups. A positive association between the havehalf and the level of fertility within cohorts and over time is obvious. In other words, lower average fertility was associated with higher concentration.

Figure 4.13 extracts four selected occupational groups and the total from *Figure 4.12*, and connects the changes over time per group. Taken as a whole (total), the cohort declines in average fertility, and in the havehalf the decreases were almost exactly proportional from the cohort married before 1905 to that of 1905–1909 and that of 1920–1924; in other words, the association was linear. For the big groups of agricultural laborers and miners, the lines of development are almost parallel to the total, but starting at different levels of fertility and concentration. The independent artists and actors as well as professors and

                                    Distributional Aspects of Human Fertility

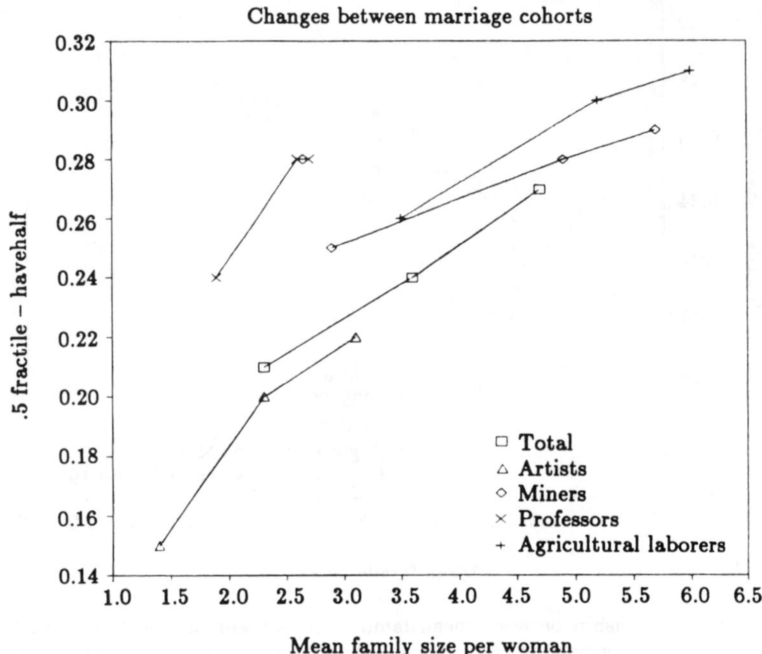

Figure 4.13. Changes in the association between concentration and the level of fertility over time for selected occupational groups for cohorts married before 1904, 1905–1909, and 1920–1924 in Germany and Austria.

university officials show a steeper increase of concentration with declining average fertility. For these groups as many as 22% (professors) and 35% (artists) of the marriage cohort 1920–1924 were childless in 1939.

Lower concentration in high-fertility groups results in a more even picture of mean family sizes from the children's perspective than from the women's perspective. For the cohort married before 1905, children of independent farmers averaged 6.5 brothers and sisters, children of church officials 4.8, children of innkeepers 5.3, and children of construction workers 5.7. Only families of physicians and professors did not follow this tendency, having both low fertility and low concentration. Consequently, on average, the child of a physician whose parents were married before 1905 had only 2.6 brothers and sisters.

Another interesting aspect that is revealed by comparing mean parity with mean sibship size is that the marital fertility transition in Germany and Austria was much less significant from the children's perspective than from the couple's point of view: while the mean number of children per couple declined by more than half between the pre-1905 and the 1920–1924 marriage cohorts, the mean family size for children declined by only 38% on the average.

The following section examines whether this pattern of increase in concentration is also true for the historical fertility transition in today's industrialized countries, or if equivalent patterns may be observed in the countries that currently experience their secular fertility transition.

4.3.2. Time series for selected less-developed countries

For countries that are still in the process of the secular fertility transition it is very difficult to find data that indicate trends in the distribution of children among mothers over the course of the fertility decline. Completed parity distributions by age are provided by official censuses for only a few less-developed countries. *Table 4.10* lists some of these countries. The data come from the special topic tables on nuptiality found in the *UN Demographic Yearbook* (1981). For Costa Rica, Republic of Korea, and Libya, the female population is broken down by place of residence; for Bolivia, Egypt, and Fiji, the data refer to the total female population. The information provided may be subject to incorrect reporting by age and by parity, which – especially for older women – might be significant. Women over age 65 might forget to mention some births, especially if the child died at a young age. Another possible bias is selectivity (by mortality) with respect to achieved fertility.

In terms of period fertility the patterns shown in these data mainly refer to the time from 1920 to the late 1960s when the women considered were in their prime childbearing ages. In all populations considered, with the exception of urban Korea, the average level of fertility seems to have increased over time at least for the age groups 60–64 and 45–49. This increase is most pronounced in Egypt and Libya where the mean completed family size increases by almost one child. From the given data it is difficult to assess whether this increase was real or a consequence of errors in reporting differential parity by age. In some populations such as urban Costa Rica and Fiji a slight decline in mean family sizes from the age groups 70–74 to 60–64 was observed. Since the underreporting of parity was expected to be most serious in the oldest age groups, such cases may be seen as evidence against a very strong effect of incorrect reporting. Still this might be different from one country to another.

It does not seem too unreasonable to assume a slight increase in fertility between about 1930 and 1950. It is often observed that before the fertility transition the average level of fertility increases somewhat because of improved health conditions, a desire for large families, and the lack of birth control (e.g., Easterlin, 1978). The onset of the fertility transition resulting in markedly lower average family sizes for women aged 45–49 compared with women aged 55–59 in 1975 is noticeable only in the case of the urban population of the Republic of Korea.

Generally, the concentration of fertility does not change dramatically over the more than 30 years, but some decrease of concentration is visible in every country considered. It is most pronounced in Egypt where the .5 fractile increases from .23 to .28, while the mean number of children per woman increases from 4.25 to 5.23. This is consistent with the finding in the previous

Table 4.10. Mean family sizes and concentration of parity distributions for women beyond reproductive age in selected LDCs.

Country, year of census	Age group	Mean/woman	Mean/child	.5 fractile
Bolivia, 1976	45–49	6.08	8.09	0.29
	50–54	5.97	8.09	0.29
	55–59	5.90	8.05	0.29
	60–64	5.58	7.82	0.28
	65+	5.42	7.73	0.27
Costa Rica, 1973	45–49	4.94	7.60	0.24
Urban	50–54	4.84	7.69	0.23
	55–59	4.80	7.69	0.23
	60–64	4.53	7.67	0.22
	65–69	4.72	8.01	0.22
	70–74	4.69	8.02	0.22
	75+	4.89	8.16	0.23
Costa Rica, 1973	45–49	7.37	9.37	0.30
Rural	50–54	7.17	9.34	0.29
	55–59	7.11	9.31	0.29
	60–64	6.82	9.20	0.28
	65–69	6.95	9.26	0.28
	70–74	6.73	9.18	0.28
	75+	6.73	9.19	0.28
Egypt, 1976	45–49	5.23	7.07	0.28
	50–54	4.81	6.98	0.26
	55–59	4.89	7.08	0.26
	60+	4.25	6.83	0.23
Fiji, 1976	45–49	7.99	9.56	0.31
	50–54	7.99	9.52	0.31
	55–59	7.77	9.37	0.31
	60–64	7.46	9.25	0.31
	65–69	7.48	9.23	0.31
	70–74	8.41	9.83	0.31

section that higher fertility is associated with lower concentration, but this time the trend goes in the other direction than that for the marital fertility transition in Germany and Austria. An explanation for this decrease in relative variation (i.e., concentration) is that differences in fecundability – the major source of variation in natural fertility populations – diminished as health conditions improved. This results in a decline in the proportion of women childless or with low completed parities. In Egypt the proportion of childless women declined from 18% (age 60+) to 9% (age 45–49). At the upper end of the spectrum women who were already close to the maximum fertility possible in the specific culture with given birth-spacing practices, etc., could hardly increase their fertility further. This made the distribution of children ever born more even and consequently reduced the concentration of reproduction.

In the case of urban Korea, (*Figure 4.14*) the beginning of the fertility transition also meant a reversal of the decreasing trend of concentration. The introduction of birth control tended to increase relative variation again.

Table 4.10. Continued.

Country, year of census	Age group	Mean/woman	Mean/child	.5 fractile
Korea, Rep. of, 1975	45–49	4.66	5.66	0.30
Urban	50–54	5.03	6.24	0.30
	55–59	5.10	6.50	0.29
	60–64	5.00	6.51	0.28
	65–69	4.79	6.40	0.28
	70–74	4.66	6.20	0.27
	75+	4.53	6.10	0.27
Korea, Rep. of, 1975	45–49	5.72	6.67	0.33
Rural	50–54	5.85	6.99	0.33
	55–59	5.72	6.95	0.32
	60–64	5.38	6.70	0.31
	65–69	5.17	6.47	0.30
	70–74	5.00	6.27	0.30
	75+	4.83	6.06	0.29
Libya, 1973	45–49	7.46	8.87	0.33
Urban	50–54	7.05	8.61	0.33
	55–59	6.99	8.55	0.33
	60–64	6.58	8.29	0.32
	65–69	6.63	8.22	0.32
	70–74	6.39	8.08	0.32
	75+	5.99	7.81	0.30
Libya, 1973	45–49	7.72	8.91	0.35
Rural	50–54	7.36	8.73	0.34
	55–59	7.26	8.62	0.34
	60–64	6.93	8.37	0.34
	65–69	6.93	8.31	0.34
	70–74	6.48	8.02	0.33
	75+	6.31	7.91	0.32

4.3.3. A cross-sectional view on 41 less-developed WFS countries

A more reliable and complete source of data than the few censuses with age-specific information on the number of children ever born is given by the WFS. A tremendous amount of work was invested (Cleland and Hobcraft, 1985) to check the consistency and accuracy of information given, making the WFS the best body of standardized information on fertility for a large number of less-developed countries.

This section analyzes the relative concentration of children ever born by ever-married women aged 40–49 at the time of the survey. The demographic transition cannot be studied in a longitudinal manner because data on only one age group and at one point in time per country were available. Instead a cross-sectional approach was taken. The basic assumption is that all countries follow a similar pattern of fertility transition but are at different stages of the transition at the time of the survey.

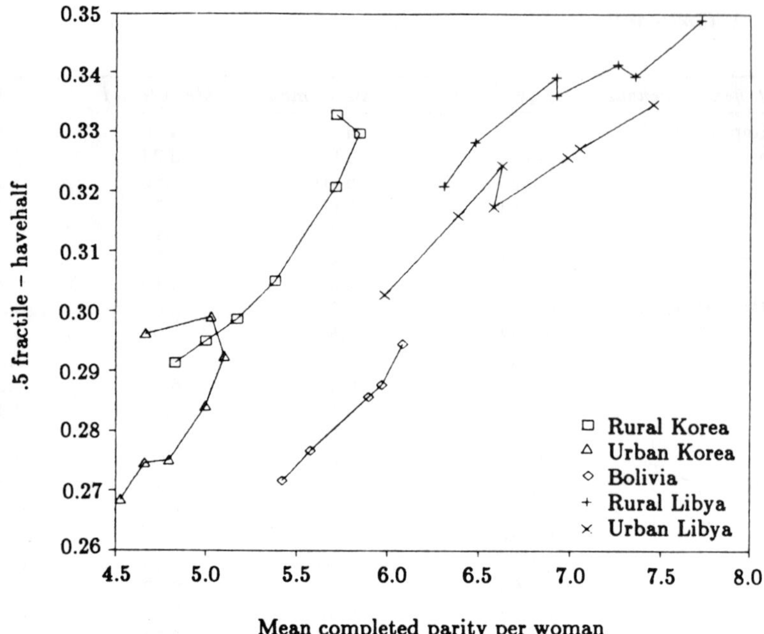

Figure 4.14. Relationship between average parity and the concentration of reproduction in five selected less-developed populations for age groups 40–49 to 75+. (For data, see *Table 4.10.*)

Figure 4.15 shows the Lorenz curves for two countries with very low concentration – Jordan and Tunisia – in which the curves are closest to the diagonal, and for two countries with high concentration – Portugal and Venezuela (only educated women were considered in Venezuela) – in which the curves are further from the diagonal. Steepness at the beginning of the curve, such as that for Portugal (considered an LDC by the WFS), indicates that a small fraction of high-parity women accounts for a large fraction of the births. The flattening of this concentration curve toward the end signifies a smaller relative contribution of low-parity women to the number of children born as compared with the other countries. This implies a very heterogeneous population in Portugal; and that the concentration is mostly due to small groups of very high-fertility women as opposed to large groups of childless and low-fertility women.

Table 4.11 lists the mean number of children per woman for the 41 less-developed countries participating in the WFS. The concentration, as measured by the .5 fractile, are inversely related; the lower a country's level of fertility the higher the concentration of reproduction. The two countries with the highest mean number of children, Jordan and Kenya, have the lowest concentration. Jordan has an average of 8.7 and Kenya an average of 7.7 children. More than 36% of all the women have half the children in these countries. Obviously, if

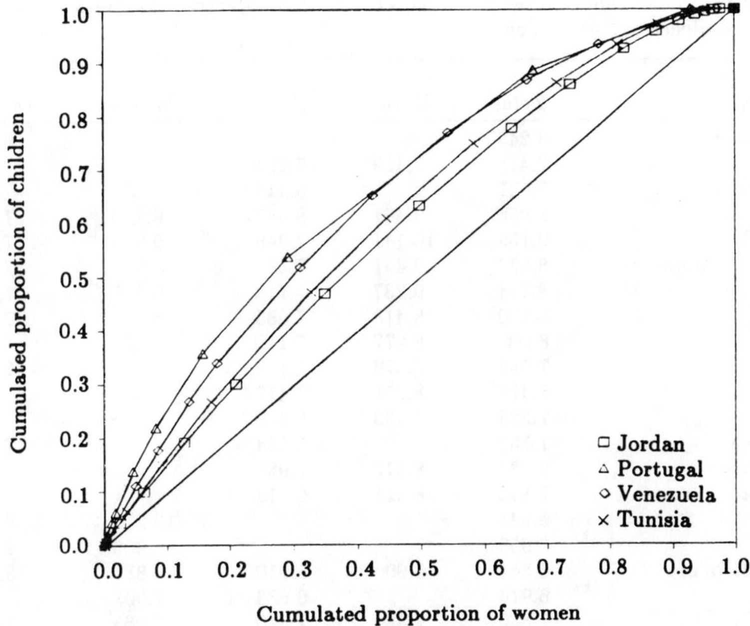

Figure 4.15. Lorenz curves for the concentration of fertility in selected WFS populations: Jordan (women without formal schooling), Portugal (all women), Venezuela (women with some schooling), and Tunisia (rural women).

50% had half, the distribution of offspring among women would be equal. Cameroon and Portugal have the lowest fertility: 4.9 and 2.9 children, respectively. These countries also have the highest concentration, with a havehalf of 26% and 24%, respectively. Furthest away from the regression line lies the Republic of Korea, with a concentration much lower than that expected from the level of fertility, and Costa Rica, with a higher concentration than the mean number of 6.9 children would imply.

The almost linear relationship between the havehalf statistic and mean fertility in these countries is even more apparent when looking at urban and rural populations separately, *Figure 4.16.* Urban fertility is generally lower than the fertility of women from rural areas. It is interesting to notice that the regression line for the relationship between the concentration and the level of fertility for rural areas is almost parallel to that for urban areas, with the urban line falling slightly below and to the left of the rural line. Country-specific characteristics seem to pertain beyond this breakdown. Korea is an outlier with the Korean rural and urban populations lying some distance above the regression line. However, urban fertility is significantly lower and more concentrated than rural, and the trajectory of these two points is parallel to that of the regression line. This is also true for most urban-rural differentials within individual countries.

Table 4.11. Mean family sizes from the children's perspective: 41 WFS countries by place of residence and education.

Country	Total	Rural	Urban	No education	Some education
Bangladesh	8.242				8.258
Benin	7.415	7.439	7.221		
Cameroon	7.527		6.118		
Colombia	8.856	9.461	8.443	9.199	7.828
Costa Rica	9.135	10.141	7.345	9.980	7.923
Dominican Republic	8.538	9.441	7.383	8.961	7.384
Ecuador	8.714	9.237	7.714	9.375	7.456
Egypt	8.120	8.413	7.685	8.175	7.989
Fiji	8.009	8.277	7.118	8.231	7.584
Ghana	7.544	7.676	7.118		7.052
Guyana	8.477	8.791	7.412	8.851	
Haiti	7.323	7.433	6.469		
Indonesia	7.152		7.334		7.418
Ivory Coast	8.324	8.372	7.985		
Jamaica	7.800	8.321	6.118		
Jordan	9.948			10.228	8.738
Kenya	8.956			8.906	9.036
Korea, Rep. of	6.341	6.906	5.610	6.887	5.777
Lesotho	6.914		6.683	7.003	
Malaysia	7.830	7.884	7.310	7.965	7.374
Mauritania	7.779	7.611	7.923	7.799	7.662
Mexico	8.944	9.348	8.560	9.356	8.677
Morocco	8.920	8.779	8.251		
Nepal	7.021				
Nigeria	7.343				
Pakistan	8.267	8.157	8.326		
Panama	7.479	8.368	6.536	8.626	6.486
Paraguay	8.456	9.440	6.386	9.306	6.818
Peru	8.435	8.875	8.046	9.084	7.703
Philippines	8.345	8.632	7.512	9.018	8.018
Portugal	4.597	5.025	3.296	5.246	3.231
Senegal	8.369	8.375	8.360		
Sri Lanka	7.325		6.554	8.010	6.954
Sudan	7.829	7.842	7.780		
Syria	9.051	9.060	9.041		7.708
Thailand	7.883		6.314	7.746	7.780
Trinidad and Tobago	7.511	7.988	7.151	7.559	
Tunisia	8.062	8.081	7.984		
Turkey	7.697	8.405	6.252	8.326	5.914
Venezuela	8.042			9.004	6.661
Yemen	7.951				

In all countries except Portugal urban concentration is higher than rural. The highest differentials between urban and rural populations are found in Latin American countries, in particular, in the Caribbean. In urban areas of the Dominican Republic, for instance, 26% of the women have half the children; whereas in the countryside, this percentage is 33%. In Africa, these differentials

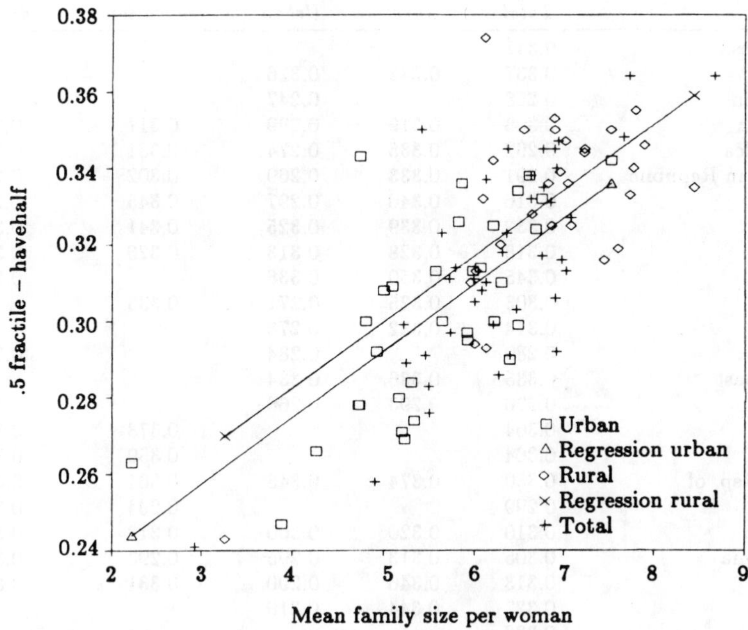

Figure 4.16. Relationship between mean completed family size per woman and .5 fractile for urban and rural women for WFS LDCs.

in concentration are less significant; the differences are only 1–3 percentage points.

It is also worth noting that in all countries except Portugal the concentration of reproduction, in the total population is not higher than that in the rural and urban segments separately *Table 4.12.* This deserves attention because concentration is not additive. If two rather homogeneous subpopulations with different fertility levels were pooled together one might expect that the aggregate is more heterogeneous than any of the subpopulations. However, these findings indicate that in almost any country family size differentials within the cities are greater than those between towns and the countryside. Only in Portugal is the concentration of reproduction higher for the total population than it is for either of the subpopulations.

For educational differentials the pattern is similar to that of the residential breakdown *Figure 4.17.* In most countries the .5 fractiles are clearly lower for women with at least some schooling. Only in Kenya, Mauritania, Lesotho, and Portugal is the concentration of reproduction higher for women without schooling. Interestingly enough, Kenya, Mauritania, and Lesotho are also the only countries where the level of fertility is lower for women without schooling. The concentration of fertility in the total population lies between the values of the

Table 4.12. The .5 fractiles for 41 WFS countries by place of residence and education.

Country	Total	Rural	Urban	No education	Some education
Bangladesh	0.347				0.358
Benin	0.337	0.342	0.326		
Cameroon	0.258		0.247		
Colombia	0.306	0.319	0.299	0.317	0.293
Costa Rica	0.292	0.335	0.274	0.331	0.269
Dominican Republic	0.291	0.333	0.269	0.302	0.277
Ecuador	0.316	0.340	0.297	0.345	0.296
Egypt	0.332	0.339	0.325	0.341	0.319
Fiji	0.318	0.328	0.313	0.326	0.319
Ghana	0.345	0.350	0.336		0.343
Guyana	0.303	0.325	0.271	0.335	
Haiti	0.314	0.332	0.278		
Indonesia	0.289		0.284		0.299
Ivory Coast	0.335	0.336	0.334		
Jamaica	0.276	0.293	0.266		
Jordan	0.364			0.378	0.335
Kenya	0.364			0.359	0.379
Korea, Rep. of	0.350	0.374	0.343	0.361	0.352
Lesotho	0.299			0.294	0.302
Malaysia	0.310	0.320	0.300	0.318	0.301
Mauritania	0.305	0.313	0.295	0.293	0.318
Mexico	0.313	0.346	0.290	0.331	0.304
Morocco	0.327	0.344	0.310		
Nepal	0.323				
Nigeria	0.291				
Pakistan	0.345	0.350	0.332		
Panama	0.297	0.325	0.292	0.328	0.296
Paraguay	0.286	0.316	0.278	0.319	0.267
Peru	0.317	0.350	0.300	0.353	0.295
Philippines	0.331	0.345	0.313	0.360	0.324
Portugal	0.241	0.243	0.263	0.246	0.272
Senegal	0.340	0.347	0.324		
Sri Lanka	0.311		0.309	0.323	0.309
Sudan	0.311	0.310	0.314		
Syria	0.348	0.355	0.342		0.323
Thailand	0.323		0.308	0.333	0.321
Trinidad and Tobago	0.283	0.294	0.280	0.326	
Tunisia	0.345	0.353	0.338		
Turkey	0.308	0.336	0.300	0.337	0.291
Venezuela	0.299			0.330	0.298
Yemen	0.338				

two separate subpopulations, except in Fiji, Korea, and Portugal, where the concentration of the total population is higher than for the two separate subpopulations.

Thus, in almost every less-developed country considered, lower fertility is associated with a higher concentration of reproduction. The slope of the regression line is around +.02, both on the aggregate level and for the subgroups. This

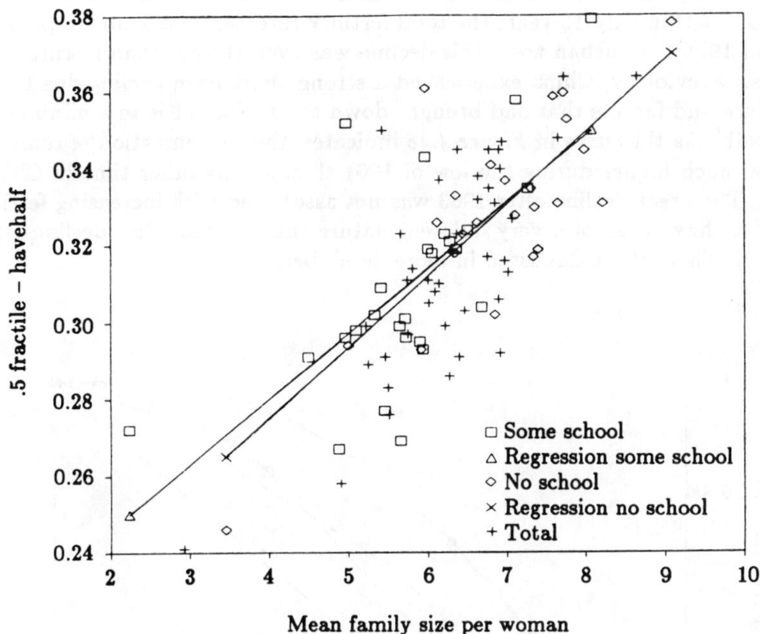

Figure 4.17. Relationship between mean completed family size per woman and .5 fractile for women with and without some formal education in WFS LDCs.

means that one child less in the average completed family size implies a .5 fractile that is two percentage points lower.

As in the historical case of Germany and Austria the relative variation between mean family sizes from the children's point of view is less than from the women's point of view. In Portugal mean sibship size is 1.6 times mean parity. In Jordan mean sibship size is only 1.15 times greater than mean parity. This discrepancy is due to the fact pointed out earlier, formula (4.5), that the difference between those two means is a function of the relative variance and consequently of the concentration of the distribution.

The strong empirical association between the level of fertility and its concentration in the case of Germany and Austria for the historical fertility transition and in the cross section of 41 LDCs participating in the WFS seems to be a universal pattern. King and Lutz (1988) recently demonstrated a similar association for cohort fertility trends in the USA for a period of more than 100 years. But there is at least one important exception from this general pattern: a very significant portion of the world population – the Chinese – experienced a secular fertility decline that was obviously not associated with increasing concentration of reproduction among women.

4.4. The Concentration of Period Fertility in China, 1955–1981

China recently experienced one of the most dramatic fertility declines ever observed. Within only 15 years the total fertility rate declined from 7.5 (in 1963) to 2.7 (in 1978). In urban areas this decline was even steeper than in rural communities. Previously, China experienced a strong short-term decline due to harvest failure and famine that had brought down the period TFR to a minimum of 3.3 in 1961. As the curve in *Figure 4.18* indicates, the concentration of reproduction was much higher during the low of 1961 than at any other time in Chinese history. The great decline after 1963 was not associated with increasing fertility. It seems to have been of a very different nature than all the other declines studied so far. This will be discussed in more detail below.

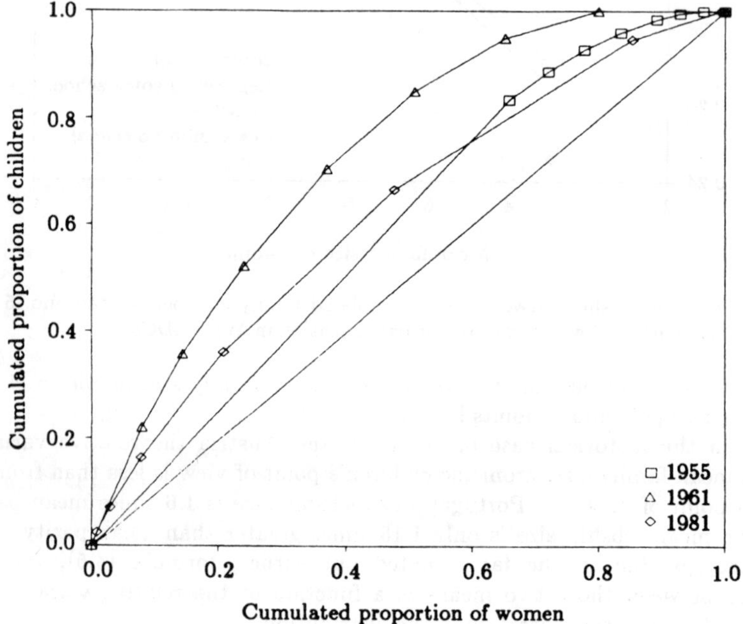

Figure 4.18. Lorenz curves for the concentration of fertility in China, 1955, 1961, and 1981.

Feeney and Yu (1987) recently presented estimates for period parity-progression ratios for China as a whole and for urban and rural areas for the period 1955–1981, based on the National One-per-Thousand Fertility Survey. The method used for estimating period parity-progression ratios is based on earlier work by Feeney (1983) and shall not be discussed here.[2] This section builds on the information given, highlighting one aspect not mentioned by

Feeney and Yu. Also this section shows that the Chinese trends, with respect to concentration of fertility, are quite distinct from most other countries in the world.

For each year completed parity distributions implied by the given period parity-progression ratios, $p(i)$, i referring to parity, were calculated by successively applying the ratios to a radix of 1,000 women, $l(0)$, starting the process of reproduction at parity zero. (The notation used here corresponds to the fertility table used in Chapters 2 and 3.) The proportion of women dropping out of the process of reproduction at parity i, $d(i)$, and hence having completed parity i is calculated by

$$d(i) = l(i)[1 - p(i)]$$

where

$$l(i) = l(i - 1)p(i - 1).$$

Figure 4.19 gives the mean family sizes of women, calculated as a weighted average of the completed parity distributions. These averages are comparable to the total fertility rates calculated from age-specific rates: both give the mean number of children of a synthetic cohort based on period observations. The mean family sizes calculated by completed parity distributions are not exact with respect to births of orders eight or more.[3] The time-series of total fertility rates and mean family sizes under a parity-specific approach cannot be expected to be identical because one approach considers the age distribution of the population while the other is based on the parity distribution. However, since age and parity are highly correlated the empirical findings should not be too different.

Feeney and Yu (1987) mention two significant empirical differences between the time-series of TFRs and the series of mean family sizes based on a parity-specific view. First, the total fertility rate is higher than the mean family size during the late 1960s and lower during the 1970s. Second, the age-specific approach implies a reversal of the long fertility decline experienced shortly before the survey, i.e., an increase from 2.24 in 1980 to 2.63 in 1981, whereas the parity-specific approach indicates a further, although somewhat slower, decline. Which indicator is correct? In a country where fertility is controlled independent of parity (such as China), the parity-specific approach is less sensitive to period fluctuations in the timing of births (e.g., women delaying first births for some reason) and hence can be expected to give a more stable picture of cohort behavior. The completed parity distributions implied by period fertility in 1980 and 1981 show that the relatively modest decline in mean family size was the result of two counteracting trends: the proportions of women with expected parities of two or more consistently decreased, but at the same time the expected proportion of childless women also decreased. Only the proportion of women expected to have one child saw significant increases. Hence, the fertility results

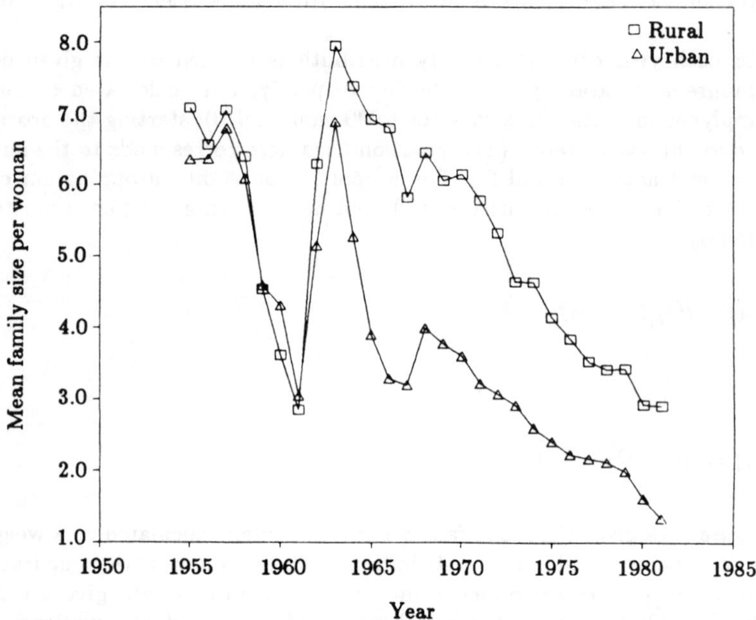

Figure 4.19. Trends in the mean family size per woman for urban and rural China, 1955–1981.

for 1981 do not necessarily mean a failure of recent birth control policies, but the parity-specific findings indicate that more women than ever before tend toward the one-child family. As mentioned earlier, *Figure 4.19* shows the mean family size as seen by the parity-specific approach for urban and rural areas separately. An initial fertility decline is noted between 1957 and 1961 and a second, larger decline, after 1963.

Figure 4.20 plots the trends in the .5 fractile or havehalf, from 1955 to 1981 for rural and urban areas. Although the level of fertility has been substantially higher in rural areas than in the cities of China since 1963, the extent of concentration in the distribution of period completed parity distributions has not differed much. Generally, about 35% of all women have had half the children since 1961. This percentage is much higher, i.e., the concentration is much lower, than in most other countries with controlled fertility. In industrialized countries with total fertility rates between 2.0 and 3.0, usually 22% to 26% of all women have half the children (see Vaupel and Goodwin, 1986; Lutz, 1987c).

Table 4.13 and *Figure 4.20* also indicate that the fertility declines experienced in China between 1957 and 1961 and those experienced since 1963 are of very different nature. An analysis of the period parity-progression ratios (not shown here) indicates that the first decline, which led to a minimum of 2.88

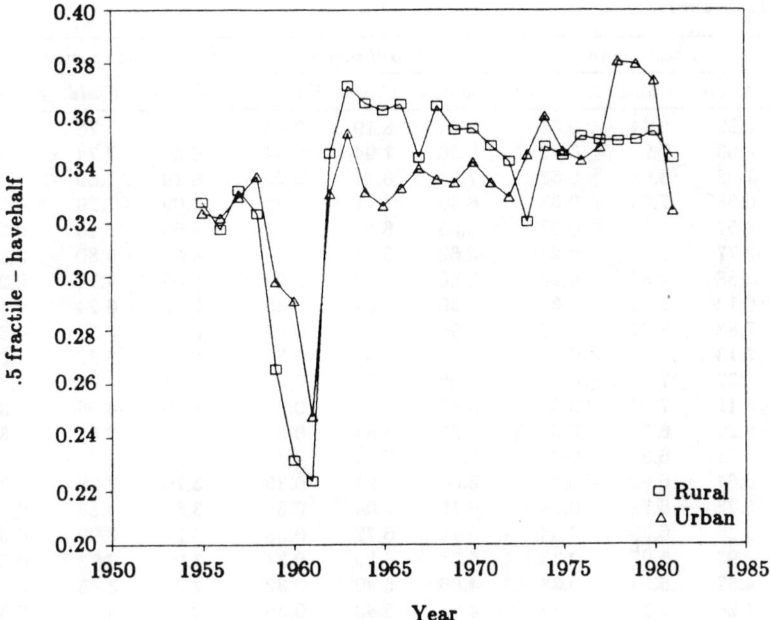

Figure 4.20. Trends in the concentration of fertility for urban and rural China, 1955–1981.

children per mother in 1961, was highly selective and did not affect all women. The decline was largely caused by an increase in women expected to remain childless. The period parity-progression ratios of 1961 imply that 20% of the women would remain childless under the observed rates, whereas other portions of the female population would still have rather high fertility. As a consequence of this unevenness the concentration of reproduction increased rapidly. In 1962 the .5 fractile jumped back up to 0.34. By 1980 and 1981 the overall level of fertility was lower than in 1961 but concentration had not increased. This means that the relative variation in the distribution remained almost stable and that the fertility decline affected practically all Chinese women, not only certain segments of the population as it did before 1961 and as it is usually observed in less-developed countries (see previous section).

A consequence of the stable level of concentration is that the mean sibship, i.e., the mean family size from the child's perspective, declined even more strongly than the mean from the women's perspective, from 8.27 in 1963 to 3.25 in 1981. Contrarily, during the extraordinary fertility decline of 1959–1961 the mean from the children's perspective declined less than from the women's perspective because of simultaneously increasing concentration. By 1981 the mean family size from the children's perspective had declined to the very low value of

Table 4.13. Mean family sizes and concentration of fertility in the People's Republic of China, 1955–1981.

Year	Total mean			Rural mean			Urban mean		
	Woman	Child	Havehalf	Woman	Child	Havehalf	Woman	Child	Havehalf
1955	6.99	8.14	0.33	7.08	8.19	0.33	6.36	7.70	0.32
1956	6.53	7.92	0.32	6.56	7.94	0.32	6.36	7.74	0.32
1957	7.02	8.08	0.33	7.04	8.11	0.33	6.79	7.89	0.33
1958	6.35	7.65	0.33	6.39	7.71	0.32	6.09	7.29	0.34
1959	4.57	6.54	0.27	4.55	6.62	0.27	4.60	6.10	0.30
1960	3.77	5.94	0.24	3.62	5.94	0.23	4.31	5.80	0.29
1961	2.88	4.86	0.23	2.86	4.88	0.22	3.05	4.74	0.25
1962	6.12	7.19	0.34	6.30	7.34	0.35	5.16	6.24	0.33
1963	7.83	8.27	0.37	7.95	8.34	0.37	6.89	7.77	0.35
1964	7.13	7.88	0.36	7.38	8.02	0.36	5.28	6.32	0.33
1965	6.37	7.33	0.35	6.92	7.72	0.36	3.91	4.77	0.33
1966	6.11	7.07	0.35	6.80	7.57	0.36	3.29	4.05	0.33
1967	5.20	6.30	0.35	5.83	6.84	0.34	3.20	3.83	0.34
1968	5.95	6.86	0.35	6.45	7.24	0.36	4.00	4.77	0.34
1969	5.64	6.62	0.34	6.06	6.94	0.35	3.79	4.59	0.34
1970	5.72	6.71	0.34	6.15	7.04	0.36	3.61	4.33	0.34
1971	5.36	6.39	0.34	5.79	6.72	0.35	3.23	3.90	0.34
1972	4.93	5.97	0.33	5.33	6.29	0.34	3.09	3.73	0.33
1973	4.57	5.55	0.33	4.66	5.80	0.32	2.93	3.45	0.35
1974	4.28	5.10	0.34	4.65	5.43	0.35	2.61	3.03	0.36
1975	3.83	4.59	0.34	4.15	4.88	0.35	2.41	2.84	0.35
1976	3.55	4.23	0.34	3.85	4.49	0.35	2.23	2.63	0.34
1977	3.29	3.92	0.34	3.53	4.14	0.35	2.17	2.55	0.35
1978	3.21	3.79	0.34	3.43	3.99	0.35	2.12	2.42	0.38
1979	3.22	3.81	0.34	3.43	4.00	0.35	2.00	2.31	0.38
1980	2.72	3.23	0.35	2.93	3.41	0.35	1.62	1.89	0.37
1981	2.66	3.25	0.33	2.92	3.47	0.34	1.62	1.89	0.37

1.89 in the cities of China. This is probably the lowest value of mean sibship size of any sizable population in the whole world including the very low-fertility cities of the FRG. The reason for this is that, even in a modern industrialized city where the total fertility rate might be lower than in Chinese cities, the mean family size from the children's perspective is greater because of higher concentration: this is mainly a consequence of high proportions of women expected to remain childless (generally more than 30%) in European cities. In sharp contrast to this the parity-specific fertility pattern of urban China in 1981 implies that only 1.4% of all women remain childless.

To compare this Chinese evolution of fertility levels and concentration in the distribution with the patterns of association described in the earlier parts of this chapter, the Chinese trends are superimposed on the cross section of WFS countries described above. *Figure 4.21* shows that the Chinese experience of 1955–1981 (the + symbol) follows the same general pattern as those countries studied by the WFS up to a level of fertility of 5 or 6 (around 1970).[4] At lower fertility China deviates from the pattern. The Chinese experience of the late 1950s fits well into the pattern of rural high-fertility societies. Even the very

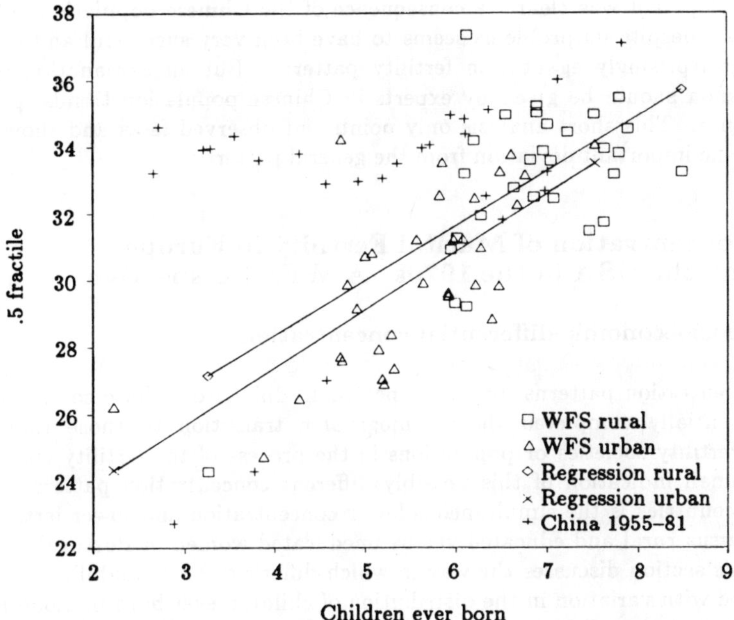

Figure 4.21. Relationship between mean completed family size and the concentration of fertility for a cross section of LDCs and China, 1955–1981.

steep fertility decline of 1959–1961 (the + symbols in the lower left corner), which was associated with highly increased concentration, followed the cross-sectional pattern of countries that had entered their secular fertility declines. The figure indicates that between 1962 and 1970 (upper middle) the Chinese association between fertility levels and fertility concentration was similar to that occurring in most other countries and was even slightly above them, i.e., China has somewhat lower concentration for the given level of fertility. After 1970, however, the steep decline in Chinese fertility levels is not associated with increased concentration, and the trend (upper left corner) deviates grossly from the general cross-sectional pattern previously observed. It also deviates significantly from the time-series of the US and European countries discussed above.

The general pattern of increasing concentration with declining fertility, as described in the previous analysis of the cross section of LDCs and of historical Europe, could be explained by the following rationale: in addition to the already existing variation due to differential fecundability and differential exposure, the introduction and differential practice of birth control brings a new source of variation into the distribution of family sizes. But why is the Chinese pattern of parity-specific fertility decline so completely different from that observed in any

other population? A strictly demographic answer would be that relative variation in the distribution did not increase because the decline affected all segments
of the population to a similar extent. It might also be said that this extraordinary development was clearly a consequence of the Chinese population policy, a
policy that despite its problems seems to have been very successful and brought
about a surprisingly egalitarian fertility pattern. But an explanation of this
phenomenon should be given by experts in Chinese population trends, policies,
and culture. This short analysis only points out observed facts and shows that
there is one important deviation from the general pattern.

4.5. Concentration of Marital Fertility in Europe and the USA in the 1970s: A WFS Perspective

4.5.1. Socioeconomic differential concentration

The concentration patterns may be expected to differ from those countries that
have essentially completed their demographic transition to those that have
natural fertility societies or populations in the process of the fertility transition.
A first small indication of this possibly different concentration pattern in low-
fertility countries is the simultaneous lower concentration and lower fertility for
urban versus rural and educated versus uneducated women in Portugal (Section
4.3). This section discusses the way in which differential fecundability is weakly
associated with variation in the distribution of children ever born in modern contraceptive societies. When – at least theoretically – everybody has access to relatively convenient methods of birth control, the determinants of unevenness in the
distribution are based, to a much higher degree, on differential intentions and
desires.

The data for this section were obtained from the European WFS.[5] In
most cases, the survey includes only ever-married women in its samples. This is
important to keep in mind because in Europe the proportion of women remaining unmarried is high.[6] Despite the relatively high incidence of non-marital fertility, average fertility of unmarried women is still much lower than that of married women. In particular, the proportion of childless women is expected to be
very high among unmarried women. Therefore, the distribution of reproduction
among married couples can be expected to be significantly more even (i.e., less
concentrated) than that of all women, for the cohorts observed in the European
WFS. Concentration analysis shows that, on average, about 30% of all married
women had half the number of children ever born to all married women aged
40–44. The concentration within the population of all women cannot be assessed
on the basis of the European WFS. This issue will be discussed in Section 4.6.

Despite the weak heterogeneity among married couples in European countries and the USA after the post–World War II baby boom, socioeconomic
differentials in fertility patterns may be detected within the populations. With
respect to the woman's place of residence it appears that for all countries considered, the average family size per woman is higher in rural areas than in cities.

The differentials range from more than one child difference in Poland to less than .1 in Belgium [see *Table 4.14(b)*].

In most countries, this lower urban fertility is associated with higher concentration [see *Tables 4.14(b), 4.15(b)*, and *4.16(b)*]. In Belgium, the higher concentration even results in a higher mean sibship for urban children versus rural children. However, in Yugoslavia, Norway, and the Netherlands, rural concentration is lower than urban. Nevertheless, in contrast to the negative association that appeared for urban and rural populations between the level of fertility and its distribution during the demographic transition in most countries, *Figure 4.22* shows that for Europe in the mid-1970s these regression lines are almost horizontal.

For female work status the pattern is similar to that of place of residence [see *Tables 4.14(b), 4.15(b)*, and *4.16(b)*]: there is a clear fertility distinction between groups, but the concentration differentials are more muddled. In all countries considered, women who had never worked had above-average mean family sizes. The causal relationship underlying this is not clear: maybe some women prefer to be housewives and to have more children, or maybe women with many children cannot work even if they would like to do so. The magnitude of the fertility differential between the two groups varies greatly from one country to another. In general, the differential is greater as the proportion of women who never worked decreases. For example, in Finland, where almost all women worked at least some time, the differential is highest, probably because of strong selection into the group of women who never worked. In other countries – like Spain – where great proportions of women are housewives, the differentials between the groups are much smaller.

The pattern of concentration is quite uneven across countries. In Denmark and Yugoslavia concentration among never-working women is highest, whereas in Belgium and Great Britain it is higher among women that had worked at one time. It can be assumed that these differentials are largely a function of differential selectivity to the respective groups in various countries.

Differences in achieved levels of education are associated with differences in fertility, but there are also concentration distinctions [see *Tables 4.14(a), 4.15 (a)*, and *4.16(a)*]. Generally, women with a higher education have a lower fertility. However, for about half of the countries observed, the best-educated women have a higher mean family size than the preceding group. This U–shape of the mean family size with respect to education appears in Belgium, Denmark, Great Britain, the Netherlands, Norway, and Spain.

There is no clear association between the level of fertility and concentration of countries *within* education groups: the regression lines are almost horizontal (*Figure 4.23*). The relationship among different educational groups within the same country, however, is clearly positive (*Figure 4.24*): higher education associated with lower average family size results in lower concentration. Such a pattern is very clear in France and Czechoslovakia but is also approximated by most other countries. This observed relationship means a reversal of the clear negative association between concentration and the level of fertility observed for populations in the process of the secular fertility transition.

Table 4.14(a). Mean family sizes per woman for ever-married women aged 40–44 in 13 WFS countries by highest completed education.

Country	Incomplete elementary	Complete elementary	Low secondary	High secondary	Post secondary
Belgium	-	2.52	2.77	2.10	2.44
Czechoslovakia	4.25	2.56	2.49	2.01	1.81
Denmark	-	2.62	2.52	2.19	2.84
Finland	3.87	2.90	2.41	2.36	2.08
France	3.42	2.57	2.43	2.38	2.16
Great Britain	3.33	2.79	2.52	2.46	2.52
Italy	3.08	2.29	2.09	1.92	1.87
Netherlands	-	1.85	1.65	1.40	1.75
Norway	-	3.16	2.68	2.59	2.69
Poland	3.80	2.96	2.53	2.11	1.77
Spain	3.22	2.90	3.24	3.03	3.39
United States	4.32	4.08	3.24	3.33	2.92
Yugoslavia	3.29	2.39	-	1.97	1.59

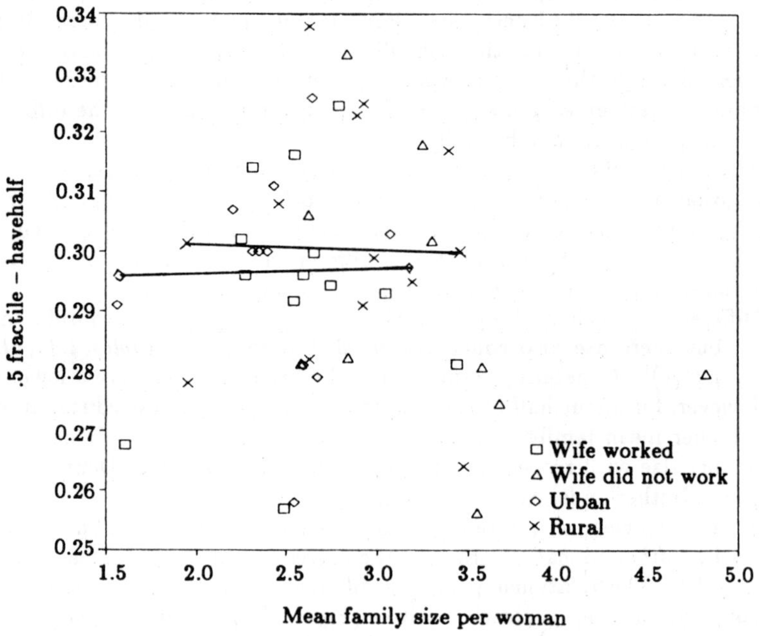

Figure 4.22. Relationship between mean family size per woman and .5 fractile for ever-married women aged 40–44 in 143 WFS countries by place of residence and work status.

Table 4.14(b). Mean family sizes per woman for ever-married women aged 40–44 in 13 WFS countries by place of residence and work status.

Country	Rural	Urban	Ever worked	Never worked
Belgium	2.63	2.54	2.49	2.84
Czechoslovakia	2.63	2.20	2.31	-
Denmark	2.93	2.43	2.54	2.58
Finland	2.99	2.40	2.65	3.55
France	2.92	2.59	2.54	3.58
Great Britain	-	-	2.60	2.83
Italy	2.46	2.31	2.25	2.62
Netherlands	1.95	1.56	1.61	-
Norway	2.89	2.64	2.79	-
Poland	3.40	2.35	2.75	3.31
Spain	3.20	3.07	3.05	3.26
United States	-	-	3.44	4.82
Yugoslavia	3.48	2.67	2.27	3.67

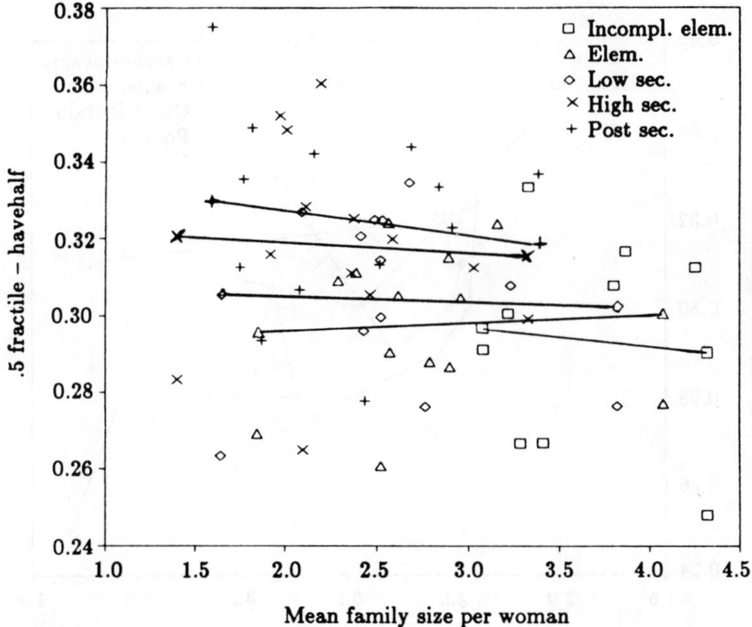

Figure 4.23. Relationship between mean family size per woman and .5 fractile for ever-married women aged 40–44 in 143 WFS countries by highest completed education.

Table 4.15(a). Mean family sizes from children's perspective (sibship size) in 13 WFS countries born to ever-married women aged 40–44 by highest completed education.

Country	Incomplete elementary	Complete elementary	Low secondary	High secondary	Post secondary
Belgium	-	3.75	3.84	3.10	3.40
Czechoslovakia	5.59	3.28	3.10	2.45	2.23
Denmark	-	3.45	3.32	2.50	3.33
Finland	4.76	3.92	3.11	3.11	2.69
France	4.82	3.45	3.37	2.99	2.71
Great Britain	4.20	3.67	3.41	3.30	3.23
Italy	4.16	2.99	2.58	2.45	2.58
Netherlands	-	2.63	2.45	2.14	2.43
Norway	-	3.94	3.26	3.26	3.21
Poland	4.79	3.82	3.24	2.68	2.27
Spain	4.26	3.69	4.17	3.83	4.05
United States	6.24	5.67	5.31	4.39	3.67
Yugoslavia	4.62	3.17	-	2.43	1.94

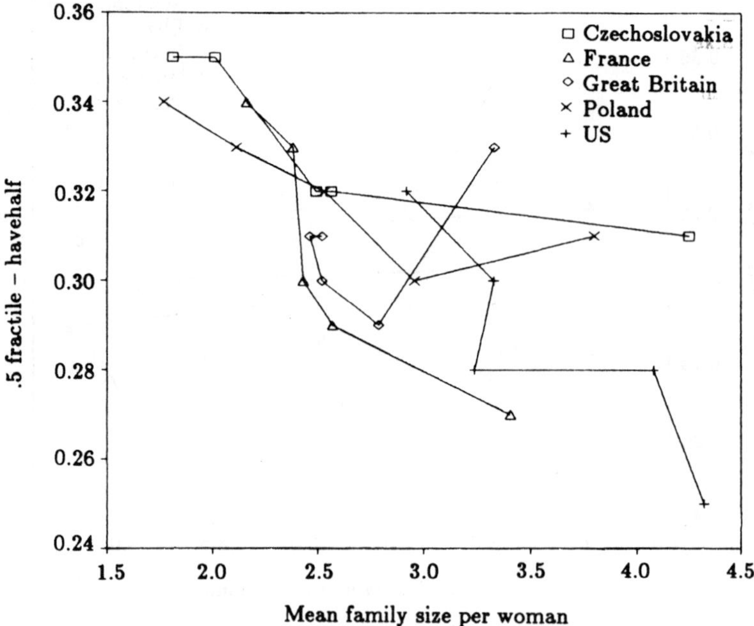

Figure 4.24. Relationship between mean family size per woman and .5 fractile for different educational groups within Czechoslovakia, France, Great Britain, Poland, and the USA.

Table 4.15(b). Mean family sizes from children's perspective (sibship size) in 13 WFS countries born to ever-married women aged 40–44 by place of residence and work status.

Country	Rural	Urban	Ever worked	Never worked
Belgium	3.53	3.87	3.81	3.85
Czechoslovakia	3.21	2.88	2.96	-
Denmark	3.64	3.18	3.29	3.68
Finland	3.64	3.26	3.57	5.08
France	3.92	3.66	3.48	4.85
Great Britain	-	-	3.50	3.41
Italy	3.26	3.14	2.97	3.56
Netherlands	2.90	2.26	2.40	-
Norway	3.56	3.33	3.46	-
Poland	4.27	3.16	3.71	4.39
Spain	4.25	4.04	4.11	4.14
United States	-	-	4.82	6.45
Yugoslavia	4.88	3.76	3.04	5.01

Table 4.16(a). The .5 fractile (havehalf) for ever-married women aged 40–44 in 13 WFS countries by highest completed education.

Country	Incomplete elementary	Complete elementary	Low secondary	High secondary	Post secondary
Belgium	-	0.26	0.28	0.27	0.28
Czechoslovakia	0.31	0.32	0.32	0.35	0.35
Denmark	-	0.31	0.31	0.36	0.33
Finland	0.32	0.29	0.32	0.31	0.31
France	0.27	0.29	0.30	0.33	0.34
Great Britain	0.33	0.29	0.30	0.31	0.31
Italy	0.29	0.31	0.33	0.32	0.29
Netherlands	-	0.27	0.26	0.28	0.31
Norway	-	0.32	0.33	0.32	0.34
Poland	0.31	0.30	0.32	0.33	0.34
Spain	0.30	0.32	0.31	0.31	0.34
United States	0.25	0.28	0.28	0.30	0.32
Yugoslavia	0.27	0.31	-	0.35	0.38

Table 4.16(b). The .5 fractile (havehalf) for ever-married women aged 40–44 in 13 WFS countries by place of residence and work status.

Country	Rural	Urban	Ever worked	Never worked
Belgium	0.28	0.26	0.26	0.28
Czechoslovakia	0.34	0.31	0.31	-
Denmark	0.32	0.31	0.32	0.28
Finland	0.30	0.30	0.30	0.26
France	0.29	0.28	0.29	0.28
Great Britain	-	-	0.30	0.33
Italy	0.31	0.30	0.30	0.31
Netherlands	0.28	0.29	0.27	-
Norway	0.32	0.33	0.32	-
Poland	0.32	0.30	0.29	0.30
Spain	0.30	0.30	0.29	0.32
United States	-	-	0.28	0.28
Yugoslavia	0.26	0.28	0.30	0.27

The occurrence of lower fertility with lower concentration levels in sub-groups of industrialized populations indicates that the association between fertility levels and concentration is determined differently in developed countries than in LDCs. It can be assumed that this has something to do with use and availability of contraception. The next section focuses on the differential use and efficiency of contraception and its consequence on the concentration of reproduction.

4.5.2. Birth control and concentration

This level of the analysis begins with a look at contraceptive use as a potential determinant of differentials in the concentration of completed parity distributions on actual fertility, on the one hand, and socioeconomic variables and intentions, on the other hand. Hence, contraceptive use has been characterized as an intermediate variable (Davis and Blake, 1956) or a proximate fertility determinant (Bongaarts, 1978). At this point the investigation turns to the question of differential use of contraception *per se*, which can help to explain the observed pattern or the level of fertility intentions with contraception playing a purely instrumental role.

There is no doubt that at the level of proximate determinants, besides the effect of differential fecundability and marriage, all variation in the distribution of children ever born is due to differential use of contraception or abortion. The lack of data on the role of induced abortion restricts the study to contraception. Hence, the problem is to measure contraceptive use in a way that is relevant to the explanation of completed parity. This turns out to be a very difficult task because it is strongly related to the timing of births. A few short periods without contraception during the long potentially reproductive span of a woman are enough to produce a few births regardless of current use or ever-use of specific methods measured by a survey. Therefore, the two usually measured indicators of contraceptive use – ever use and current use – can only partly explain the *how* and, to much lesser extent, the *why* of the resulting completed parity distribution.

Data from the European WFS make it possible to focus explicitly on the relationship between contraceptive use and the distribution of reproduction. The data refer to ever-married women up to age 44. The three categories of contraceptive use predefined by the WFS are efficient methods, inefficient methods, and no methods. For most of the countries this information is available for current use of contraception as well as for ever use. The fertility concentration in the three categories can be compared nationally or internationally.

For countries where contraceptives are not universally available the expectation – based on the previous analysis – is that the group of women not using contraception has higher average fertility and shows a lower degree of concentration than the total. For the users of modern contraceptions the result is expected to depend largely on the desired family sizes. Hence, on an aggregate level that includes both groups, concentration turned out to be relatively high. When explicitly studying the role of contraception in the concentration of the fertility distribution in low-fertility industrialized countries, two factors must be considered.

First, caution must be taken when analyzing current use of contraception. The analysis should not include women who otherwise use efficient methods but at the time of the survey were trying to become pregnant. To avoid problems of this kind the analysis was restricted to women who do not want additional children. For this group of women the pattern of association is given in *Table 4.17* for two selected countries with a relatively high percentage of nonusers, namely, Poland and Spain.

Second, when analyzing the number of children ever born to women currently using efficient methods, it is necessary to keep in mind that these women might have started to use efficient methods fairly recently because the availability and social acceptance of such methods changed in recent years. If we study ever use of contraception instead of current use, the differentials should be affected less by selectivity. Since it is not influenced by current circumstances, ever use is a better indicator of a woman's attitude toward birth control at a time when it was relevant for her level of fertility. For these reasons, the discussion turns to the study of ever use of contraceptives and its associations with variable fertility and concentration. However, the direct technical link is lost between use or nonuse of contraception at a given time and the conception of a birth during that period when referring only to ever use. Hence, ever use is more of an attitudinal indicator than a proximate determinant.

In this context the distribution of children ever born by age groups of ever-married women and by ever use of contraception is studied for seven European countries. The mean completed family sizes (for women age 40–44) range from 1.92 in the Netherlands to 2.32 in Spain. The other countries, namely, Belgium, Great Britain, Italy, Norway, and Poland, have mean completed family sizes between 2.5 and 2.9, *Table 4.18*.

Figure 4.25 shows the relationship between the mean number of children ever born and the .5 fractile in the distribution of children for women age 40–44 (the oldest age group in the European WFS surveys) in all countries except Hungary (which has no data for age group 40–44). The three lines indicate the regression lines for the bivariate relationships of women using efficient, inefficient, or no contraception. The group of women that is not using contraception is the most highly concentrated one, although there is some variance in the degree of concentration. The reason for this variance might be found in selectivity. In Spain, where more than half of the women in the group do not use contraception, concentration is lower, whereas, for example, in Poland, where only a quarter uses no contraceptives, concentration in the group of nonusers is higher (see also *Table 4.17*). The international comparison suggests that the lower the proportion of women that do not use contraception, the higher the proportion of subfecund women, which results in a lower level of average fertility. This is most extreme in Belgium. Nevertheless, some women in the nonuser group have very high fertility. The result is that as the group of nonusers becomes proportionately smaller, it becomes more heterogeneous, and hence more concentrated.

Table 4.17. Concentration and current use of contraception in Poland and Spain (only women with no additional children expected).

Method	Age group	n	Mean number of children ever born	.5 fractile (Havehalf)
Poland				
Efficient method	40-44	361	2.43	0.32
Inefficient method	40-44	851	2.85	0.32
No method	40-44	417	3.04	0.27
Efficient method	35-39	400	2.49	0.34
Inefficient method	35-39	828	2.75	0.34
No method	35-39	282	2.85	0.28
Spain				
Efficient method	40-44	150	3.51	0.34
Inefficient method	40-44	410	2.30	0.26
No method	40-44	583	3.01	0.30
Efficient method	35-39	171	2.23	0.28
Inefficient method	35-39	354	1.95	0.28
No method	35-39	345	2.74	0.31

Although current contraceptive use and ever use are similar indicators, there are a number of disadvantages to current use.

Table 4.18. Mean family sizes and concentration of parity distribution for women aged 40–44 in seven European countries by ever-use of contraception.

	Country	Mean		.5 fractile
		Mother	Child	
Wife ever-used	Belgium	3.06	4.29	0.28
efficient method	Great Britain	2.70	3.50	0.31
	Italy	2.58	3.34	0.32
	Netherlands	1.95	2.55	0.30
	Norway	2.94	3.56	0.33
	Poland	2.53	3.24	0.32
	Spain	3.56	4.39	0.33
Wife ever-used	Belgium	2.25	3.24	0.29
inefficient method	Great Britain	2.57	3.70	0.28
	Italy	2.44	3.12	0.32
	Netherlands	1.82	2.70	0.24
	Norway	2.49	2.96	0.35
	Poland	2.86	3.66	0.31
	Spain	3.21	4.02	0.32
All women together	Belgium	2.55	3.82	0.26
(includes no use)	Great Britain	2.60	3.50	0.30
	Italy	2.38	3.19	0.30
	Netherlands	1.69	2.46	0.27
	Norway	2.78	3.46	0.32
	Poland	2.78	3.76	0.29
	Spain	3.12	4.12	0.30

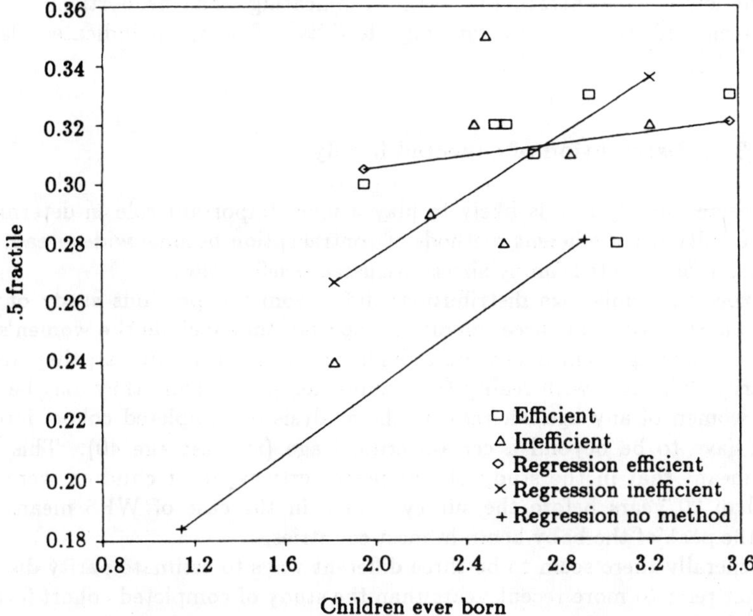

Figure 4.25. Relationship between the mean number of children ever born and the concentration of the distribution for married women between 40 and 44 ever-using efficient, inefficient, or no methods of birth control in Belgium, Great Britain, Italy, the Netherlands, Norway, Poland, and Spain.

It is interesting to notice that the regression line for women using inefficient methods is parallel to that of women using no methods. The line for women that had ever-used efficient methods in their life is almost horizontal. In other words, for the population of women that used modern means of contraception, changes in the average level of fertility do not bring about any significant change in the extent of concentration. The main reason for this is that the range of completed parities is much smaller for these "modern" women than for women using traditional methods. This corresponds to the finding (see Gisser, 1985) that the distribution of desired family sizes shows much less variance than the distribution of actual family sizes. And for women that use efficient contraceptive methods, actual family size is more likely to correspond to desired family size.

Another aspect of the groups of women using efficient methods of contraception worth noting. In a number of countries, the average fertility of these groups is *higher* than in the other groups (see *Table 4.18*). A possible explanation for this apparent paradox is that the difference in fertility levels is not so much caused by unwanted pregnancies but by differentials in the desire for children. In Spain only 12% of the women age 40 to 44 used efficient methods, which leads to the assumption that this group is some kind of elite that also wanted more children than other strata of the population. These women also show the lowest concentration of fertility, indicating small proportions of child-less women and women with very high fertility. This again indicates planned fertility.

4.5.3. The distribution of expected family size

The expected family size is likely to play a more important role in determining actual fertility when efficient methods of contraception become widespread. The distribution of expected family size is discussed briefly below.

Expected family size distributions differ from the previous study of completed cohort fertility in three important aspects: they include the women's own intentions, making them indicators of higher psychological interest; they are not necessarily congruent with reality (real completed parity); and they may be studied for women of any age whereas, in the analysis of completed cohort fertility, women have to be beyond a certain critical age (at least age 40). This third aspect meant that in the study of completed fertility, most children were born more than 20 years before the survey, which in the case of WFS means even before the peak of the baby boom in most countries.

Generally there seem to be three different ways to estimate parity distributions that refer to more recent years than the study of completed cohort fertility. One method is to estimate completed parity distributions for synthetic cohorts, which is presented in Chapter 3. Another way is to analyze real cohorts and estimate the still incomplete reproductive performance of younger cohorts up to the age of 45 by using some fertility model. A third approach is to take the statements made by women on expected family sizes as an estimator of future fertility, most often done with surveys. This analysis is based on this last approach.

Expected family size distributions for ten European WFS countries were looked at using three selected marriage cohorts: women who married before 1956, between 1961 and 1965, and after 1971. *Figure 4.26* plots the relationship between average expected family size and the coefficient of concentration, the .5 fractile, of the expected family size distributions.

A comparison of *Figure 4.25* and *Figure 4.26* reveals that expected family size distributions tend to be more even than the empirical distributions of achieved fertility. This is because most married couples do not want to remain childless and very few want to have more than four children. Consequently, concentration is very low, ranging from 30% to 43% of all women having half the children. *Figure 4.26* also reveals a clear change in the structure of the relationship over time. For the earlier marriage cohorts the negative association between fertility and concentration appears, which was derived before in the case of completed cohort fertility. However, for women married after 1960 the association is reversed. This trend continues, and for women married after 1971 the cross-sectional pattern shows lower concentration associated with lower fertility. A look at the distributions shows that for younger cohorts the range of expected family sizes seems to have become smaller.

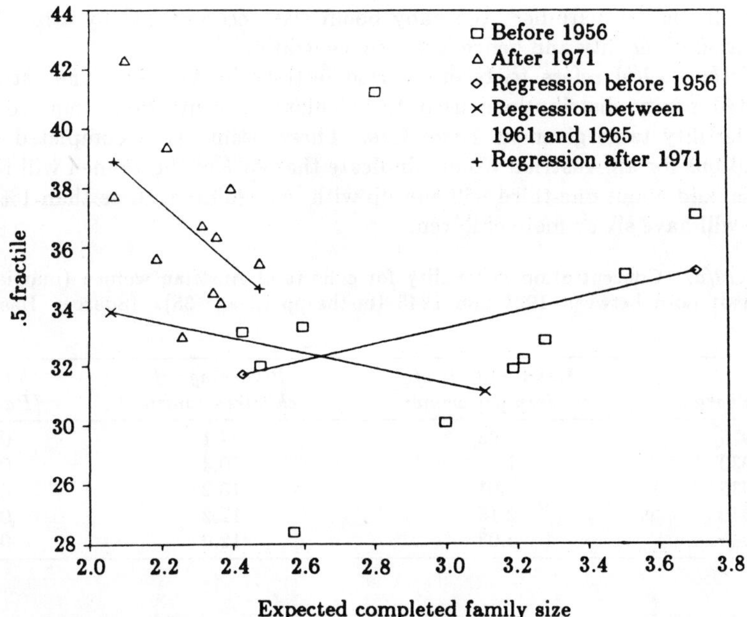

Figure 4.26. Relationship between average expected family size and concentration for cohorts of women that married before 1956, between 1961 and 1965, and after 1971 in ten European WFS countries.

4.6. The Concentration of Overall Fertility in Austria

So far this analysis has focused on marital fertility. This was mainly determined by the design of the WFS, which did not include unmarried women from most countries. The major difference between unmarried and married women with respect to concentration analysis is that the prevalence of completed parity zero is much higher among unmarried women. For this reason any analysis finds that concentration tends to be higher in overall fertility than in marital fertility. In countries where marriages at a young age are almost universal, however, this difference is not very significant.

Austria is an example of a country with high illegitimacy rates (more than 30%). *Table 4.19(a)* presents fertility and concentration measure for cohorts of Austrian women born between 1921 and 1945. Because the survey was taken in 1981, only births up to age 35 could be considered. To make the figures comparable across cohorts, this age limit was kept for all birth cohorts. During these 25 years, roughly covering the period from immediately after the war to shortly after the peak of the baby boom, concentration of reproduction decreased significantly. One major reason for this was the strong decrease in childlessness. Almost a quarter of all women born between 1921 and 1925 remained childless up to age 35, whereas for the cohort born between 1941 and 1945 the comparable figure is only 12%. This phenomenon has been observed throughout Europe, and, in all countries studied, the baby boom was accompanied by a more even distribution of fertility and hence lower concentration.

Table 4.19(b) refers to recent period fertility in Austria. The estimated completed parity distributions used to calculate concentration stem from the period fertility table given in *Table 3.10*. These estimates of completed parity distributions for all Austrian women indicate that 28% of the women will remain childless, and about one-third will end up with two children. Less than 1% of all women will have six or more children.

Table 4.19(a). Concentration of fertility for cohorts of Austrian women (married and unmarried) born between 1921 and 1945 (births up to age 35). (Source: Haslinger, 1985.)

Cohorts born	Mean number of children per woman	Percentage of childless women	.5 fractile (Havehalf)
1921–1925	1.65	24.1	0.21
1926–1930	1.82	20.4	0.23
1931–1935	2.01	16.2	0.26
1936–1940	2.15	12.2	0.28
1941–1945	2.03	12.0	0.27

Table 4.19(b). Concentration of fertility by educational groups for synthetic cohorts of Austrian women, 1977–1980; estimates based on period parity-specific fertility rates. (Source: Lutz, 1985.)

	Mean number of children per woman	Percentage of childless women	.5 fractile (Havehalf)
Austria total	1.62	27.9	0.23
Education			
Primary	1.62	33.6	0.22
Vocational	1.62	20.6	0.27
Secondary	1.52	28.2	0.22
University	1.95	34.0	0.19

This distribution results in a mean number of children per woman of 1.62 and a .5 fractile of 0.23. This degree of concentration is significantly higher than that for cohorts participating in the baby boom. The estimation shows that the concentration of completed parity implied by the behavior that took place between 1977 and 1980 will be equivalent to that of the birth cohorts born between 1926 and 1930. Despite these similarities in the extent of concentration, the distributions are quite different: for the 1926–1930 cohort the relative variance originated to a greater extent from women with larger families, whereas for current period fertility the high proportion of childless women raises concentration.

Breakdowns of the Austrian female population by educational levels reveal an interesting pattern. Fertility is least concentrated for women that went to a vocational school because of the relatively low proportion (20%) of childless women in that group; it is most concentrated among women with university degrees. Although caution should be taken because of the few women with such degrees in the sample ($n = 252$), these women show an almost dichotomous behavior: on the one hand, they have the highest percentage of childlessness (34%) among all groups; on the other hand, once they decide to have children, they have significantly more than average. This results in a concentration coefficient indicating that only 19% of all women have half the children.

Hence, the results for overall period fertility in Austria may lead to the assumption that recent fertility patterns, again, show a higher degree of concentration than those during the time of the post–World War II baby boom. This increase in relative variance is due not to certain segments of the population with increased fertility but to a consequence of greater proportions of childless women.

4.7. Conclusions

Until a certain late stage of the demographic transition process, it has been found that lower fertility is associated with a higher degree of concentration of reproduction among women. The most likely explanation for this empirical finding is that the introduction of birth control into a fertility regime that used to be determined mainly by fecundability tends to increase the relative variance in the distribution. Aside from China, which followed a different path, all of the 41 WFS countries studied in Section 4.3 seem to follow the pattern exhibited in Portugal, which has the lowest fertility and the highest concentration. But already in Portugal rural-urban differentials indicate a reversal of the otherwise consistent positive association between the havehalf and the mean number of children per woman.

Portugal already shows the "new" pattern that is found in all modern European societies. In these societies the distribution of family sizes desired has gained a leading role in determinating concentration. And since the distribution of family sizes is generally rather even in modern societies, this tends to result in lower concentration if desire and reality are not too far apart. Here, contraception plays an instrumental role. Without contraception (and possibly abortion as another means of birth control) actual fertility would deviate substantially from the rather homogeneous desired family size distribution. In other words, birth control in certain segments of society leads first to increased concentration, but, once contraception becomes almost universal and highly efficient, concentration tends to decline because of an approximation of actual family size to desired family size, at least from the side of excess fertility. Nevertheless, sub-fecundity and involuntary childlessness – further reasons for increased concentration – are not directly linked to contraception. This means that the future trend of concentration in reproduction will largely depend on two factors: the prevalence of voluntary and involuntary childlessness.

Notes

[1]   Vaupel and Goodwin (1986) extend Preston's algebra a bit by giving the mean ratio:

$$\rho = \frac{\bar{x}}{\bar{c}} = \frac{1}{I+1}$$

where I is the square of the coefficient of variation of the distribution of women by number of children, that is,

$$I = \frac{\sigma_x^2}{\bar{x}^2}.$$

I was introduced by Crow (1958) for a summary measure of unevenness of a distribution.

[2]   The parity-progression ratios given by Feeney and Yu (1987) seem to refer only to married women. But since marriage is almost universal (progression to first marriage is between 0.98 and 0.99 over most of the period) this need not be of much concern and we may speak of total fertility instead of marital fertility.

[3]   Since the parity-progression ratios given by Feeney and Yu (1987) ended at parity eight, one must make adjustments for higher-order births. In this chapter it is assumed that women with eight or more births have, on the average, nine births.

[4]   It is always problematic to compare trends directly over time and variations in a cross section. But if we consider the case in the cross section as standing for different stages of a process (demographic transition), this combination may be justified. With respect to age, demographers do this all the time when constructing synthetic cohorts.

[5]   This study is based on data extracted from the standard recode files at Economic Commission for Europe in Geneva. I am grateful for the permission to use those data.

[6]   Current nuptiality patterns imply proportions of women remaining unmarried of about 30% in several European countries. For the cohorts interviewed in the survey these percentages were probably still lower.

Epilogue

Consequences of Fertility Distribution and Concentration

The birth of a child is not only of most fundamental importance to the new individual, it also affects the life of the parents and of their peers, and has impacts on the society, economy, and environment. Every birth has far-reaching consequences, and the nature of the consequences also depends on the circumstances of the birth: Was the child born in a slum of Calcutta or in a Scandinavian hospital? Was it the first child or the fifth? Is the mother a teenager or over 30? Do the parents live together? Do they have regular employment? All these factors matter primarily for the child's survival probability, physical and mental development, and opportunities in life. But the circumstances of the birth of this new person also have consequences for the rest of the world: he or she probably alters the family's life-style, may change the employment pattern of the mother, may raise new demands for housing and consumer goods, may require schooling and social benefits, may take part in politics, may invent new technologies, may give life to his or her own children, may even destroy the life of others, and in many cases may be the only person to care for elderly parents.

This study looked at these phenomena from a specifically demographic perspective. The focus was on the distribution of births along various demographic dimensions. The quantum and the tempo of fertility by parity, the influence of marriage and marital duration, and some socioeconomic variables – mostly education and residence – were studied. The section on the distribution of reproduction results from the belief that specific distributional aspects of fertility have a wide range of consequences. These are different from and often independent of the consequences of the average level of fertility.

Most of this study was descriptive; some sections looked at possible causes. This epilogue briefly discusses the consequences of uneven fertility distributions. This is important for two different reasons: first, as with almost every study, the significance of the implications and consequences of the subject determine the relevance of the study; second, demographers have traditionally ignored distributional aspects of fertility, which is a subject well worth further exploration.

Fertility Levels in the Next Generation

One demographic consequence of fertility concentration in one generation is the influence it may have on the level of fertility in the next generation if there is at least a small positive association between the family sizes of mothers and daughters on an individual level. Vast empirical evidence indicates a slight but positive correlation of family sizes across generations. A recent survey of such evidence (Anderton *et al.*, 1988) summarizes that family sizes of successive generations are positively but weakly related. In this context it is preferable not to think in terms of *correlation* but rather to look at the degree of *orientation*. Orientation is preferred here because correlation coefficients are insensitive to constant absolute changes in the individual level of fertility. A case in which every daughter had one child less than her mother would yield a correlation coefficient of one, whereas the degree of orientation is clearly less than in the case of exact replication.

Assuming that daughters orient their family size to a certain extent on the sibship size they experienced during their childhood, and assuming heterogeneity in the distribution of family sizes in their mothers' generation (resulting in a difference between mean parity and mean sibship size), this would *ceteris paribus* tend to increase the average level of fertility in the next generation. In the extreme case that every daughter has exactly as many children as her mother – i.e., exactly replicates the sibship size of her childhood (disregarding mortality) – then the level of fertility would *ceteris paribus* increase from one generation to the next by exactly the difference between mean parity of the mothers and mean sibship size from the children's perspective. This assumption of exact replication is applied to three selected parity distributions. This exercise shows that in the case of replication the degree of concentration in the fertility distribution has a greater effect on future levels of fertility than in the initial level of fertility.

Tables E.1 and *E.2* give the examples of two cohorts of American women born between 1901 and 1905 and between 1931 and 1935 and a synthetic cohort of Austrian women in 1981. Almost one-quarter of women in the 1901–1905 cohort remained childless, a fact resulting in the very low level of average fertility (only 2.28 children per woman). Fertility in the 1901–1905 cohort was highly concentrated with only 18% of all women having half the children. Conversely, in the 1931–1935 cohort, which participated in the peak of the baby boom, 27% of all women had half the number of children born by the cohort, hence indicating a relatively homogeneous fertility pattern. Austrian period data of 1981 show yet another pattern of fertility distribution: a very high incidence of childlessness together with a relatively homogeneous low level of fertility pattern of mothers. This results in an average parity of only 1.62 and a moderate degree of concentration.

Table E.1. Three selected completed parity distributions.

| Cohort | Completed parity distribution in percent | | | | | | | Mean | | | |
	0	1	2	3	4	5	6	Parity	Sibship size	Variation coefficient	Concentration .5 fractile
US 1901–1905	24	18	20	13	7	4	2	2.27	4.48	2.20	.18
US 1931–1935	11	9	21	22	15	8	5	3.03	4.39	1.36	.27
Austria, synthetic 1981	28	17	32	15	5	2	1	1.62	2.75	1.13	.23

The completed parity distribution of the synthetic cohort for Austria, 1981, is estimated in *Table 3.10.* (US data source: King and Lutz, 1988.)

Table E.2. Two models of replication of mother's family size over two generations for three selected completed parity distributions.

| Cohort | Exact replication of mother's family size | | Replication, but 30% become childless | |
	Mean parity	Mean sibship	Mean parity	Mean sibship
US 1901–1905	2.28	4.48	2.28	4.48
Second generation	4.48	5.95	3.14	5.95
Third generation	5.95	7.12	4.16	7.12
US 1931–1935	3.03	4.39	3.03	4.39
Second generation	4.39	5.38	3.10	5.38
Third generation	5.38	6.32	3.89	6.32
Austria synthetic 1981	1.62	2.75	1.62	2.75
Second generation	2.75	3.28	1.93	3.28
Third generation	3.28	3.80	2.30	3.80

Table E.2 shows the implications of the three fertility distributions on future fertility levels under the very restrictive model of exact replication of mother's family size. In all three cases the level of fertility increases significantly over two generations, and it increases more sharply in the more concentrated populations. This is clear from the comparison of the two American cohorts. In the rather homogeneous distribution of the 1931–1935 cohort, fertility increases at a slower rate than in the distribution of the 1901–1905 cohort. On the basis of the Austrian distribution implied by 1981 parity-specific period fertility, the mean parity of women would also double in two generations.

There is no doubt that exact replication of family size is a very unrealistic model. One of the reasons is that in the mothers' generation some women have no children but in the daughters' generation this is not possible. A relaxation of the assumption would allow a certain percentage of women in each generation to remain childless. These childless women would be drawn randomly from all women of the daughters' generation regardless of sibship size. *Table E.2* shows that even in this case, as many as 30% of the women of each generation were childless; if the others had exactly their mothers' family size, mean parity would significantly increase over two generations because of the variance in the parity distributions. The percentage of childless women does not affect the mean sibship size in the next generation, so that the right columns in *Table E.2* remain unchanged.

Exact replication of mother's family size – even when allowing for a certain proportions of the daughters to remain childless – is not realistic. It is only used to illustrate the point in an extreme case. The deterministic assumption of replication can be replaced by the notion of stochastic association between mother's and daughter's family size. This is a more general model that allows us to vary the degree of linear association. The mathematics of this relationship are described in Lutz *et al.* (1988). Two major conclusions can be drawn from both the deterministic and the stochastic description of the mechanism:

(1) Greater heterogeneity in the family size distribution implies *ceteris paribus* higher fertility in the next generation if there is some (even tiny) positive association of family sizes between mothers and daughters.
(2) If the variance in the parity distribution is greater than zero, a higher degree of association between family sizes results *ceteris paribus* in a higher level of fertility in the subsequent generation.

Such conclusions might seem strange in light of declining fertility rates, in most countries. Since it has been shown that variation exists in parity distribution and some positive association between family sizes exists, it is likely that the assumption on constant levels of the fertility distributions based on sibship size is wrong in the real world. In other words, the trend of declining fertility due to all the other factors is much stronger than the tiny positive effect induced by this mechanism.

Conversely, if there were no intergenerational correlation between family sizes together with heterogeneity in the parity distribution, fertility levels would have declined even faster. And, future changes in the concentration of reproduction or in the degree of cross-generational association will be relevant factors – among many others – affecting future fertility levels.

Kin Availability for Elderly

Fertility distributions also affect the distributions of available kin to care for the elderly. Population aging is one of the major social problems in industrialized countries and increasingly also in less-developed nations. The proportion of young people will further decrease while the portion of elderly people will increase. As a consequence the old-age dependency ratio increases, implying an increased economic burden on the economically active. On a macro-level the ratio of young to old depends largely on total fertility levels and not on the distribution of fertility, but on a micro-level distributional aspects clearly matter.

When looking at the way in which individual elderly people are cared for, one must distinguish between two important sources of care: the public care and family care. For most of today's elderly (especially in less-developed countries) support by children or the wider kinship network is by far the most important source of care. In most industrialized countries elderly persons receive most of their economic support from pensions, public health care, and other institutions. But this does not cover the probably much more important side of social and emotional contact.

It is obvious that for the family relations of elderly people, distributional aspects of fertility are very important. Even at fixed levels of fertility it makes a big difference if every elderly person had two children or if half remained childless and the others had four children. To illustrate this point *Table E.3* gives the results of three simple model calculations for different parity distributions.

Case 1 considers a situation in which every woman has exactly two children. The mean parity of the women will be identical to the mean sibship size, and there will be no concentration havehalf of .5. Case 2 assumes a more realistic situation in which 20% of the women have zero, one, two, three, and four children each. In this case the mean parity will be also 2.0, but the mean sibship size will increase to 3.0 due to the concentration in the distribution in which 27% of the women have half the children. Case 3 assumes an extreme in the other direction: half of the women remains childless, and the other half has four children each. Again, the mean parity will be 2.0, but the mean sibship size rises to 4.0 as a consequence of even higher concentration.

Table E.3. Distribution of expected numbers of living siblings and living children for a 75-year-old woman under three hypothetical parity distributions. For siblings the survival probability was assumed to be .58 and for children .93.

| | *Case 1* | *Case 2* | | | | | *Case 3* | |
| | *100% has* | *20% has* | | | | | *50% has* | |
Parity distribution	*2*	*0*	*1*	*2*	*3*	*4*	*0*	*4*
Mean parity	2.0			2.0				2.0
Mean sibship size	2.0			3.0				4.0
.5 fractile	.5			.27				.25
Number of living siblings								
None	.420			.418				.074
One	.580			.344				.307
Two	–			.190				.424
Three	–			.049				.195
Number of living children								
None	.005			.215				.500
One	.130			.215				.001
Two	.865			.215				.009
Three	–			.206				.114
Four	–			.150				.375

The consequences of these three hypothetical distributions are considered for the average number of living siblings of a 75-year-old woman. For this it is assumed that the average age of the potential siblings is also 75 and that the survival probability for men and women up to age 75 is .58 (from the Finnish life table of 1984). For case 1, where each woman had two children, 42% of the 75-year-old women will have no living sibling, whereas 58% will have one. For the more realistic distribution in case 2, the percentage of women without living siblings will be similar (42%), but there will also be some women with two or three siblings. In case 3 only 7% of the women are expected to have no living siblings because the sibship size for every woman was four, and the distribution of living siblings is due to mortality only. In summary, the fertility distributions of the mothers have only a relatively minor impact (except for the extreme case 3) on the numbers of living siblings for daughters when they are 75.

The picture is very different when looking at the impact the three hypothetical fertility distributions have on the number of living children of 75-year-old women. For this model it was assumed that children are, on the average, 25 years younger than their mothers and have a survival probability of .93 up to age 50. In case 1 less than 1% has no living children, whereas it is 22% in case 2 and 50% in case 3. These great differences arise from distributions that have the same level of fertility. A decrease in fertility levels would further increase the proportion of women without living children.

These simple calculations illustrate the consequences of higher fertility concentration on the kin availability of elderly women even if fertility remains constant. Since recent fertility trends in many industrialized countries imply that up to one-third of all women can be expected to remain childless, it can be anticipated that the problem of the elderly without living kin will become much more serious in the future. Public services probably will try to fill part of the gap. It is already doubtful that they can take the place of kin in practical support, but they certainly cannot in emotional terms.

Dampening of Possible Fertility Cycles

Heterogeneity in the reproductive performance of a cohort also has consequences on one of the most prominent hypotheses in fertility analysis, namely, Easterlin's relative income argument (e.g., Easterlin, 1980). Briefly summarized, the relative income hypothesis states that a mechanism of self-generating fluctuations exists in fertility levels. The mechanism should work as follows: generation one has low relative income and therefore low fertility. This results in a small cohort for generation 2. Generation 2 grows up with low aspirations for wealth but finds advantageous conditions in the job market because of few competitors. Therefore, the children in generation 2 have a higher income than their parents. This higher income together with the low aspirations result in a higher relative income. This will encourage generation 2 to have many children. The children in generation 3 then is a large cohort with high aspirations because they grow up in wealth. They experience higher competition and therefore low income. This low income relative to the aspirations will cause generation 3 to have low fertility again, and so forth.

Aside from all other substantive points of criticism on this hypothesis, it also contains two unrealistic assumptions: all mothers bear their children at roughly the same age and all families have about the same number of children. The first assumption of very low variance in the age distribution of births is necessary to keep the generations distinguishable from each other. If some children are born to teenage mothers and others to mothers above age 40, then soon members of different generations will have children during the same historical time. This mixing of generations would confuse the cohort effects and destroy the mechanism of self-generating cycles. As shown in the study, however, there is considerable distribution of births over age.

The second implicit assumption refers to the identity of family sizes. If we relax the assumption and allow for heterogeneity in the distribution of family size at any point of the process, this will seriously affect the cyclical mechanism. Consider, for example, that in the case of the cohort with low average fertility a certain portion of couples has significantly larger families than others. Their children experience large sibship sizes and will not share the pattern of income and aspirations supposed to be characteristic for their generation because the unusually large family size reduced the family's per capita income. This would at least significantly dampen the cycles from one generation to the next.

It would be interesting to discuss the effect of heterogeneity on this hypothesis and other economic models of fertility in more detail. At this point it suffices to emphasize that the assumption of heterogeneity in the family size distribution may upset fertility theories based on average fertility behavior.

Housing Demand

Considering that most children grow up with their parents, it is obvious that the distribution of family sizes is an important determinant of the distribution of household sizes. The distribution of fertility is possibly the most important factor influencing the distribution of household sizes. Two other factors influence this distribution, namely, patterns of formations and dissolutions of unions (not necessarily always marriages) and general trends in the level of fertility.

The distribution of household sizes has several consequences on society and on the economy. One consequence is the structure of the demand for appropriate housing. A distribution in which all women have two children would require a large number of average-size apartments, whereas a strong concentration of fertility would result in the demand for some very large housing units and a large number of small units.

Another complication is that the distribution of incomes does not match with the distribution of family sizes. That is, people with large families tend to have the smaller incomes and vice versa. Also, regardless of the level of family income, a larger number of children means a smaller income per person in the family. This inequality is reinforced by the fact that after the birth of a child the mother usually stays out of paid employment for some time. Unless the government has specific policies to ease the burden, large families often cannot afford the larger homes they need. Meanwhile, persons with no or few children have, on average, more resources available and can afford larger homes than they actually need.

Consumer Goods

The structure of consumer goods demanded also depends on the distribution of family sizes. A significant number of durable consumer goods is directed to children (toys, buggies, clothes, children's furniture, etc.). It makes a big difference if every woman or man has to purchase these things or if childless people do not need them while others with children buy them once and use them for all of their children.

Also the fact that fertility distributions themselves influence the distribution of disposable per capita income affects the structure of consumer goods demanded, as mentioned above. These factors result in considerable inequalities in the per capita income distributions between high- and low-fertility families, and this in turn influences the structure of demands: the families with many children will tend to be striving to meet their basic needs, while childless or one-child families have money to spend on sports cars, long-distance trips, and other luxury goods. A possible future increase in fertility concentration would make these differences even more pronounced.

Social Mobility

The unequal distribution of fertility can be one of the reasons that upward social mobility seems more common than downward mobility. This can be made more explicit by a simple model: let us assume, first, an economy with fixed proportions of well-paid and poorly paid positions; second, that social standing is generally inherited from one generation to the next; and third, that fertility is concentrated in the lower social strata. As the upper classes – due to their low fertility – cannot fill all the high-status jobs, children from the lower social groups may become upwardly mobile.

Although this model is simplified, its assumptions are not unrealistic for present industrialized societies. It illustrates that socioeconomic inequalities in the fertility distribution are a driving force for social mobility. Of course, this is only one mechanism among many others.

Socialization

Every person is primarily formed and socialized in his or her family. Psychologists of various schools agree that the experiences of a child during the first years are of utmost importance for character and social skills development. Siblings are certainly an important factor during these early phases of formation. It is practically common knowledge that single children carry this attribute with them throughout their life. Similarly, children from large families tend to have characteristic patterns of experiences and aspirations. It might have far-reaching consequences for the future of the society whether the majority of children comes from larger families or a great proportion grows up in a one-child family.

Family size distributions have also indirect effects on a child's socialization through the channels of socioeconomic inequality. Children from large families with low per capita income might be exposed to additional forms of stress: in LDCs this could be malnutrition for younger children or excessively hard work to help the family survive for older children. In most industrialized societies the situation is less extreme, but children from large families may have less opportunities for a good education and an otherwise more difficult start in life.

Equity Issues

These points now bring us fully into the field of social equity issues and values. The different consequences of fertility concentration pointed out above allude to the equity not only among children but also among parents with different numbers of children.

Is low-fertility concentration better or worse than high-fertility concentration? This question is extremely difficult to answer. Even in rather homogeneous European populations the answer might be different depending on whether one takes a micro- or macro-level perspective – whether one puts more weight on economic aspects or on social questions– and depending especially on the value that is attributed to the emotional relationship to children. On a global scale the question becomes even more complex. In some countries a surplus of new children is one of the greatest problems, whereas in other countries a lack of children causes severe problems for the age structure and for the future payment of pensions.

Besides the issues of equity among offspring and parents one might also look at the equity between the sexes. There is a lot of evidence from different continents and cultures that the total amount of work involved in raising children is extremely unequally distributed between the sexes. Even when considering the fact that men are more involved in external economic activities, the discrepancy remains. In Austria, for example, figures on the daily time budgets show that the total time spent on economic, household, and child-care activities is on the average significantly higher for women than for men (see Lutz and Vaupel, 1987). This probably also holds for most other countries. Also it was found that the greater the number of children, the less the father helps in the household and with child care. This might be explained by the fact that *traditional* families have both more children and less involvement of the father than the modern couples that try to divide the labor more equally.

Scientific analysis, in general, can hardly provide answers to such questions, and this demographic perspective provides even less. Answers must be found by the people concerned in the specific cultures and value systems. Demographic analysis, however, may be helpful in describing the existing distributions, pointing out interesting differences when comparing various distributions, and making society aware of some of the consequences that follow from various degrees of concentration and inequality. If this study contributes to this understanding and if it helps to convince some demographers to give more attention to distributional aspects of fertility, then it may be considered a worthwhile effort.

Appendix A

Completed parity distributions of ever-married women aged 40–49 at the time of the survey for 41 LDC-World Fertility Surveys (including Portugal) and 13 European World Fertility Surveys (including USA). These data are the only necessary input to calculate the cohort parity tables as discussed in Chapter 2.

Table A.1. *D(i)* for all countries.

Country	F(0)	Completed parity distribution (per 1000)															
		0	1	2	3	4	5	6	7	8	9	10	11	12	13	14	15
AFRICA																	
Benin	6.14	32	25	62	70	105	89	120	143	141	106	51	38	9	3		
Cameroon	4.91	154	96	71	76	62	71	89	101	92	78	43	30	17	6	4	1
Egypt	6.64	38	32	45	48	72	104	118	131	118	103	91	38	31	11	7	5
Ghana	6.38	23	19	51	66	94	99	134	138	135	110	77	32	5	9	0	
Ivory Coast	6.78	40	51	42	43	62	76	96	107	135	146	82	71	22	10	6	2
Kenya	7.73	31	24	23	31	33	56	85	118	146	155	132	78	47	22	9	4
Lesotho	5.22	52	71	94	99	103	101	118	114	97	73	40	15	12	5		
Mauritania	6.01	47	48	70	83	89	102	100	125	76	106	54	42	36	10	4	
Morocco	7.08	69	37	39	40	47	57	95	97	124	119	108	63	57	20	11	9
Nigeria	5.41	73	53	73	94	114	107	108	101	88	74	54	27	20	14		
Senegal	6.92	35	40	43	46	71	68	85	117	139	128	95	88	35	6		
Sudan	6.00	75	50	67	66	69	76	96	118	130	87	89	44	21	5		
Tunisia	6.78	36	21	29	48	71	106	126	133	123	133	72	47	30	9	7	0
AMERICAS																	
Colombia	6.90	28	38	55	86	84	91	83	94	93	77	80	70	39	29	26	18
Costa Rica	6.92	28	35	71	105	89	72	88	76	80	72	68	54	58	42	20	34
Dominican Rep.	6.39	49	60	58	78	109	80	102	58	84	73	64	75	58	37	8	
Ecuador	6.98	18	26	58	74	94	97	96	96	97	96	72	57	50	32	14	18
Guyana	6.46	54	64	46	73	65	84	101	98	103	93	77	47	47	22	12	7
Haiti	5.80	34	61	61	87	101	110	114	108	110	97	62	34	11	3		
Jamaica	5.51	73	86	91	73	106	82	74	101	97	60	60	39	34	12	10	4
Mexico	7.03	37	37	55	61	76	82	91	97	94	107	75	61	46	37	16	21
Panama	5.74	33	41	91	106	102	134	105	95	83	55	59	43	31	10	4	
Paraguay	6.27	29	74	122	208	95	107	86	56	71	44	35	32	26	8		
Peru	6.76	22	35	51	82	86	92	104	107	98	97	71	60	47	19	10	11
Trinidad & Tobago	5.50	58	66	78	104	110	97	117	90	85	50	48	36	29	20	3	
USA	4.48	57	72	228	233	152	115	54	36	21	15	12	2	2	1		
Venezuela	6.21	20	43	102	84	99	104	93	99	67	78	81	61	34	17	11	

Table A.1. Continued.

Country	F(0)	Completed parity distribution (per 1000)														
		0	1	2	3	4	5	6	7	8	9	10	11	12	13	14	15
ASIA AND PACIFIC																	
Bangladesh	6.95	25	27	40	55	49	87	112	153	128	127	87	51	30	10	7	4
Fiji	6.31	51	39	55	69	69	100	111	124	114	94	77	45	21	8	7	8
Indonesia	5.25	66	84	83	91	94	98	114	105	97	64	44	32	17	3	1	
Jordan	8.66	23	9	21	27	43	42	74	90	87	141	136	111	73	61	32	24
Korea	5.42	15	38	48	77	147	187	167	149	95	39	20	9	3	1		
Malaysia	6.13	29	50	68	88	95	103	103	109	101	84	70	47	28	8	5	5
Nepal	5.65	39	36	76	73	127	123	119	131	107	87	42	21	10	3		
Pakistan	6.91	36	28	35	50	57	87	97	149	141	117	95	47	32	13	5	3
Philippines	6.86	24	31	43	66	81	87	111	107	112	119	90	55	34	20	6	6
Sri Lanka	5.73	36	52	76	89	98	104	140	117	90	78	50	35	14	8	3	1
Syria	7.66	36	13	23	41	44	72	108	104	139	114	106	83	54	26	16	12
Thailand	6.36	25	40	56	69	99	101	116	118	106	100	76	36	27	11	5	5
Turkey	6.08	27	17	76	102	117	129	100	112	81	82	56	40	25	12	10	5
Yemen	6.65	21	23	38	71	95	109	109	128	128	100	66	59	28	16	2	
EUROPE																	
Belgium	2.56	74	212	291	195	106	52	38	18	4	5	3	1	3			
Czechoslovakia	2.31	39	165	451	212	85	30	13	2	4							
Denmark	2.53	61	116	370	242	147	32	19	8	4							
Finland	2.67	48	145	336	244	118	60	22	13	5	5	3	1				
France	2.69	60	158	308	228	122	54	36	23	3	3	5					
Great Britain	2.58	60	139	354	217	136	49	28	13	4							
Italy	2.38	58	170	387	228	94	36	10	7	4	5						
Netherlands*	1.67	171	289	303	184	39	13										
Norway	2.75	48	100	299	281	175	77	20									
Poland	2.78	31	140	357	223	125	58	33	14	7	8	1	1	1	1		
Portugal	2.01	58	182	312	161	102	56	44	31	19	9	8	7	3	2		
Spain	3.10	40	80	295	254	166	76	42	22	10	6	3	3	1			
Yugoslavia	3.05	43	121	351	183	110	56	52	40	21	22						

*In this context the Dutch data are not strictly comparable to the other countries because they are restricted to the marriage cohorts 1963–1973.

Table A.2. *D(i)* for all countries, some schooling.

Country	F(0)	Completed parity distribution (per 1000)															
		0	1	2	3	4	5	6	7	8	9	10	11	12	13	14	15
AFRICA																	
Egypt	6.37	40	38	61	68	67	110	119	118	102	104	72	38	31	10	10	3
Ghana	5.97	25	19	76	44	141	96	153	115	141	128	44	12				
Kenya	8.10	14	17	11	28	28	53	99	99	176	164	124	90	51	28	11	
Lesotho	5.34	46	75	84	96	107	101	113	119	105	75	32	17	19	5		
Mauritania	6.06	46	52	64	73	67	99	111	149	99	96	67	38	20	11		
AMERICAS																	
Colombia	5.94	32	54	80	109	105	98	98	102	76	58	72	47	36	18	7	
Costa Rica	5.68	37	45	103	156	128	78	88	75	75	47	45	25	42	20	12	17
Dominican Rep.	5.48	45	58	91	111	143	84	156	32	58	52	84	25				
Ecuador	5.73	26	35	102	120	113	120	91	102	85	72	41	30	30	21	4	
Mexico	6.70	35	47	65	76	79	84	104	89	83	106	66	57	39	32	11	20
Panama	4.97	43	47	112	129	125	162	98	84	80	43	43	24	6			
Paraguay	4.91	29	74	122	208	95	107	86	56	71	44	35	32	26	8		
Peru	5.93	21	45	75	125	117	113	106	98	72	71	47	51	17	14	10	10
USA	4.33	52	76	238	248	152	120	46	32	17	10	10					
Venezuela	5.11	28	51	136	113	125	119	113	130	45	51	34	39	11			
ASIA AND PACIFIC																	
Bangladesh	7.13	13	20	53	60	33	60	107	174	127	174	53	67	46	6		
Fiji	6.01	56	40	66	66	68	110	122	136	107	94	71	35	11	7	4	
Indonesia	5.65	58	55	72	90	92	116	114	94	111	63	51	48	24	4		
Jordan	7.29	23	9	37	61	94	61	142	104	75	127	104	37	47	52	18	
Korea	4.98	10	43	61	101	177	217	162	130	55	22	13	2				
Malaysia	5.72	27	59	91	101	103	107	103	94	68	75	36	22	5			
Philippines	6.53	23	35	52	73	98	97	121	114	101	99	75	51	30	15	4	5
Sri Lanka	5.41	43	49	86	98	115	107	141	123	87	56	43	30	7	7	1	
Syria	6.21	53	29	23	88	76	142	147	71	136	71	65	59	29	5		
Thailand	6.29	23	43	59	73	97	115	113	116	99	93	79	37	31	11	4	
Turkey	4.51	37	37	146	183	158	141	91	62	52	42	24	17	4			

Table A.2. Continued.

Country	F(0)	Completed parity distribution (per 1000)															
		0	1	2	3	4	5	6	7	8	9	10	11	12	13	14	15
EUROPE																	
Belgium	2.51	83	184	307	201	112	45	43	16	5	3						
Czechoslovakia	2.21	33	190	485	187	67	21	15	3								
Denmark	2.36	23	121	494	241	80	29	11									
Finland	2.33	51	172	389	245	102	26	4	4	2	2	2					
France	2.37	72	152	348	290	80	29	14	14								
Great Britain	2.47	73	137	347	238	131	36	22	12	2							
Italy	3.01	84	189	441	217	63	7										
Netherlands*	1.58	220	240	300	220	20											
Norway	2.63	50	112	320	276	161	71	9									
Poland	2.17	30	223	471	179	57	21	11	3	2	3						
Portugal	2.22	70	239	373	159	79	31	26	8	6	2	1					
Spain	3.16	26	74	286	265	169	95	58	5	11	5	5					
Yugoslavia	1.86	69	224	552	121	17	9	9									

*In this context the Dutch data are not strictly comparable to the other countries because they are restricted to the marriage cohorts 1963–1973.

Table A.9. *D(i)* for all countries, no schooling.

Country	F(0)	Completed parity distribution (per 1000)															
		0	1	2	3	4	5	6	7	8	9	10	11	12	13	14	15
AFRICA																	
Egypt	6.82	37	28	35	35	75	101	117	139	128	102	103	39	31	11	5	5
Kenya	7.59	37	26	27	32	34	57	80	125	136	151	135	73	46	20	9	3
Mauritania	5.92	47	44	78	95	116	105	88	98	51	119	40	47	54	10		
AMERICAS																	
Colombia	7.37	26	30	43	75	74	89	75	91	102	87	85	83	41	36	36	20
Costa Rica	8.27	18	25	38	54	49	67	87	77	85	98	93	85	74	64	28	51
Dominican Rep.	6.87	51	61	40	61	92	78	75	71	98	85	71	71	75	54	9	
Ecuador	8.01	11	18	20	36	77	77	100	91	108	117	100	81	68	41	22	24
Guyana	7.33	29	37	29	44	59	66	133	96	140	96	88	59	59	37	22	
Mexico	7.68	40	18	38	34	72	78	68	110	114	108	92	70	60	46	24	22
Panama	7.14	16	32	52	64	60	84	119	119	92	79	91	80	79	23	3	
Paraguay	7.43	27	42	60	60	55	78	60	93	103	93	98	85	60	37	17	25
Peru	7.79	23	23	23	31	49	67	102	118	130	128	99	70	83	26	10	11
Trinidad & Tobago	6.21	40	40	32	96	80	104	120	193	48	64	96	48	31			
USA	5.12	81	40	212	131	152	81	111	61	51	51	30					
Venezuela	7.39	12	36	66	54	72	90	72	66	90	108	132	84	60	36	17	
ASIA AND PACIFIC																	
Fiji	6.64	43	40	37	78	72	83	95	104	132	98	92	66	43	11		
Jordan	9.12	23	10	15	15	25	35	50	86	92	146	148	138	82	65	37	25
Korea	4.75	19	47	64	121	191	216	143	105	58	19	8	2				
Malaysia	6.35	30	44	56	80	90	101	104	113	106	95	67	55	32	10	4	4
Philippines	7.73	28	22	22	49	37	60	86	89	141	170	128	67	44	33	11	6
Sri Lanka	6.46	21	59	56	68	62	97	137	106	95	126	67	48	29	10	7	3
Thailand	6.36	32	35	53	62	103	77	124	124	124	118	74	35	20	11		
Turkey	7.00	21	5	36	56	93	123	106	142	98	106	75	53	36	19	15	7

Table A.3. Continued.

Country	F(0)	Completed parity distribution (per 1000)															
		0	1	2	3	4	5	6	7	8	9	10	11	12	13	14	15
EUROPE																	
Belgium	2.52	66	241	277	192	102	54	34	19	2	7	5					
Czechoslovakia	2.53	54	102	367	279	136	54	7									
Denmark	2.61	80	112	310	241	181	34	23	11	6							
Finland	2.94	46	126	291	244	130	88	36	21	8	8	4					
France	2.87	52	161	286	194	145	69	48	28	4	4	8					
Great Britain	2.79	28	146	363	170	146	80	42	14	9							
Italy	2.50	49	164	369	232	105	46	13	9	6	7						
Netherlands*	1.84	77	385	308	115	77	38										
Norway	2.88	44	71	257	310	221	97										
Poland	3.14	32	88	287	252	168	82	48	21	11	11	2					
Portugal	3.44	48	136	264	163	121	76	58	49	30	14	14	10	6	3		
Spain	3.06	43	81	293	257	167	74	40	26	10	6	3					
Yugoslavia	3.17	41	112	332	188	118	62	56	44	23	24						

*In this context the Dutch data are not strictly comparable to the other countries because they are restricted to the marriage cohorts 1963–1973.

Table A.4. *D(i)* for all countries, rural.

Country	F(0)	Completed parity distribution (per 1000)															
		0	1	2	3	4	5	6	7	8	9	10	11	12	13	14	15
AFRICA																	
Benin	6.22	28	30	52	72	92	98	120	138	152	112	56	34	10	1		
Egypt	6.98	42	29	37	35	64	92	94	136	125	118	111	49	34	14	9	3
Ghana	6.57	21	13	43	65	84	107	139	131	133	116	86	37	6	10	1	
Ivory Coast	6.85	43	47	40	40	61	81	92	105	138	143	89	71	23	10	7	2
Mauritania	6.03	36	46	64	83	90	114	111	135	75	109	44	46	36	5		
Morocco	7.65	59	15	36	34	44	58	77	89	138	124	117	72	72	28	18	12
Senegal	7.02	33	31	40	53	63	65	87	114	142	140	99	95	27	4		
Sudan	5.98	79	54	74	59	61	69	101	123	130	91	83	44	19	7		
Tunisia	6.90	36	23	18	43	65	96	131	138	118	156	80	55	33	3		
AMERICAS																	
Colombia	7.63	27	27	44	57	64	91	88	94	84	84	84	94	44	44	40	27
Costa Rica	8.49	21	21	29	42	53	66	84	76	92	92	95	87	74	71	37	53
Dominican Rep.	7.75	33	23	37	61	71	52	94	66	80	104	85	123	94	52	18	
Ecuador	7.81	13	18	28	50	63	84	108	104	99	117	89	71	65	42	18	24
Guyana	7.10	37	48	37	48	48	87	115	95	128	97	83	60	56	33	13	7
Haiti	6.12	28	55	39	73	89	110	131	115	125	115	70	36	7			
Jamaica	6.15	72	60	82	52	82	75	75	115	100	77	85	57	22	12	17	7
Mexico	7.91	30	21	23	37	57	62	84	101	118	124	106	91	62	43	23	11
Panama	6.87	26	13	53	83	70	104	90	144	87	80	87	73	60	20	3	
Paraguay	7.48	27	54	59	66	39	38	66	98	91	91	86	93	76	36	17	27
Peru	7.54	29	30	21	34	48	75	109	110	127	133	92	79	71	19	9	4
Trinidad & Tobago	6.01	58	62	68	58	100	100	117	103	65	79	68	62	24	27	3	

Table A.4. Continued.

Country	F(0)	Completed parity distribution (per 1000)															
		0	1	2	3	4	5	6	7	8	9	10	11	12	13	14	15
ASIA AND PACIFIC																	
Fiji	6.66	54	32	45	59	59	82	105	121	131	118	83	50	30	7	9	7
Korea	6.13	10	29	31	28	99	156	194	197	137	61	32	16	5			
Malaysia	6.30	32	48	61	73	84	103	100	117	110	93	82	54	26	9	3	
Pakistan	6.91	31	22	37	51	52	97	96	158	146	119	93	40	31	14	4	
Philippines	7.25	26	27	35	52	57	74	115	104	118	140	105	65	37	24	7	6
Syria	7.80	24	11	31	37	44	57	102	128	138	125	95	89	61	27	13	11
Turkey	7.07	20	11	28	64	85	130	104	109	105	113	89	62	33	16	17	6
EUROPE																	
Belgium	2.63	44	186	336	168	124	88	44	9								
Czechoslovakia	2.62	32	77	423	288	103	38	32	6								
Denmark	2.89	50	124	174	331	231	50	41									
Finland	3.00	40	102	284	273	138	89	31	24	7	7	2	2				
France	2.87	60	121	259	267	147	60	60	26								
Italy	2.40	45	178	374	243	112	16	16	4	2	8						
Netherlands*	1.95	190	238	143	286	143											
Norway	2.87	51	83	273	269	209	91	24									
Poland	3.39	21	66	237	276	183	97	66	25	16	12						
Portugal	3.25	51	151	277	175	115	66	51	43	24	12	11	10	5	3		
Spain	3.21	65	75	239	259	154	90	60	35	20	5						
Yugoslavia	3.47	42	104	276	178	133	74	74	51	31	37						

*In this context the Dutch data are not strictly comparable to the other countries because they are restricted to the marriage cohorts 1963–1973.

Table A.5. *D(i)* for all countries, urban.

Country	F(0)	Completed parity distribution (per 1000)															
		0	1	2	3	4	5	6	7	8	9	10	11	12	13	14	15
AFRICA																	
Benin	5.83	44	12	95	63	146	63	121	159	108	89	38	50	6			
Cameroon	3.89	148	151	111	97	1	61	129	86	83	68	0					
Egypt	6.24	33	35	56	64	81	119	148	125	109	84	67	24	28	6	5	6
Ghana	5.87	29	37	74	67	123	78	119	156	141	93	55	18	3			
Ivory Coast	6.50	32	64	50	55	69	60	111	115	129	157	60	74	18			
Mauritania	5.93	64	52	80	84	88	84	84	112	80	104	72	36	36	20	0	
Morocco	6.30	83	66	44	49	51	55	122	109	107	113	96	51	36	10	2	
Senegal	6.69	39	62	51	28	90	73	79	125	130	96	85	68	56	11		
Sudan	6.10	64	38	51	84	90	97	84	103	129	77	103	45	25			
Tunisia	6.63	36	19	41	54	79	117	122	128	128	112	66	41	28	14	8	1
AMERICAS																	
Colombia	6.51	29	45	62	103	96	92	80	94	98	72	78	56	37	21	17	13
Costa Rica	5.36	35	50	112	167	125	80	92	77	70	54	45	25	44	14	4	
Dominican Rep.	5.23	63	92	75	92	143	105	109	50	88	46	46	33	25	25	0	
Ecuador	5.94	24	35	95	104	131		113	82	86	95	71	53	42	33	20	8
Guyana	5.21	87	94	62	118	97	80	80	104	59	87	66	24	31	3		
Haiti	4.76	50	79	123	130	137	115	72	94	72	50	43	28				
Jamaica	4.28	76	132	108	108	148	96	76	84	96	36	24	11				
Mexico	6.43	42	48	78	79	90	96	96	94	77	94	53	41	35	32	10	27
Panama	4.94	38	61	117	122	124	156	115	63	81	38	40	22	11	4		
Paraguay	4.74	30	61	126	206	116	119	80	49	86	46	49	21	6			
Peru	6.25	17	38	71	115	112	104	101	105	79	72	56	46	31	19	10	15
Trinidad & Tobago	5.18	58	69	85	133	117	96	117	82	98	32	34	19	32	15	4	

Table A.5. Continued.

Country	F(0)	Completed parity distribution (per 1000)															
		0	1	2	3	4	5	6	7	8	9	10	11	12	13	14	15
ASIA AND PACIFIC																	
Fiji	5.59	46	53	74	87	87	133	125	130	89	56	69	38	7			
Indonesia	5.32	82	76	85	74	105	91	94	119	85	65	56	37	19	5		
Korea	4.75	19	47	64	121	191	216	143	105	58	19	8	2				
Malaysia	5.67	23	55	85	118	117	107	112	96	86	70	50	36	33	6		
Pakistan	6.77	52	45	31	49	70	59	101	126	129	115	101	66	38	10		
Philippines	6.00	21	40	61	96	131	115	104	114	100	74	57	36	26	13	4	
Sri Lanka	5.11	26	72	121	101	89	112	179	104	80	49	34	23	5			
Syria	7.53	48	16	14	46	44	87	113	80	141	104	117	78	46	24	20	13
Thailand	5.02	19	64	103	84	214	110	116	90	77	71	32	12				
Turkey	4.82	35	24	138	153	159	130	97	118	49	43	14	12	14	8		
EUROPE																	
Belgium	2.54	79	216	283	200	103	46	37	19	4	6	3	1	3			
Czechoslovakia	2.21	42	201	461	180	78	26	5	0	5	0	3					
Denmark	2.42	64	114	431	215	121	27	12	10	2	0	2					
Finland	2.41	55	180	378	220	102	36	15	4	4	4	4					
France	2.59	59	175	331	212	112	52	26	22	4	0	7					
Italy	2.31	69	167	403	220	82	36	5	9	6	3						
Netherlands*	1.47	164	309	364	145												
Norway	2.65	42	121	332	295	126	58	16	0	11							
Poland	2.36	38	188	436	190	88	33	13	7	1	5	2	0	1			
Portugal	2.21	71	247	385	133	76	36	28	6	8	1	3					
Spain	3.01	36	81	306	255	168	74	39	20	8	6	4	3	0	1		
Yugoslavia	2.67	44	137	419	187	89	40	32	31	12	8						

*In this context the Dutch data are not strictly comparable to the other countries because they are restricted to the marriage cohorts 1963–1973.

Appendix B

Mean ages at birth of certain orders (i) for women with completed parity (j) and standard deviations in parentheses under the means: cohorts of ever-married women aged 40–49 in 41 LDC-World Fertility Surveys (including Portugal). For details see discussion in Section 2.3.

Bangladesh

Birth of order i

Completed parity j	1	2	3	4	5	6	7	8	9	10	11	12	13	14	15
1	22.2 (7.8)														
2	19.8 (4.9)	24.7 (6.0)													
3	19.6 (4.9)	23.9 (5.3)	29.3 (6.4)												
4	19.0 (4.2)	22.5 (4.6)	26.1 (4.6)	30.7 (5.4)											
5	18.3 (3.6)	21.9 (4.0)	25.5 (4.6)	28.9 (4.9)	33.3 (4.7)										
6	18.5 (3.8)	21.6 (4.2)	24.8 (4.3)	27.9 (4.3)	31.4 (4.6)	35.0 (4.4)									
7	18.1 (3.5)	20.9 (3.7)	23.8 (3.8)	26.7 (4.2)	29.7 (4.3)	32.8 (4.1)	36.1 (4.2)								
8	17.8 (3.3)	20.7 (3.4)	23.3 (3.6)	25.8 (3.8)	28.5 (3.9)	31.1 (4.1)	33.9 (3.9)	37.3 (3.5)							
9	17.5 (3.3)	20.0 (3.3)	22.5 (3.5)	25.1 (3.7)	27.4 (3.6)	30.0 (3.6)	32.5 (3.5)	34.9 (3.6)	37.8 (3.6)						
10	16.5 (2.2)	19.1 (2.5)	21.7 (2.5)	24.4 (2.9)	27.1 (3.2)	29.6 (3.5)	31.8 (3.5)	34.0 (3.5)	36.3 (3.1)	39.1 (2.9)					
11	15.9 (2.1)	18.0 (2.2)	20.2 (2.2)	22.4 (2.4)	24.7 (2.3)	26.8 (2.4)	29.2 (2.5)	31.5 (2.5)	33.7 (2.8)	35.8 (3.0)	38.7 (3.2)				
12	15.8 (2.0)	17.6 (2.4)	19.6 (2.9)	21.8 (3.1)	23.9 (3.5)	26.3 (3.9)	28.3 (3.8)	30.5 (3.4)	32.6 (3.5)	35.0 (3.4)	37.3 (3.3)	39.6 (3.2)			
13	16.4 (1.8)	18.4 (1.8)	20.6 (2.4)	22.4 (2.5)	24.1 (2.8)	26.9 (2.8)	29.0 (2.8)	30.8 (2.6)	32.5 (2.5)	34.3 (2.1)	35.8 (2.0)	38.3 (2.3)	40.7 (2.7)		
14	15.7 (2.5)	17.3 (2.9)	18.9 (3.2)	21.1 (3.4)	22.7 (3.3)	24.5 (3.6)	26.5 (4.2)	27.5 (4.2)	29.2 (4.3)	31.1 (4.7)	34.2 (2.4)	36.8 (1.9)	39.7 (2.0)	42.0 (2.1)	
15	14.6 (1.4)	15.5 (1.3)	17.3 (2.0)	19.1 (2.3)	21.1 (3.0)	22.9 (3.5)	24.6 (3.7)	26.8 (3.2)	29.1 (2.8)	31.2 (2.0)	33.3 (1.3)	35.5 (1.7)	38.1 (1.9)	40.0 (2.5)	41.9 (3.5)

Benin

Birth of order i

Completed parity j	1	2	3	4	5	6	7	8	9	10	11	12	13
1	25.2 (8.5)												
2	25.7 (7.1)	30.3 (7.8)											
3	23.7 (5.9)	27.6 (5.4)	31.9 (6.4)										
4	22.1 (4.7)	25.4 (4.5)	28.8 (4.8)	33.0 (5.3)									
5	21.1 (4.1)	24.1 (4.0)	27.6 (4.4)	30.7 (4.7)	34.3 (5.0)								
6	19.4 (4.0)	22.6 (3.9)	25.4 (4.3)	28.6 (4.2)	32.1 (4.3)	35.6 (4.6)							
7	20.5 (3.0)	23.1 (3.2)	25.9 (3.4)	28.5 (3.5)	31.2 (3.7)	34.1 (3.8)	37.3 (4.0)						
8	20.1 (3.3)	22.6 (3.3)	25.0 (3.3)	27.7 (3.5)	30.2 (3.6)	32.9 (3.7)	35.8 (3.6)	39.1 (3.7)					
9	19.6 (2.6)	22.3 (2.6)	24.7 (2.8)	27.2 (3.1)	29.7 (3.3)	32.0 (3.5)	34.6 (3.5)	37.2 (3.4)	40.1 (3.3)				
10	18.5 (2.5)	21.1 (2.8)	23.2 (2.8)	25.6 (3.1)	27.6 (3.6)	29.9 (4.0)	32.3 (4.3)	34.8 (4.6)	37.2 (4.8)	39.6 (4.5)			
11	17.9 (3.5)	20.3 (3.3)	22.5 (3.2)	24.6 (3.1)	27.0 (3.0)	29.2 (3.1)	32.1 (2.6)	34.5 (2.6)	36.9 (2.8)	39.2 (3.2)	42.2 (2.9)		
12	20.0 (3.5)	22.6 (3.5)	24.7 (4.1)	26.8 (4.8)	28.8 (5.1)	30.9 (5.4)	32.8 (4.5)	34.6 (4.5)	36.2 (3.7)	37.8 (4.0)	40.2 (3.8)	41.8 (2.8)	
13	20.8 (4.5)	22.7 (2.9)	24.0 (2.1)	25.8 (2.9)	28.5 (.9)	30.1 (.1)	32.1 (.1)	33.4 (.8)	35.0 (1.4)	36.5 (2.3)	37.3 (1.2)	40.3 (1.1)	42.5 (.7)

Cameroon

Birth of order i

Completed parity j	1	2	3	4	5	6	7	8	9	10	11	12	13	14
1	23.8 (7.1)													
2	23.2 (7.0)	27.3 (7.5)												
3	22.2 (6.5)	25.9 (6.8)	29.8 (7.1)											
4	23.2 (6.6)	26.0 (6.7)	29.3 (6.6)	33.1 (7.0)										
5	22.4 (6.2)	25.7 (6.4)	28.7 (6.2)	31.7 (6.4)	35.1 (6.5)									
6	21.7 (4.9)	24.7 (5.2)	27.6 (5.1)	30.8 (5.2)	33.7 (5.3)	37.3 (5.3)								
7	20.2 (4.4)	22.9 (4.3)	25.7 (4.8)	28.3 (5.0)	31.1 (5.2)	33.8 (5.3)	37.3 (5.2)							
8	20.0 (4.4)	22.5 (4.4)	25.2 (4.7)	27.8 (4.6)	30.2 (4.7)	32.7 (4.7)	35.6 (5.0)	39.1 (5.1)						
9	19.1 (3.8)	21.9 (4.0)	24.4 (3.8)	26.9 (4.2)	29.4 (4.3)	31.9 (4.4)	34.3 (4.4)	36.6 (4.5)	39.5 (4.5)					
10	18.6 (2.9)	20.8 (3.1)	23.2 (3.2)	25.7 (3.2)	28.0 (3.2)	30.2 (3.4)	32.4 (3.6)	34.5 (3.8)	36.8 (4.2)	39.7 (4.2)				
11	18.2 (3.0)	20.2 (3.2)	22.4 (3.4)	24.4 (3.5)	26.8 (3.7)	28.6 (3.8)	30.7 (4.0)	32.9 (4.0)	35.0 (4.4)	37.3 (4.8)	40.0 (4.5)			
12	17.9 (3.0)	19.9 (3.2)	21.6 (3.1)	23.6 (3.1)	26.3 (3.2)	28.8 (3.4)	30.8 (3.5)	33.2 (3.4)	35.5 (2.8)	37.7 (2.9)	39.8 (2.8)	42.2 (2.7)		
13	17.7 (3.8)	19.9 (3.6)	21.6 (3.6)	23.3 (3.5)	25.1 (3.3)	26.9 (3.4)	29.0 (3.1)	30.8 (3.1)	32.9 (2.8)	34.5 (2.7)	36.6 (2.9)	38.4 (3.0)	41.4 (3.6)	
14	19.4 (2.8)	21.2 (2.9)	22.8 (2.6)	24.5 (2.6)	26.4 (2.6)	27.8 (2.8)	29.6 (2.6)	31.3 (2.5)	33.1 (2.4)	34.7 (3.1)	36.8 (3.7)	37.8 (3.7)	39.2 (3.7)	42.9 (3.5)

Colombia

Birth of order i

Completed parity j	1	2	3	4	5	6	7	8	9	10	11	12	13	14	15
1	27.5 (7.3)														
2	25.3 (5.8)	29.4 (5.8)													
3	23.0 (5.2)	26.7 (5.5)	31.0 (6.1)												
4	23.6 (5.2)	26.2 (5.2)	29.4 (5.8)	33.5 (6.0)											
5	23.3 (4.9)	25.8 (4.9)	28.3 (4.7)	31.1 (4.9)	34.7 (5.3)										
6	21.4 (4.3)	23.6 (4.1)	25.8 (4.4)	28.1 (4.8)	30.7 (5.0)	34.7 (4.8)									
7	21.5 (4.3)	23.6 (4.3)	25.7 (4.6)	27.8 (4.5)	30.2 (4.5)	32.7 (4.7)	35.5 (4.8)								
8	21.5 (3.2)	23.6 (3.2)	25.4 (3.3)	27.5 (3.3)	29.7 (3.6)	31.8 (3.6)	34.1 (3.4)	37.5 (3.7)							
9	20.7 (3.3)	23.0 (3.5)	24.9 (3.5)	26.7 (3.4)	28.5 (3.4)	30.3 (3.5)	32.3 (3.7)	34.5 (3.8)	37.3 (4.1)						
10	20.1 (3.1)	22.1 (3.0)	24.0 (3.1)	25.8 (3.1)	28.0 (3.0)	29.9 (2.9)	31.6 (2.9)	33.7 (3.2)	35.8 (3.4)	38.6 (3.4)					
11	19.9 (2.5)	21.5 (2.8)	23.3 (2.7)	25.2 (2.8)	27.0 (2.9)	28.9 (3.1)	30.7 (3.2)	32.6 (3.5)	34.8 (3.4)	36.7 (3.4)	38.9 (3.6)				
12	18.5 (3.9)	20.3 (3.8)	22.1 (3.8)	23.8 (3.7)	25.5 (3.6)	27.2 (3.7)	29.1 (3.5)	30.8 (3.4)	32.7 (3.5)	34.9 (3.2)	36.8 (3.3)	39.2 (3.2)			
13	17.7 (3.0)	19.6 (3.2)	21.1 (3.4)	22.9 (3.7)	24.6 (3.9)	26.7 (3.9)	28.3 (3.8)	30.4 (3.8)	32.3 (3.6)	34.2 (3.8)	36.0 (3.3)	38.0 (3.6)	40.4 (3.3)		
14	17.7 (2.6)	19.3 (2.5)	20.8 (2.7)	22.2 (2.8)	23.8 (2.9)	25.3 (2.9)	27.1 (2.9)	28.6 (3.1)	30.3 (3.2)	31.9 (3.1)	33.9 (3.6)	35.7 (3.1)	37.5 (3.0)	40.4 (2.8)	
15	17.6 (2.6)	19.0 (2.4)	20.4 (2.4)	21.7 (2.4)	23.0 (2.4)	24.4 (2.6)	25.7 (2.7)	27.2 (2.7)	28.7 (2.7)	29.9 (2.8)	31.3 (3.1)	33.1 (3.2)	34.6 (3.1)	36.5 (2.9)	38.3 (3.3)

Costa Rica

Birth of order i

Completed parity j	1	2	3	4	5	6	7	8	9	10	11	12	13	14
1	26.0 (5.7)													
2	24.7 (4.5)	28.1 (4.6)												
3	23.5 (4.1)	26.0 (4.1)	28.9 (4.2)											
4	22.6 (3.7)	24.7 (3.8)	26.9 (3.6)	30.0 (3.8)										
5	21.8 (3.8)	24.0 (3.7)	26.2 (3.8)	28.6 (3.9)	31.4 (3.9)									
6	22.4 (3.9)	24.5 (4.0)	26.4 (3.8)	28.6 (3.8)	31.0 (3.8)	33.7 (3.5)								
7	20.5 (3.0)	22.3 (3.3)	24.3 (3.3)	26.2 (3.3)	28.3 (3.3)	30.3 (3.3)	32.6 (3.6)							
8	20.6 (3.0)	22.6 (2.8)	24.5 (2.8)	26.5 (3.0)	28.7 (3.3)	30.5 (3.4)	32.5 (3.4)	34.8 (3.7)						
9	20.0 (2.3)	22.0 (2.3)	23.6 (2.3)	25.4 (2.2)	27.1 (2.4)	29.1 (2.4)	30.9 (2.4)	33.1 (2.4)	35.2 (2.5)					
10	19.9 (2.5)	21.8 (2.3)	23.7 (2.7)	25.5 (2.5)	27.3 (2.4)	29.2 (2.3)	31.3 (2.4)	33.2 (2.6)	35.1 (2.8)	37.2 (2.8)				
11	19.7 (2.3)	21.5 (2.7)	23.0 (2.7)	24.6 (2.7)	26.3 (2.8)	28.0 (2.8)	29.8 (2.8)	31.5 (2.9)	33.3 (2.9)	35.4 (3.0)	37.3 (2.6)			
12	19.3 (2.7)	20.8 (2.8)	22.2 (2.8)	24.0 (2.7)	25.5 (2.6)	27.1 (2.6)	28.8 (2.7)	30.4 (2.8)	32.1 (2.8)	34.0 (2.9)	35.6 (2.9)	37.4 (3.1)		
13	18.2 (1.6)	19.9 (1.9)	21.4 (2.1)	23.0 (2.0)	24.7 (2.2)	26.4 (2.4)	27.7 (2.6)	29.1 (2.6)	30.8 (2.8)	32.7 (2.3)	34.6 (2.5)	36.2 (2.5)	38.3 (2.1)	
14	18.3 (1.5)	19.9 (1.6)	21.3 (1.9)	22.7 (1.9)	24.1 (1.9)	25.5 (1.9)	26.9 (1.9)	28.2 (1.9)	29.5 (1.9)	31.0 (2.1)	32.6 (1.9)	33.9 (2.2)	35.5 (2.1)	37.1 (2.2)

Dominican Republic

Birth of order i

Completed parity j	1	2	3	4	5	6	7	8	9	10	11	12	13	14	15
1	23.8 (6.8)														
2	23.0 (4.9)	26.4 (6.0)													
3	24.1 (5.9)	27.2 (6.1)	30.5 (6.1)												
4	21.1 (4.8)	24.0 (5.3)	28.0 (5.1)	31.7 (5.5)											
5	19.5 (3.0)	22.3 (3.7)	25.3 (4.6)	27.8 (4.9)	31.0 (5.6)										
6	21.3 (4.4)	23.8 (4.8)	26.4 (4.5)	29.2 (4.4)	31.5 (4.4)	34.6 (5.1)									
7	21.7 (4.1)	24.8 (4.9)	26.9 (5.0)	29.4 (5.2)	31.9 (4.8)	34.6 (5.0)	37.6 (5.6)								
8	20.2 (3.9)	22.4 (4.1)	24.7 (4.0)	27.1 (3.8)	29.4 (4.0)	31.7 (4.1)	34.0 (4.2)	37.1 (3.6)							
9	19.9 (3.1)	22.4 (3.1)	24.4 (3.2)	26.7 (3.2)	28.8 (3.0)	31.2 (3.3)	33.3 (3.5)	35.6 (3.4)	37.9 (3.3)						
10	18.3 (2.0)	20.1 (2.4)	22.1 (2.8)	24.1 (3.0)	26.1 (3.2)	28.2 (2.9)	30.5 (2.7)	33.2 (3.1)	35.1 (3.3)	37.6 (3.3)					
11	18.3 (2.6)	20.1 (3.0)	22.1 (2.9)	24.2 (2.9)	26.3 (2.9)	28.0 (3.0)	29.8 (2.9)	32.5 (2.8)	34.3 (2.5)	36.6 (2.5)	39.2 (2.9)				
12	18.1 (3.2)	20.2 (3.5)	22.2 (3.8)	23.9 (3.7)	25.8 (3.8)	27.5 (3.8)	29.3 (3.6)	31.1 (3.5)	32.7 (3.4)	34.9 (3.3)	36.7 (3.3)	38.8 (3.6)			
13	17.8 (2.4)	19.5 (2.3)	21.5 (2.5)	23.6 (2.6)	25.4 (2.4)	27.3 (2.8)	29.1 (3.0)	30.9 (2.8)	32.8 (2.8)	34.3 (2.9)	36.2 (2.8)	37.6 (2.9)	40.1 (2.3)		
14	18.6 (2.9)	20.5 (2.9)	22.2 (3.2)	24.0 (3.9)	26.2 (4.7)	27.7 (4.5)	29.1 (4.4)	30.9 (3.8)	32.9 (4.6)	34.4 (4.2)	35.9 (3.8)	36.8 (3.8)	38.5 (3.8)	40.8 (4.5)	
15	18.5 (3.0)	20.0 (2.9)	21.3 (2.9)	22.7 (2.6)	24.1 (2.7)	25.6 (3.0)	27.8 (2.8)	29.1 (3.1)	30.9 (3.1)	32.3 (3.0)	34.1 (3.3)	35.3 (3.2)	37.0 (3.3)	38.5 (3.4)	40.1 (3.8)

Ecuador

Completed parity j	Birth of order i														
	1	2	3	4	5	6	7	8	9	10	11	12	13	14	15
1	28.6 (6.1)														
2	25.1 (5.8)	29.1 (6.2)													
3	25.1 (4.6)	28.5 (4.5)	32.3 (4.8)												
4	23.2 (4.8)	25.8 (5.0)	29.1 (5.1)	32.9 (5.6)											
5	22.2 (4.1)	24.9 (4.3)	27.5 (4.5)	30.8 (4.4)	34.7 (4.6)										
6	21.9 (4.2)	24.0 (4.5)	26.5 (4.6)	29.2 (4.6)	31.9 (4.6)	35.0 (4.9)									
7	21.3 (3.6)	23.5 (3.2)	25.9 (3.3)	28.1 (3.4)	30.6 (3.5)	32.9 (3.7)	36.3 (3.9)								
8	19.9 (3.6)	22.3 (3.5)	24.5 (3.6)	26.9 (3.8)	29.3 (4.0)	31.7 (4.0)	34.2 (4.2)	37.5 (4.6)							
9	20.0 (3.1)	22.0 (3.3)	24.2 (3.3)	26.5 (3.3)	28.7 (3.5)	31.1 (3.6)	33.3 (3.6)	35.9 (3.8)	38.9 (3.6)						
10	19.4 (3.0)	21.3 (3.1)	23.3 (3.2)	25.3 (3.3)	27.2 (3.5)	29.3 (3.5)	31.3 (3.6)	33.7 (3.6)	36.1 (3.5)	39.0 (3.6)					
11	19.0 (3.1)	21.0 (3.1)	22.9 (2.9)	24.8 (2.8)	26.8 (2.9)	28.6 (3.0)	30.5 (3.1)	32.3 (3.0)	34.3 (3.1)	36.8 (3.3)	39.6 (3.1)				
12	18.3 (3.0)	20.3 (2.8)	22.3 (2.7)	24.0 (2.8)	25.8 (2.7)	27.9 (2.6)	30.0 (2.6)	31.7 (2.7)	33.8 (2.7)	35.7 (2.7)	38.0 (2.5)	40.5 (2.6)			
13	17.0 (2.1)	18.9 (2.0)	20.7 (2.0)	22.6 (2.1)	24.3 (2.1)	26.2 (2.3)	28.2 (2.2)	30.0 (2.3)	31.7 (2.3)	33.8 (2.5)	35.6 (2.7)	37.8 (2.4)	40.8 (3.3)		
14	16.4 (2.1)	18.3 (2.3)	20.0 (2.3)	21.9 (2.3)	23.8 (2.8)	25.5 (2.8)	27.3 (2.9)	29.2 (3.0)	31.2 (2.8)	32.8 (3.1)	35.0 (3.2)	37.0 (3.0)	39.0 (2.8)	41.1 (2.8)	
15	16.6 (2.1)	18.3 (2.6)	19.5 (2.6)	21.0 (2.9)	22.5 (3.0)	23.8 (2.9)	25.1 (2.9)	26.9 (2.9)	28.4 (3.0)	30.2 (2.8)	32.3 (3.2)	34.0 (3.5)	35.5 (3.6)	37.6 (3.8)	39.8 (3.0)

Egypt

Completed parity j	Birth of order i														
	1	2	3	4	5	6	7	8	9	10	11	12	13	14	15
1	25.9 (8.2)														
2	24.5 (5.9)	29.4 (6.3)													
3	23.7 (5.8)	26.7 (5.8)	30.9 (5.8)												
4	21.7 (4.7)	24.6 (5.1)	27.5 (5.2)	31.3 (5.7)											
5	20.9 (3.9)	23.5 (4.0)	26.1 (4.2)	29.0 (4.6)	32.9 (4.8)										
6	20.0 (3.7)	22.4 (3.8)	24.8 (4.0)	27.2 (4.0)	30.0 (4.3)	33.5 (4.5)									
7	19.1 (3.1)	21.3 (3.2)	23.7 (3.4)	26.1 (3.5)	28.7 (3.8)	31.3 (4.0)	34.8 (4.1)								
8	18.5 (3.0)	20.9 (3.5)	23.2 (3.5)	25.5 (3.5)	27.7 (3.5)	30.0 (3.7)	32.8 (3.9)	36.4 (4.2)							
9	18.3 (2.9)	20.4 (3.0)	22.4 (3.3)	24.6 (3.3)	26.7 (3.4)	28.9 (3.5)	31.1 (3.5)	33.7 (3.8)	37.0 (4.0)						
10	17.7 (2.7)	19.6 (2.7)	21.6 (2.7)	23.6 (3.0)	25.7 (3.3)	27.8 (3.5)	29.9 (3.6)	32.1 (3.8)	34.4 (4.0)	37.4 (3.9)					
11	17.5 (2.7)	19.3 (2.6)	21.2 (2.8)	22.9 (2.8)	24.7 (3.1)	26.7 (3.3)	28.6 (3.5)	30.6 (3.8)	32.8 (4.0)	35.3 (4.2)	38.2 (4.2)				
12	17.3 (2.1)	19.1 (2.1)	20.8 (2.2)	22.6 (2.6)	24.5 (2.6)	26.4 (2.7)	28.2 (2.7)	30.2 (2.9)	32.2 (2.8)	34.3 (3.0)	36.6 (3.3)	39.2 (3.5)			
13	16.2 (1.9)	17.6 (2.1)	19.3 (2.3)	21.3 (2.6)	23.2 (2.8)	25.0 (3.1)	27.0 (3.3)	28.6 (3.6)	30.1 (3.7)	31.9 (3.8)	33.5 (4.0)	35.8 (3.8)	38.0 (4.3)		
14	16.9 (2.3)	18.7 (2.7)	20.3 (2.7)	21.9 (3.4)	23.3 (3.7)	24.5 (3.7)	26.3 (3.9)	27.9 (3.8)	30.0 (4.2)	31.3 (4.1)	32.7 (4.4)	34.2 (4.4)	36.6 (4.8)	38.9 (5.1)	
15	15.7 (1.6)	16.8 (1.8)	18.1 (2.0)	19.6 (2.4)	21.5 (3.0)	22.6 (3.1)	24.0 (3.4)	25.3 (3.6)	26.1 (3.5)	27.7 (3.5)	29.3 (3.4)	30.9 (3.2)	32.3 (3.2)	34.3 (3.0)	37.0 (3.7)

222

Fiji

<table>
<tr><td colspan="16">Birth of order i</td></tr>
<tr><td>Completed
parity j</td><td>1</td><td>2</td><td>3</td><td>4</td><td>5</td><td>6</td><td>7</td><td>8</td><td>9</td><td>10</td><td>11</td><td>12</td><td>13</td><td>14</td><td>15</td></tr>
<tr><td>1</td><td>24.4
(6.5)</td><td></td><td></td><td></td><td></td><td></td><td></td><td></td><td></td><td></td><td></td><td></td><td></td><td></td><td></td></tr>
<tr><td>2</td><td>22.6
(4.7)</td><td>27.9
(5.9)</td><td></td><td></td><td></td><td></td><td></td><td></td><td></td><td></td><td></td><td></td><td></td><td></td><td></td></tr>
<tr><td>3</td><td>21.2
(4.1)</td><td>24.6
(4.4)</td><td>30.0
(6.0)</td><td></td><td></td><td></td><td></td><td></td><td></td><td></td><td></td><td></td><td></td><td></td><td></td></tr>
<tr><td>4</td><td>22.5
(4.4)</td><td>25.6
(4.8)</td><td>28.7
(5.3)</td><td>32.7
(5.7)</td><td></td><td></td><td></td><td></td><td></td><td></td><td></td><td></td><td></td><td></td><td></td></tr>
<tr><td>5</td><td>22.1
(4.3)</td><td>24.8
(4.4)</td><td>27.1
(4.6)</td><td>29.7
(4.8)</td><td>33.4
(5.0)</td><td></td><td></td><td></td><td></td><td></td><td></td><td></td><td></td><td></td><td></td></tr>
<tr><td>6</td><td>20.5
(3.8)</td><td>23.2
(4.2)</td><td>25.7
(4.2)</td><td>28.3
(4.3)</td><td>31.2
(4.3)</td><td>34.6
(4.5)</td><td></td><td></td><td></td><td></td><td></td><td></td><td></td><td></td><td></td></tr>
<tr><td>7</td><td>19.7
(3.5)</td><td>22.1
(3.6)</td><td>24.4
(3.8)</td><td>26.9
(4.0)</td><td>29.2
(4.0)</td><td>32.1
(4.0)</td><td>35.2
(4.1)</td><td></td><td></td><td></td><td></td><td></td><td></td><td></td><td></td></tr>
<tr><td>8</td><td>19.4
(3.0)</td><td>21.5
(3.2)</td><td>23.8
(3.4)</td><td>26.2
(3.4)</td><td>28.3
(3.5)</td><td>30.5
(3.5)</td><td>33.1
(3.7)</td><td>36.3
(3.8)</td><td></td><td></td><td></td><td></td><td></td><td></td><td></td></tr>
<tr><td>9</td><td>18.6
(3.4)</td><td>20.6
(3.4)</td><td>22.7
(3.5)</td><td>24.9
(3.8)</td><td>27.1
(3.7)</td><td>29.2
(3.8)</td><td>31.7
(4.1)</td><td>34.0
(4.3)</td><td>37.4
(4.5)</td><td></td><td></td><td></td><td></td><td></td><td></td></tr>
<tr><td>10</td><td>18.0
(3.1)</td><td>20.1
(3.1)</td><td>22.1
(3.1)</td><td>23.9
(3.3)</td><td>25.8
(3.6)</td><td>27.8
(3.6)</td><td>30.0
(3.1)</td><td>32.2
(3.5)</td><td>34.7
(3.8)</td><td>37.7
(4.4)</td><td></td><td></td><td></td><td></td><td></td></tr>
<tr><td>11</td><td>17.3
(3.0)</td><td>19.4
(3.0)</td><td>21.4
(3.2)</td><td>23.3
(3.1)</td><td>25.0
(3.3)</td><td>26.8
(3.5)</td><td>28.8
(3.4)</td><td>31.1
(3.5)</td><td>33.1
(3.7)</td><td>35.2
(3.7)</td><td>37.8
(4.0)</td><td></td><td></td><td></td><td></td></tr>
<tr><td>12</td><td>17.3
(2.9)</td><td>19.5
(3.0)</td><td>21.4
(3.1)</td><td>23.4
(2.9)</td><td>25.3
(3.4)</td><td>27.0
(3.1)</td><td>28.9
(3.2)</td><td>30.6
(3.3)</td><td>32.5
(3.1)</td><td>34.1
(3.2)</td><td>36.2
(3.5)</td><td>38.8
(3.7)</td><td></td><td></td><td></td></tr>
<tr><td>13</td><td>17.2
(2.4)</td><td>18.9
(2.5)</td><td>20.2
(2.4)</td><td>21.7
(2.2)</td><td>23.7
(2.4)</td><td>25.9
(2.1)</td><td>28.3
(3.2)</td><td>29.9
(2.7)</td><td>32.0
(3.1)</td><td>33.2
(2.7)</td><td>34.6
(2.9)</td><td>36.7
(2.9)</td><td>38.3
(2.5)</td><td></td><td></td></tr>
<tr><td>14</td><td>18.3
(2.3)</td><td>19.7
(2.4)</td><td>21.8
(2.8)</td><td>24.0
(3.1)</td><td>25.7
(2.8)</td><td>27.0
(2.8)</td><td>28.2
(2.9)</td><td>29.7
(3.0)</td><td>31.4
(2.8)</td><td>32.8
(2.9)</td><td>34.1
(3.0)</td><td>36.1
(3.4)</td><td>37.6
(3.2)</td><td>40.0
(3.1)</td><td></td></tr>
<tr><td>15</td><td>16.0
(2.2)</td><td>17.9
(2.5)</td><td>19.2
(2.7)</td><td>20.9
(1.9)</td><td>23.0
(1.6)</td><td>24.2
(1.5)</td><td>25.6
(1.1)</td><td>27.5
(1.7)</td><td>29.1
(1.7)</td><td>30.6
(1.6)</td><td>32.3
(2.5)</td><td>33.7
(2.9)</td><td>35.1
(2.7)</td><td>36.6
(2.8)</td><td>38.8
(2.8)</td></tr>
</table>

Ghana

<table>
<tr><td colspan="14">Birth of order i</td></tr>
<tr><td>Completed
parity j</td><td>1</td><td>2</td><td>3</td><td>4</td><td>5</td><td>6</td><td>7</td><td>8</td><td>9</td><td>10</td><td>11</td><td>12</td><td>13</td></tr>
<tr><td>1</td><td>24.1
(6.8)</td><td></td><td></td><td></td><td></td><td></td><td></td><td></td><td></td><td></td><td></td><td></td><td></td></tr>
<tr><td>2</td><td>24.2
(6.7)</td><td>29.1
(6.7)</td><td></td><td></td><td></td><td></td><td></td><td></td><td></td><td></td><td></td><td></td><td></td></tr>
<tr><td>3</td><td>24.1
(5.7)</td><td>27.7
(5.8)</td><td>32.3
(6.1)</td><td></td><td></td><td></td><td></td><td></td><td></td><td></td><td></td><td></td><td></td></tr>
<tr><td>4</td><td>23.4
(4.6)</td><td>26.7
(4.5)</td><td>30.8
(4.7)</td><td>35.5
(4.9)</td><td></td><td></td><td></td><td></td><td></td><td></td><td></td><td></td><td></td></tr>
<tr><td>5</td><td>22.0
(4.6)</td><td>25.3
(4.7)</td><td>28.5
(4.9)</td><td>32.2
(4.9)</td><td>35.8
(5.1)</td><td></td><td></td><td></td><td></td><td></td><td></td><td></td><td></td></tr>
<tr><td>6</td><td>21.3
(4.2)</td><td>24.4
(4.4)</td><td>27.5
(4.5)</td><td>30.9
(4.4)</td><td>34.1
(4.4)</td><td>37.8
(4.4)</td><td></td><td></td><td></td><td></td><td></td><td></td><td></td></tr>
<tr><td>7</td><td>20.2
(3.4)</td><td>22.8
(3.6)</td><td>26.0
(3.8)</td><td>28.7
(4.0)</td><td>31.7
(4.0)</td><td>34.7
(4.1)</td><td>38.3
(3.9)</td><td></td><td></td><td></td><td></td><td></td><td></td></tr>
<tr><td>8</td><td>19.8
(3.1)</td><td>22.5
(3.2)</td><td>25.2
(3.3)</td><td>27.9
(3.4)</td><td>30.5
(3.6)</td><td>33.2
(3.6)</td><td>36.0
(3.5)</td><td>39.0
(3.5)</td><td></td><td></td><td></td><td></td><td></td></tr>
<tr><td>9</td><td>19.2
(3.1)</td><td>21.8
(3.2)</td><td>24.3
(3.1)</td><td>26.9
(3.2)</td><td>29.5
(3.5)</td><td>32.1
(3.5)</td><td>34.7
(3.4)</td><td>37.4
(3.4)</td><td>40.4
(3.4)</td><td></td><td></td><td></td><td></td></tr>
<tr><td>10</td><td>18.6
(2.8)</td><td>20.7
(3.1)</td><td>23.0
(2.9)</td><td>25.4
(3.0)</td><td>28.0
(3.2)</td><td>30.7
(3.5)</td><td>33.0
(3.6)</td><td>35.6
(3.6)</td><td>38.2
(3.4)</td><td>40.8
(3.4)</td><td></td><td></td><td></td></tr>
<tr><td>11</td><td>18.2
(2.9)</td><td>20.5
(3.4)</td><td>22.7
(3.4)</td><td>24.9
(3.9)</td><td>27.2
(4.1)</td><td>29.6
(4.4)</td><td>31.8
(4.5)</td><td>34.2
(4.0)</td><td>36.6
(4.1)</td><td>38.9
(3.9)</td><td>41.3
(3.6)</td><td></td><td></td></tr>
<tr><td>12</td><td>18.5
(4.7)</td><td>21.3
(4.7)</td><td>23.6
(4.5)</td><td>25.5
(4.7)</td><td>27.3
(4.8)</td><td>29.0
(4.7)</td><td>30.8
(4.2)</td><td>32.4
(4.1)</td><td>34.3
(3.9)</td><td>36.3
(4.3)</td><td>39.5
(4.3)</td><td>41.4
(5.0)</td><td></td></tr>
<tr><td>13</td><td>16.8
(1.8)</td><td>18.3
(1.9)</td><td>20.2
(2.0)</td><td>23.0
(3.3)</td><td>24.7
(3.2)</td><td>26.1
(3.7)</td><td>28.0
(3.7)</td><td>30.3
(3.8)</td><td>32.8
(3.7)</td><td>35.0
(3.5)</td><td>36.8
(3.5)</td><td>39.7
(2.7)</td><td>41.6
(2.7)</td></tr>
</table>

Guyana

Birth of order i

Completed parity j	1	2	3	4	5	6	7	8	9	10	11	12	13	14	15
1	23.5 (7.5)														
2	22.8 (5.8)	26.8 (7.3)													
3	22.9 (5.6)	25.8 (6.4)	30.3 (6.6)												
4	21.3 (3.8)	23.5 (4.1)	26.5 (4.3)	30.8 (5.8)											
5	21.5 (3.9)	24.3 (4.3)	26.6 (4.7)	29.5 (5.2)	33.6 (5.7)										
6	20.7 (3.7)	23.3 (4.0)	25.7 (4.1)	28.0 (4.1)	30.7 (4.3)	34.1 (4.6)									
7	20.3 (3.3)	22.8 (3.6)	25.1 (3.6)	27.4 (3.7)	29.8 (3.9)	32.3 (4.5)	35.3 (4.6)								
8	19.2 (3.4)	21.5 (3.7)	23.6 (3.7)	25.5 (3.8)	27.7 (4.0)	29.8 (4.0)	32.2 (4.0)	35.2 (4.3)							
9	18.4 (2.2)	20.6 (2.8)	22.9 (2.8)	25.0 (3.1)	27.1 (3.2)	39.8 (9.9)	42.0 (9.9)	44.5 (9.9)	47.3 (9.9)						
10	19.3 (2.4)	21.4 (2.5)	23.1 (2.6)	25.0 (2.4)	26.8 (2.3)	29.0 (2.4)	31.0 (2.5)	33.1 (2.7)	35.3 (2.8)	37.9 (3.0)					
11	17.7 (2.4)	20.2 (2.5)	22.2 (2.5)	23.9 (2.3)	25.8 (2.5)	27.9 (2.3)	30.0 (2.5)	31.8 (2.5)	33.8 (2.8)	36.2 (2.8)	38.3 (2.9)				
12	17.5 (2.3)	19.3 (2.3)	21.4 (2.4)	23.1 (2.5)	24.8 (2.6)	26.5 (2.5)	28.4 (2.4)	30.3 (2.6)	32.3 (2.4)	34.1 (2.2)	36.2 (2.4)	38.4 (2.4)			
13	17.2 (1.7)	19.0 (1.5)	20.6 (1.5)	22.4 (2.1)	23.9 (2.2)	25.5 (2.5)	27.4 (2.6)	28.9 (2.7)	30.7 (2.7)	32.3 (2.7)	34.0 (3.1)	35.9 (3.2)	38.2 (3.6)		
14	18.2 (2.5)	19.9 (2.3)	21.6 (2.4)	23.2 (2.2)	24.9 (2.5)	26.3 (2.5)	27.7 (2.5)	29.2 (2.6)	30.7 (2.7)	32.6 (3.4)	34.9 (3.6)	36.5 (2.8)	38.2 (2.8)	40.4 (2.8)	
15	17.9 (1.1)	19.7 (1.2)	21.2 (1.0)	22.8 (1.6)	24.2 (1.7)	25.1 (1.7)	26.6 (1.5)	28.0 (1.8)	29.3 (2.1)	30.6 (2.4)	31.8 (2.3)	32.9 (2.9)	34.0 (3.2)	35.4 (3.3)	36.8 (3.9)

Haiti

Birth of order i

Completed parity j	1	2	3	4	5	6	7	8	9	10	11	12	13
1	24.3 (7.9)												
2	25.1 (6.5)	30.5 (7.1)											
3	24.7 (4.9)	28.0 (4.6)	32.5 (5.4)										
4	24.2 (5.0)	27.1 (4.7)	30.1 (5.1)	34.0 (5.4)									
5	23.0 (5.3)	25.9 (5.0)	28.8 (5.3)	32.1 (5.4)	35.6 (5.3)								
6	22.7 (4.6)	25.5 (4.6)	28.3 (4.9)	30.9 (5.0)	33.5 (5.1)	37.4 (5.3)							
7	21.6 (3.8)	24.4 (3.7)	27.1 (4.0)	29.5 (4.0)	32.1 (4.2)	34.8 (3.9)	37.9 (4.2)						
8	22.1 (3.3)	24.4 (3.2)	26.7 (3.4)	29.0 (3.5)	31.2 (3.7)	33.7 (3.7)	36.5 (3.8)	39.7 (3.5)					
9	21.0 (3.3)	23.0 (3.3)	25.5 (3.7)	27.6 (3.5)	30.0 (3.6)	32.5 (3.9)	34.6 (4.0)	36.9 (4.1)	40.4 (4.1)				
10	20.6 (2.8)	22.9 (2.8)	25.1 (2.9)	27.1 (3.1)	29.2 (3.3)	31.2 (3.3)	33.6 (3.4)	36.1 (3.6)	38.2 (3.9)	41.3 (3.5)			
11	20.8 (3.4)	22.5 (3.4)	24.5 (3.6)	26.7 (3.5)	28.5 (3.3)	30.6 (3.2)	32.5 (3.3)	34.8 (3.3)	37.0 (3.4)	39.1 (3.4)	41.9 (3.2)		
12	19.7 (3.6)	22.4 (2.2)	24.1 (2.0)	25.6 (2.1)	27.2 (2.0)	29.2 (2.3)	31.6 (3.2)	33.5 (3.1)	35.2 (3.1)	36.9 (2.8)	38.9 (2.9)	41.3 (3.0)	
13	17.8 (1.7)	19.6 (.9)	22.2 (1.2)	24.5 (.2)	26.8 (1.4)	29.7 (1.6)	30.6 (2.8)	32.8 (2.5)	34.6 (2.5)	36.5 (2.0)	37.6 (1.8)	39.3 (.9)	41.1 (.5)

Indonesia

Completed parity j	Birth of order i														
	1	2	3	4	5	6	7	8	9	10	11	12	13	14	15
1	23.1 (7.0)														
2	21.9 (5.7)	27.0 (6.7)													
3	21.9 (5.2)	25.9 (5.6)	30.6 (6.3)												
4	20.6 (4.9)	24.1 (5.0)	27.9 (5.2)	32.2 (5.7)											
5	20.3 (4.6)	23.7 (4.7)	27.1 (5.1)	30.4 (5.0)	34.3 (5.2)										
6	20.2 (3.9)	23.3 (4.1)	26.2 (4.3)	29.2 (4.6)	32.1 (4.7)	35.5 (4.8)									
7	19.6 (3.5)	22.4 (3.7)	25.1 (3.8)	27.7 (3.8)	30.4 (3.8)	33.1 (3.7)	36.4 (4.0)								
8	18.7 (3.3)	21.2 (3.4)	23.8 (3.7)	26.5 (3.8)	29.2 (4.0)	31.9 (4.0)	34.6 (4.0)	37.9 (4.2)							
9	18.2 (3.2)	20.6 (3.1)	23.1 (3.2)	25.3 (3.5)	27.8 (3.6)	30.4 (3.7)	32.8 (3.8)	35.2 (3.7)	38.3 (3.9)						
10	17.8 (3.0)	20.0 (3.0)	22.1 (3.2)	24.2 (3.2)	26.4 (3.2)	28.7 (3.6)	30.8 (3.7)	33.1 (3.8)	35.7 (3.9)	38.4 (4.1)					
11	17.3 (2.9)	19.6 (2.9)	21.9 (3.3)	24.0 (3.3)	25.9 (3.2)	28.0 (3.5)	29.8 (3.3)	32.3 (3.3)	34.7 (3.4)	37.1 (3.1)	39.7 (3.1)				
12	16.7 (2.4)	18.9 (2.0)	20.9 (2.2)	23.1 (2.6)	25.2 (3.0)	27.6 (3.4)	29.6 (3.4)	31.5 (3.5)	33.3 (3.4)	35.1 (3.5)	37.2 (3.5)	39.3 (3.5)			
13	16.8 (2.2)	18.5 (2.6)	20.7 (3.0)	23.2 (3.3)	24.9 (3.4)	27.2 (3.4)	29.2 (3.4)	30.8 (3.3)	32.1 (3.5)	33.8 (3.7)	35.4 (4.5)	38.1 (4.8)	40.5 (4.5)		
14	15.2 (2.5)	16.9 (2.2)	17.9 (2.6)	18.7 (3.3)	20.2 (3.6)	21.6 (4.1)	22.7 (3.9)	24.6 (4.5)	25.9 (5.0)	27.3 (5.6)	28.9 (6.4)	30.4 (6.9)	31.4 (6.8)	33.7 (8.2)	
15	16.6 (3.6)	18.8 (3.6)	20.2 (3.0)	23.2 (3.5)	24.7 (3.1)	26.9 (3.5)	28.3 (3.4)	29.7 (3.1)	31.7 (2.5)	32.6 (2.8)	34.0 (2.5)	36.4 (2.4)	37.2 (2.3)	38.4 (1.8)	42.2 (2.4)

Ivory Coast

Completed parity j	Birth of order i														
	1	2	3	4	5	6	7	8	9	10	11	12	13	14	15
1	23.5 (7.0)														
2	22.8 (5.7)	27.6 (6.7)													
3	23.5 (6.5)	26.6 (6.9)	30.6 (6.5)												
4	21.5 (4.5)	25.5 (5.1)	29.1 (5.2)	33.8 (4.9)											
5	20.9 (4.0)	24.2 (4.4)	27.6 (4.7)	31.4 (4.9)	35.9 (5.1)										
6	21.1 (4.4)	24.2 (4.8)	27.1 (4.8)	30.0 (4.8)	33.0 (4.8)	36.7 (4.3)									
7	20.4 (3.5)	23.2 (3.8)	26.0 (3.9)	28.8 (4.1)	31.7 (4.2)	34.5 (4.5)	37.7 (4.3)								
8	19.9 (3.2)	22.5 (3.3)	25.3 (3.3)	27.9 (3.5)	30.7 (3.5)	33.4 (3.5)	36.1 (3.7)	39.3 (3.8)							
9	19.2 (3.2)	21.8 (3.3)	24.4 (3.4)	26.8 (3.4)	29.3 (3.6)	31.8 (3.7)	34.2 (3.7)	36.8 (3.5)	39.8 (3.6)						
10	18.2 (2.6)	20.5 (2.7)	22.8 (2.7)	25.1 (2.9)	27.5 (3.3)	30.0 (3.6)	32.6 (3.7)	35.0 (3.6)	37.4 (3.6)	40.4 (3.5)					
11	18.2 (2.9)	20.4 (3.0)	22.5 (3.2)	24.8 (3.4)	27.2 (3.4)	29.7 (3.4)	31.4 (3.3)	33.7 (3.6)	36.1 (3.6)	38.5 (3.6)	41.2 (3.7)				
12	18.0 (2.5)	20.0 (3.0)	22.1 (3.2)	24.3 (3.4)	26.3 (3.1)	28.1 (3.3)	30.3 (3.3)	32.4 (3.3)	34.4 (2.9)	36.5 (3.2)	38.7 (3.0)	41.1 (3.3)			
13	17.4 (3.0)	19.6 (2.7)	21.6 (2.9)	23.5 (2.7)	25.7 (2.8)	28.1 (2.7)	30.3 (2.9)	31.8 (2.7)	33.5 (2.4)	35.5 (3.2)	37.2 (3.0)	39.4 (3.0)	41.3 (3.5)		
14	16.5 (1.5)	19.1 (1.8)	20.8 (2.0)	22.6 (2.1)	24.3 (2.2)	26.2 (2.1)	28.4 (2.6)	30.3 (2.8)	32.5 (2.8)	34.0 (2.5)	36.4 (2.2)	39.0 (2.3)	41.3 (2.0)	44.0 (2.0)	
15	17.8 (1.9)	19.8 (1.5)	21.2 (1.8)	22.2 (2.3)	23.8 (3.0)	25.3 (3.9)	26.7 (3.2)	29.5 (1.9)	31.3 (2.6)	33.1 (2.4)	35.4 (2.9)	37.0 (2.6)	38.8 (3.4)	40.2 (3.5)	40.6 (2.9)

Jamaica

Birth of order i

Completed parity j	1	2	3	4	5	6	7	8	9	10	11	12	13	14	15
1	23.5 (6.4)														
2	22.7 (5.7)	28.1 (6.2)													
3	22.8 (5.4)	27.0 (5.8)	30.2 (6.4)												
4	21.7 (4.9)	24.9 (4.9)	27.9 (5.1)	32.4 (5.5)											
5	21.4 (4.4)	24.6 (4.4)	27.4 (4.3)	30.1 (4.7)	33.4 (5.0)										
6	21.9 (4.4)	24.7 (4.3)	27.4 (4.1)	30.4 (3.8)	32.9 (4.0)	36.3 (4.2)									
7	21.1 (4.1)	24.0 (4.0)	26.6 (3.8)	29.1 (3.7)	31.2 (3.9)	33.9 (3.8)	37.1 (4.1)								
8	20.7 (3.5)	23.0 (3.5)	25.4 (3.6)	27.8 (3.5)	29.8 (3.6)	32.0 (3.8)	34.6 (4.1)	37.4 (4.0)							
9	20.3 (3.6)	22.6 (3.5)	24.8 (3.7)	26.8 (3.7)	29.0 (3.6)	31.4 (3.6)	33.5 (3.8)	35.6 (3.8)	38.2 (4.0)						
10	18.7 (2.9)	21.5 (3.3)	23.4 (3.6)	25.4 (3.7)	27.1 (3.7)	29.2 (3.7)	31.4 (3.6)	33.3 (3.6)	35.4 (3.6)	38.0 (3.8)					
11	19.0 (3.1)	21.5 (2.7)	23.4 (2.4)	25.5 (2.5)	27.5 (2.5)	29.6 (2.6)	31.5 (2.6)	33.2 (2.5)	34.9 (2.4)	37.0 (2.2)	39.6 (2.6)				
12	19.2 (2.7)	20.9 (2.7)	22.8 (2.6)	24.4 (2.7)	26.4 (2.5)	28.3 (2.4)	30.3 (2.9)	31.8 (2.9)	33.7 (2.9)	35.5 (3.0)	37.5 (3.4)	40.2 (3.9)			
13	18.9 (2.9)	20.6 (2.9)	22.5 (2.4)	24.1 (2.0)	25.9 (2.1)	27.5 (2.3)	30.1 (2.1)	31.2 (1.9)	32.7 (2.1)	34.3 (1.9)	37.0 (1.7)	38.5 (1.8)	42.1 (2.6)		
14	15.8 (2.5)	17.3 (2.9)	19.8 (3.2)	21.9 (3.3)	24.2 (3.3)	25.7 (3.2)	27.6 (3.1)	30.0 (2.0)	31.4 (2.1)	33.2 (1.7)	34.9 (1.6)	36.6 (2.0)	39.2 (2.7)	41.6 (2.8)	
15	17.0 (2.4)	18.4 (1.4)	19.9 (2.0)	21.6 (1.6)	23.2 (2.2)	24.6 (2.6)	26.3 (2.0)	28.1 (2.2)	29.5 (2.6)	30.6 (2.9)	32.6 (3.2)	33.1 (3.2)	34.1 (3.3)	35.3 (3.1)	36.2 (3.4)

Jordan

Birth of order i

Completed parity j	1	2	3	4	5	6	7	8	9	10	11	12	13	14	15
1	23.5 (8.4)														
2	27.2 (7.2)	30.4 (7.3)													
3	22.9 (3.8)	25.0 (4.1)	28.9 (5.1)												
4	23.6 (5.8)	25.4 (5.8)	28.8 (6.0)	32.5 (6.1)											
5	22.8 (5.1)	25.1 (5.0)	27.4 (4.9)	30.5 (4.5)	34.2 (4.7)										
6	22.0 (5.1)	24.3 (5.4)	26.5 (5.1)	29.0 (4.9)	31.7 (4.9)	34.3 (4.9)									
7	20.5 (3.7)	22.5 (3.7)	25.3 (3.7)	27.6 (3.6)	30.3 (3.4)	32.9 (3.4)	36.5 (3.8)								
8	19.5 (3.5)	21.5 (3.6)	23.7 (3.7)	26.0 (3.7)	28.1 (3.7)	30.6 (3.6)	33.1 (4.0)	36.4 (4.0)							
9	19.5 (3.5)	21.6 (3.5)	23.7 (3.5)	25.7 (3.4)	27.8 (3.4)	29.9 (3.4)	32.0 (3.5)	34.3 (3.3)	37.3 (3.3)						
10	19.1 (3.2)	21.0 (3.2)	23.0 (3.1)	25.4 (3.2)	27.3 (3.2)	29.4 (3.0)	31.4 (2.9)	33.6 (2.7)	35.9 (2.8)	38.5 (2.8)					
11	18.7 (3.2)	20.4 (3.2)	22.3 (3.2)	24.5 (3.1)	26.6 (3.0)	28.7 (2.9)	30.8 (2.7)	33.1 (2.6)	35.1 (2.6)	37.4 (2.7)	40.1 (2.8)				
12	18.1 (2.9)	20.0 (2.9)	21.7 (3.0)	23.8 (3.0)	25.8 (3.1)	27.7 (2.9)	29.5 (2.8)	31.4 (3.0)	33.3 (2.9)	35.4 (3.1)	37.5 (2.8)	40.0 (2.6)			
13	17.4 (2.9)	19.0 (3.0)	20.6 (3.0)	22.2 (3.0)	24.1 (3.1)	25.8 (3.2)	27.5 (3.0)	29.4 (3.1)	31.0 (3.2)	32.7 (3.1)	35.1 (2.4)	37.2 (2.3)	39.6 (2.5)		
14	16.2 (2.0)	17.9 (2.2)	19.5 (2.3)	21.6 (2.6)	23.5 (2.8)	25.2 (2.7)	27.0 (2.9)	28.7 (2.9)	30.5 (2.8)	32.3 (2.9)	34.0 (3.0)	36.1 (3.1)	38.2 (2.7)	40.0 (2.9)	
15	16.5 (1.9)	18.1 (1.9)	19.6 (2.0)	21.3 (2.0)	22.8 (2.1)	24.2 (2.2)	25.5 (2.3)	27.3 (1.9)	28.8 (2.1)	30.3 (2.3)	32.2 (2.5)	33.9 (2.8)	35.7 (2.9)	37.7 (3.3)	39.2 (3.5)

Kenya

Birth of order i

Completed parity j	1	2	3	4	5	6	7	8	9	10	11	12	13	14	15
1	25.5 (7.1)														
2	23.1 (7.1)	26.6 (7.0)													
3	23.2 (6.7)	27.4 (7.0)	31.5 (7.5)												
4	24.0 (6.0)	27.4 (5.6)	30.9 (5.7)	34.5 (5.3)											
5	23.0 (5.5)	25.2 (5.5)	28.7 (5.8)	31.6 (5.9)	35.8 (5.7)										
6	21.6 (4.5)	24.2 (4.7)	26.9 (4.8)	29.7 (4.7)	33.0 (4.6)	36.5 (4.6)									
7	21.2 (4.4)	24.1 (4.4)	27.0 (4.6)	29.9 (4.7)	32.8 (4.4)	35.7 (4.4)	39.1 (4.5)								
8	19.9 (3.6)	22.3 (3.4)	24.9 (3.6)	27.4 (3.9)	30.0 (3.7)	32.8 (3.8)	35.5 (3.9)	38.6 (4.1)							
9	19.7 (3.3)	22.2 (3.5)	24.5 (3.4)	27.2 (3.4)	29.6 (3.3)	31.9 (3.4)	34.5 (3.5)	36.9 (3.5)	40.0 (3.6)						
10	19.6 (4.0)	22.0 (3.9)	24.4 (4.1)	26.7 (4.1)	29.0 (4.1)	31.2 (4.1)	33.4 (4.0)	35.6 (4.1)	38.0 (3.9)	40.8 (3.8)					
11	18.5 (3.2)	20.6 (3.3)	22.6 (3.3)	24.9 (3.2)	27.0 (3.6)	29.2 (3.3)	31.3 (3.3)	33.4 (3.3)	35.7 (3.1)	38.0 (3.2)	40.7 (3.2)				
12	17.9 (2.5)	20.0 (2.7)	21.9 (2.9)	23.9 (2.9)	26.0 (2.9)	28.0 (2.9)	29.9 (2.7)	32.1 (2.5)	34.1 (2.5)	36.3 (2.6)	38.9 (2.7)	41.5 (3.0)			
13	17.6 (2.7)	19.7 (3.2)	21.9 (3.0)	24.0 (2.8)	26.2 (3.3)	28.3 (3.2)	30.5 (3.3)	32.6 (3.2)	34.3 (3.3)	36.3 (2.8)	38.3 (2.6)	40.7 (2.5)	42.8 (2.4)		
14	18.4 (2.1)	20.0 (2.1)	21.6 (2.4)	23.5 (2.6)	25.4 (2.5)	26.8 (2.7)	28.7 (2.9)	30.8 (2.6)	32.6 (2.7)	34.3 (2.7)	36.8 (2.4)	38.7 (2.3)	40.6 (2.7)	43.3 (3.3)	
15	18.3 (2.7)	20.0 (2.5)	21.5 (2.5)	23.0 (3.2)	24.6 (3.8)	26.5 (4.1)	28.6 (3.9)	30.4 (3.9)	32.0 (3.5)	33.8 (3.9)	35.5 (3.0)	36.8 (3.1)	38.5 (3.5)	40.3 (3.6)	42.6 (3.7)

Republic of Korea

Birth of order i

Completed parity j	1	2	3	4	5	6	7	8	9	10	11	12	13
1	25.2 (7.1)												
2	23.7 (5.0)	28.1 (6.1)											
3	22.7 (3.4)	26.5 (3.8)	30.7 (4.7)										
4	22.5 (3.2)	25.9 (3.3)	29.3 (3.6)	33.2 (4.1)									
5	21.5 (2.7)	24.7 (2.9)	27.7 (2.9)	30.7 (3.2)	34.2 (3.6)								
6	20.8 (2.5)	23.8 (2.6)	26.5 (2.6)	29.4 (2.7)	32.2 (3.0)	35.5 (3.3)							
7	20.0 (2.1)	22.7 (2.2)	25.7 (2.4)	28.3 (2.5)	31.0 (2.7)	33.7 (2.8)	37.0 (3.2)						
8	19.3 (1.9)	22.1 (2.0)	24.8 (2.3)	27.4 (2.3)	30.0 (2.3)	32.7 (2.5)	35.4 (2.7)	38.6 (2.9)					
9	19.2 (1.9)	21.8 (2.0)	24.4 (2.1)	27.0 (2.0)	29.6 (2.1)	32.0 (2.1)	34.5 (1.9)	37.0 (1.9)	39.7 (2.0)				
10	18.5 (1.7)	21.0 (1.7)	23.5 (2.0)	26.0 (2.1)	28.6 (2.3)	30.8 (2.5)	33.2 (2.6)	35.7 (2.8)	38.6 (2.4)	41.3 (2.7)			
11	18.3 (.9)	20.4 (1.1)	22.6 (1.5)	25.1 (1.8)	27.5 (1.6)	29.3 (1.6)	31.5 (1.6)	33.8 (1.9)	36.1 (2.4)	38.6 (2.4)	41.5 (2.5)		
12	17.4 (1.7)	19.8 (2.0)	22.1 (1.9)	24.5 (2.5)	26.3 (2.0)	28.2 (2.3)	30.8 (2.1)	33.4 (1.7)	35.3 (2.2)	37.6 (2.6)	41.2 (2.0)	42.9 (2.1)	
13	18.4 (1.8)	20.2 (1.9)	21.9 (2.8)	23.8 (2.7)	25.7 (3.2)	28.3 (3.3)	31.0 (2.4)	32.9 (2.6)	35.1 (2.2)	36.9 (2.7)	38.5 (3.7)	40.5 (4.1)	42.7 (4.7)

Lesotho

Birth of order i

Completed parity j	1	2	3	4	5	6	7	8	9	10	11	12	13
1	22.5 (6.0)												
2	23.5 (5.8)	28.2 (6.6)											
3	22.7 (5.1)	26.5 (5.8)	30.8 (6.3)										
4	23.1 (4.1)	26.7 (4.4)	30.2 (4.7)	34.2 (5.0)									
5	21.6 (4.3)	25.2 (4.5)	28.8 (4.8)	32.4 (5.0)	36.2 (5.0)								
6	21.2 (3.4)	24.2 (3.5)	27.4 (3.3)	30.8 (3.2)	34.1 (3.5)	37.7 (3.6)							
7	21.0 (3.1)	24.0 (3.1)	26.8 (3.3)	30.0 (3.6)	32.8 (3.7)	35.5 (3.9)	39.2 (4.1)						
8	20.3 (2.8)	22.8 (2.7)	25.3 (2.8)	28.0 (2.8)	30.9 (3.0)	33.7 (3.0)	36.4 (2.8)	39.5 (2.7)					
9	19.2 (2.3)	21.7 (2.4)	24.6 (2.8)	27.2 (2.9)	29.7 (2.7)	32.1 (2.6)	34.7 (2.6)	37.7 (2.7)	40.4 (2.2)				
10	18.3 (2.2)	20.8 (2.5)	23.4 (2.9)	25.8 (3.2)	28.3 (3.1)	30.8 (2.6)	33.2 (2.5)	35.7 (2.6)	38.2 (2.5)	41.1 (2.8)			
11	18.3 (2.0)	20.7 (2.1)	22.9 (2.0)	25.1 (2.4)	27.3 (2.6)	29.5 (2.2)	31.9 (2.2)	34.1 (2.5)	36.7 (2.3)	39.0 (3.0)	42.2 (3.1)		
12	19.0 (2.2)	22.7 (1.7)	25.0 (1.7)	26.8 (2.0)	28.2 (1.8)	29.4 (1.8)	31.3 (2.1)	33.2 (2.1)	35.1 (2.6)	37.4 (2.6)	39.7 (3.0)	41.8 (2.8)	
13	20.2 (1.1)	22.6 (.9)	25.3 (1.2)	27.4 (1.2)	29.1 (1.5)	31.3 (1.4)	33.2 (1.4)	34.2 (1.7)	35.9 (2.5)	37.5 (3.0)	40.2 (2.0)	41.9 (1.8)	44.0 (1.5)

Malaysia

Birth of order i

Completed parity j	1	2	3	4	5	6	7	8	9	10	11	12	13	14	15
1	24.6 (7.9)														
2	23.8 (7.0)	29.6 (6.3)													
3	21.8 (5.5)	25.2 (5.6)	30.0 (5.8)												
4	20.8 (4.4)	23.9 (4.6)	27.3 (4.8)	32.0 (5.2)											
5	20.4 (3.9)	23.1 (3.9)	26.0 (4.1)	28.9 (4.3)	32.9 (4.6)										
6	20.1 (3.6)	22.6 (3.6)	25.2 (3.8)	27.9 (3.9)	30.9 (4.0)	34.8 (4.3)									
7	19.8 (3.3)	22.1 (3.4)	24.4 (3.5)	26.9 (3.6)	29.5 (3.7)	32.3 (3.8)	36.0 (4.2)								
8	19.2 (3.1)	21.3 (3.0)	23.8 (3.1)	26.0 (3.2)	28.4 (3.3)	30.9 (3.5)	33.4 (3.5)	36.8 (3.8)							
9	18.8 (3.2)	21.1 (3.1)	23.3 (3.2)	25.4 (3.3)	27.6 (3.4)	29.9 (3.3)	32.3 (3.3)	34.7 (3.6)	37.8 (3.8)						
10	18.6 (2.9)	20.6 (2.8)	22.7 (2.9)	24.8 (3.0)	27.0 (3.0)	29.2 (3.2)	31.3 (3.3)	33.4 (3.5)	35.7 (3.6)	38.7 (3.7)					
11	18.0 (3.3)	20.2 (2.5)	22.4 (2.6)	24.5 (2.6)	26.7 (2.6)	28.7 (2.6)	30.6 (2.6)	32.7 (2.6)	34.8 (2.8)	37.2 (2.8)	40.0 (2.9)				
12	18.0 (2.1)	19.7 (2.0)	21.6 (1.9)	23.4 (2.2)	25.4 (2.3)	27.1 (2.5)	28.9 (2.7)	30.6 (2.7)	32.5 (2.7)	34.4 (2.9)	36.4 (2.9)	39.1 (3.2)			
13	18.2 (2.3)	20.3 (2.4)	22.0 (2.4)	23.9 (2.3)	25.4 (2.4)	27.3 (2.1)	29.0 (2.2)	30.7 (2.2)	32.5 (2.4)	34.1 (2.4)	36.4 (2.5)	38.2 (2.7)	41.0 (2.6)		
14	18.8 (3.6)	19.9 (3.6)	21.8 (2.3)	23.4 (2.8)	25.3 (2.8)	26.6 (2.7)	28.4 (2.4)	29.6 (2.3)	31.2 (2.4)	33.1 (2.7)	34.5 (2.9)	35.8 (3.0)	37.8 (3.3)	39.6 (3.8)	
15	17.9 (1.5)	19.4 (2.0)	21.1 (2.2)	22.9 (2.6)	24.1 (2.5)	25.3 (2.6)	26.9 (2.9)	28.5 (3.1)	30.0 (2.9)	31.7 (3.0)	32.7 (3.0)	34.6 (2.9)	36.2 (3.0)	38.1 (3.0)	39.7 (3.3)

Mauritania

Birth of order i

Completed parity j	1	2	3	4	5	6	7	8	9	10	11	12	13	14	15
1	28.3 (9.9)														
2	22.3 (7.1)	27.8 (7.3)													
3	21.9 (5.7)	26.6 (5.7)	31.0 (6.6)												
4	24.9 (6.5)	27.9 (7.1)	31.1 (6.8)	35.3 (6.3)											
5	21.8 (6.1)	26.2 (6.2)	29.5 (6.0)	32.8 (5.5)	36.0 (5.1)										
6	19.5 (6.5)	23.2 (6.5)	26.2 (6.1)	29.0 (6.0)	31.8 (5.7)	35.0 (5.7)									
7	20.6 (4.9)	23.1 (5.1)	25.7 (5.1)	28.4 (5.2)	30.8 (5.2)	33.5 (5.2)	36.6 (5.2)								
8	19.4 (5.2)	21.9 (5.4)	24.2 (5.6)	26.7 (5.4)	29.3 (5.2)	31.7 (5.0)	34.4 (4.9)	37.5 (4.8)							
9	18.4 (4.7)	21.0 (5.1)	23.4 (5.2)	25.9 (5.0)	28.5 (4.9)	30.8 (5.0)	33.2 (5.0)	35.6 (4.6)	38.4 (4.4)						
10	17.7 (3.9)	20.2 (4.1)	22.5 (4.2)	24.7 (4.2)	26.9 (4.2)	29.0 (4.3)	31.4 (4.2)	33.8 (4.3)	36.1 (4.6)	39.6 (4.8)					
11	16.9 (4.9)	19.4 (5.4)	21.4 (5.2)	23.5 (5.2)	25.9 (5.1)	28.1 (5.0)	30.7 (4.6)	33.0 (4.3)	35.1 (4.3)	37.7 (4.5)	40.2 (4.2)				
12	16.1 (3.4)	18.7 (3.6)	20.7 (3.5)	22.6 (3.4)	24.8 (3.5)	27.0 (3.7)	29.7 (3.4)	31.9 (3.5)	34.0 (3.8)	35.9 (3.9)	37.9 (4.2)	40.2 (4.3)			
13	17.3 (2.6)	19.6 (2.6)	21.6 (2.9)	23.5 (3.3)	25.7 (3.6)	27.6 (3.7)	29.7 (4.2)	31.6 (4.5)	33.6 (5.1)	35.5 (5.6)	37.2 (5.4)	39.0 (5.2)	42.3 (5.7)		
14	16.3 .3)	17.8 .0)	21.4 (2.0)	22.6 (1.5)	24.6 (1.9)	26.4 (1.7)	28.7 (2.5)	30.4 (2.8)	31.9 (3.2)	33.4 (3.5)	35.3 (3.9)	36.9 (3.7)	39.3 (3.8)	40.8 (4.2)	
15	13.5 (5.8)	14.7 (5.3)	15.5 (6.6)	17.1 (7.7)	18.1 (9.3)	19.7 (9.8)	21.5 (9.9)	24.0 (9.2)	26.6 (8.9)	29.1 (7.8)	32.0 (7.0)	33.9 (6.3)	36.8 (5.0)	39.1 (4.2)	41.3 (4.7)

Mexico

Birth of order i

Completed parity j	1	2	3	4	5	6	7	8	9	10	11	12	13	14	15
1	26.6 (7.9)														
2	25.1 (6.4)	29.8 (6.9)													
3	24.1 (6.0)	27.2 (6.1)	31.3 (6.8)												
4	22.7 (4.8)	25.4 (4.9)	28.4 (5.4)	32.9 (5.5)											
5	21.5 (4.3)	24.3 (4.3)	27.0 (4.4)	30.2 (4.5)	34.0 (4.8)										
6	21.4 (3.8)	23.9 (3.9)	26.2 (3.8)	28.7 (3.9)	31.6 (4.0)	35.4 (4.5)									
7	20.9 (3.6)	23.4 (4.0)	25.5 (4.1)	28.0 (4.1)	30.4 (4.1)	33.5 (4.2)	36.7 (4.1)								
8	20.0 (3.3)	22.2 (3.2)	24.5 (3.5)	26.7 (3.6)	29.1 (3.6)	31.7 (3.5)	34.4 (3.5)	37.6 (3.7)							
9	19.9 (3.1)	22.2 (3.1)	24.4 (3.1)	26.5 (3.1)	28.6 (3.2)	30.9 (3.4)	33.3 (3.3)	35.9 (3.4)	39.2 (3.7)						
10	19.4 (3.1)	21.6 (3.3)	23.8 (3.0)	25.8 (2.9)	27.9 (2.9)	29.9 (2.9)	32.1 (3.0)	34.4 (3.0)	36.7 (2.8)	39.5 (3.1)					
11	18.3 (2.5)	20.0 (2.4)	21.9 (2.4)	24.0 (2.5)	26.1 (2.8)	28. (2.9)	30.3 (2.9)	32.7 (2.8)	34.7 (2.9)	37.1 (2.9)	39.9 (3.1)				
12	18.2 (2.3)	19.9 (2.3)	21.9 (2.4)	23.9 (2.4)	25.7 (2.4)	27.8 (2.5)	29.8 (2.3)	31.9 (2.5)	33.9 (2.3)	35.7 (2.3)	37.8 (2.4)	40.4 (2.7)			
13	18.3 (2.3)	19.9 (2.2)	21.7 (2.3)	23.4 (2.3)	25.3 (2.4)	27.2 (2.6)	29.0 (2.7)	30.8 (2.8)	32.6 (2.5)	34.5 (2.7)	36.3 (2.8)	38.4 (2.9)	40.9 (2.7)		
14	17.1 (2.3)	18.6 (2.4)	20.5 (2.3)	22.3 (2.3)	24.1 (2.1)	25.9 (2.1)	27.5 (2.3)	29.3 (2.4)	31.1 (2.4)	33.0 (2.5)	34.4 (2.4)	36.2 (2.4)	38.2 (2.2)	40.5 (2.8)	
15	17.4 (2.9)	19.0 (2.8)	20.5 (2.9)	22.2 (3.0)	23.8 (3.3)	25.4 (3.2)	26.7 (3.3)	28.1 (3.5)	29.6 (3.5)	31.2 (3.6)	32.6 (3.7)	34.2 (4.1)	35.7 (4.2)	37.5 (4.3)	39.1 (4.4)

Morocco

Birth of order i

Completed parity j	1	2	3	4	5	6	7	8	9	10	11	12	13	14	15
1	22.9 (7.7)														
2	21.7 (6.8)	26.1 (7.7)													
3	22.1 (6.5)	25.3 (5.9)	28.6 (6.0)												
4	21.2 (5.4)	24.0 (5.4)	26.9 (5.9)	30.8 (6.4)											
5	20.6 (4.8)	23.2 (5.1)	25.9 (5.5)	28.9 (5.6)	32.4 (6.0)										
6	20.0 (3.7)	22.8 (3.6)	25.4 (4.0)	28.0 (4.1)	30.8 (4.4)	34.1 (4.8)									
7	20.2 (4.2)	22.7 (4.4)	25.4 (4.7)	27.8 (4.7)	30.5 (4.7)	33.4 (4.7)	36.7 (4.7)								
8	19.5 (3.5)	21.8 (3.7)	24.0 (3.9)	26.4 (4.0)	28.8 (4.1)	31.3 (4.2)	34.1 (4.2)	37.3 (4.2)							
9	18.5 (3.0)	20.8 (3.1)	23.0 (3.3)	25.0 (3.2)	27.2 (3.2)	29.6 (3.2)	32.0 (3.6)	34.7 (3.6)	37.8 (3.7)						
10	18.6 (3.2)	20.6 (3.1)	22.6 (3.2)	24.7 (3.4)	26.9 (3.6)	29.1 (3.9)	31.3 (3.8)	33.8 (3.9)	36.6 (3.8)	39.6 (3.6)					
11	18.1 (2.9)	20.1 (3.0)	22.2 (3.3)	24.3 (3.7)	26.4 (3.6)	28.4 (3.6)	30.4 (3.6)	32.5 (3.5)	34.8 (3.5)	36.9 (3.4)	39.8 (3.6)				
12	17.4 (3.1)	19.2 (3.0)	21.0 (3.3)	22.8 (3.6)	24.7 (3.9)	26.5 (4.0)	28.7 (4.0)	30.7 (4.0)	32.6 (4.0)	34.9 (3.8)	37.4 (3.5)	40.0 (3.5)			
13	17.6 (3.4)	19.5 (3.3)	20.9 (3.4)	22.8 (3.4)	24.7 (3.3)	26.7 (3.3)	28.6 (3.4)	30.2 (3.6)	32.2 (3.8)	34.1 (3.9)	36.3 (3.9)	38.6 (4.0)	41.1 (3.9)		
14	16.6 (2.2)	18.2 (2.2)	20.1 (2.1)	21.6 (2.1)	23.3 (2.3)	24.6 (2.2)	26.5 (2.3)	28.3 (2.3)	30.5 (2.7)	32.1 (3.1)	33.8 (3.0)	35.5 (3.6)	38.1 (2.7)	40.7 (3.2)	
15	15.9 (2.3)	17.2 (2.3)	18.5 (2.5)	20.2 (3.4)	21.5 (3.5)	22.9 (3.3)	24.3 (3.2)	25.4 (3.2)	26.8 (3.5)	28.2 (3.3)	30.2 (3.5)	32.3 (3.3)	33.9 (3.4)	35.9 (3.2)	38.0 (2.8)

Nepal

Birth of order i

Completed parity j	1	2	3	4	5	6	7	8	9	10	11	12	13
1	24.7 (6.7)												
2	25.0 (5.8)	30.4 (6.1)											
3	23.5 (5.1)	27.6 (5.5)	32.7 (6.1)										
4	22.7 (4.6)	26.3 (4.9)	30.2 (4.7)	34.7 (4.9)									
5	22.0 (4.2)	25.1 (4.4)	28.2 (4.8)	31.7 (4.7)	35.5 (4.7)								
6	21.5 (3.6)	24.4 (3.9)	27.3 (4.2)	30.2 (4.2)	33.2 (4.1)	36.8 (4.2)							
7	20.6 (3.4)	23.2 (3.5)	25.9 (3.5)	28.7 (3.6)	31.5 (3.7)	34.2 (3.8)	37.6 (3.9)						
8	20.3 (3.5)	23.1 (3.7)	25.8 (4.0)	28.2 (4.1)	30.8 (4.1)	33.4 (4.1)	35.9 (4.2)	38.8 (4.0)					
9	19.6 (2.7)	22.1 (2.9)	24.4 (2.9)	26.8 (2.9)	29.2 (3.0)	31.7 (3.1)	33.9 (3.2)	36.5 (3.3)	39.4 (3.2)				
10	19.6 (3.2)	21.6 (3.4)	23.8 (3.6)	25.9 (3.7)	27.9 (3.6)	29.9 (3.9)	32.0 (3.5)	34.5 (3.5)	37.2 (3.4)	40.2 (3.3)			
11	18.2 (1.5)	20.1 (1.8)	22.0 (2.3)	24.1 (2.6)	26.1 (3.0)	28.1 (3.4)	30.2 (3.8)	32.0 (3.7)	34.2 (3.6)	36.4 (3.5)	38.9 (3.6)		
12	18.2 (2.7)	19.8 (2.6)	21.4 (2.8)	23.4 (2.7)	25.0 (2.8)	27.3 (3.1)	29.4 (3.1)	31.4 (3.3)	33.6 (3.7)	35.4 (4.0)	38.2 (3.8)	40.4 (3.6)	
13	20.5 (4.4)	22.4 (4.6)	25.0 (5.1)	26.7 (5.3)	28.3 (5.4)	29.9 (5.0)	31.8 (5.0)	33.5 (4.5)	34.8 (4.3)	36.2 (4.1)	38.2 (4.8)	40.6 (5.1)	43.2 (4.1)

Nigeria

Completed parity j	Birth of order i												
	1	2	3	4	5	6	7	8	9	10	11	12	13
1	25.9 (8.0)												
2	25.6 (7.7)	30.5 (7.5)											
3	24.7 (6.6)	28.6 (6.7)	32.7 (6.7)										
4	22.2 (5.1)	26.1 (5.3)	29.7 (5.4)	33.8 (5.2)									
5	22.7 (5.8)	26.3 (6.3)	29.2 (6.1)	32.2 (5.8)	35.7 (5.6)								
6	22.2 (5.1)	25.3 (4.9)	27.9 (5.0)	30.8 (5.0)	33.6 (5.0)	36.9 (5.0)							
7	21.2 (4.3)	24.0 (4.3)	26.4 (4.2)	28.8 (4.4)	31.6 (4.5)	34.5 (4.5)	37.5 (4.5)						
8	20.1 (4.6)	22.6 (4.6)	25.0 (4.5)	27.7 (4.6)	30.1 (4.7)	32.5 (4.7)	34.9 (4.4)	38.1 (4.6)					
9	18.0 (3.6)	20.6 (3.7)	22.8 (3.9)	24.8 (4.0)	27.4 (4.3)	29.6 (4.4)	32.2 (4.4)	34.4 (4.7)	37.1 (4.6)				
10	18.6 (3.6)	20.8 (3.6)	23.3 (4.0)	25.1 (4.2)	27.3 (4.2)	29.4 (4.3)	31.5 (4.4)	33.7 (4.5)	35.7 (4.7)	38.3 (5.0)			
11	18.8 (4.5)	21.1 (4.6)	23.0 (4.3)	25.1 (4.5)	26.8 (4.5)	29.1 (4.5)	31.2 (4.4)	33.3 (4.7)	35.1 (5.0)	37.2 (5.1)	39.8 (4.5)		
12	17.8 (4.0)	19.8 (4.2)	21.7 (4.2)	23.5 (4.6)	25.6 (4.8)	27.5 (4.8)	29.8 (4.2)	32.0 (3.3)	35.0 (2.7)	36.8 (2.7)	38.7 (2.7)	41.5 (3.3)	
13	16.4 (3.4)	17.8 (3.7)	19.6 (2.8)	21.6 (2.5)	23.2 (2.7)	24.6 (2.8)	26.6 (2.9)	28.5 (2.9)	30.2 (3.7)	32.2 (3.6)	34.4 (3.6)	36.5 (3.9)	38.4 (4.2)

Pakistan

Completed parity j	Birth of order i														
	1	2	3	4	5	6	7	8	9	10	11	12	13	14	15
1	21.3 (5.8)														
2	23.3 (6.6)	28.0 (6.8)													
3	21.8 (5.3)	25.2 (5.5)	29.1 (6.4)												
4	20.8 (4.4)	23.9 (4.5)	27.8 (5.0)	32.0 (5.1)											
5	21.2 (4.7)	24.4 (4.8)	27.6 (5.2)	30.8 (5.2)	35.0 (5.1)										
6	19.3 (3.5)	22.4 (4.0)	25.5 (3.9)	28.6 (3.9)	31.8 (4.1)	35.6 (4.3)									
7	18.9 (3.4)	21.9 (3.6)	24.7 (3.7)	27.5 (3.7)	30.4 (3.8)	33.4 (3.8)	36.7 (4.0)								
8	18.4 (2.9)	21.0 (3.1)	23.5 (3.3)	26.1 (3.3)	28.9 (3.3)	31.5 (3.2)	34.3 (3.5)	37.5 (3.6)							
9	18.5 (3.0)	20.9 (3.0)	23.2 (3.1)	25.8 (3.3)	28.3 (3.2)	30.7 (3.1)	33.2 (3.1)	35.7 (3.1)	38.6 (3.1)						
10	17.7 (2.6)	19.8 (2.7)	22.2 (2.9)	24.4 (3.0)	26.8 (2.9)	29.2 (2.9)	31.4 (2.9)	33.8 (2.9)	36.3 (2.9)	39.0 (2.9)					
11	17.9 (2.4)	20.1 (2.6)	22.2 (2.6)	24.2 (2.7)	26.5 (3.0)	28.5 (2.9)	30.8 (2.9)	33.1 (2.5)	35.4 (2.6)	37.8 (2.6)	40.4 (2.7)				
12	17.6 (2.1)	19.6 (2.2)	21.6 (2.6)	23.6 (2.7)	25.5 (2.8)	27.6 (2.9)	29.6 (3.0)	31.4 (3.0)	33.6 (2.8)	36.0 (2.7)	38.0 (2.7)	40.6 (2.5)			
13	17.9 (2.5)	20.3 (2.8)	22.0 (2.8)	23.8 (2.8)	25.8 (2.8)	27.8 (2.7)	29.4 (2.8)	31.3 (2.6)	33.4 (2.7)	35.4 (2.2)	37.4 (1.7)	39.5 (1.7)	41.4 (1.9)		
14	16.3 (1.9)	18.6 (2.3)	20.1 (2.3)	22.1 (2.4)	24.1 (2.5)	26.1 (3.4)	27.8 (3.9)	29.5 (4.5)	31.1 (4.7)	32.5 (4.8)	34.0 (5.0)	35.6 (5.0)	37.4 (5.7)	40.2 (6.7)	
15	15.5 (1.0)	17.3 (1.1)	18.3 (1.1)	19.5 (.9)	20.8 (.5)	22.3 (.4)	24.2 (1.1)	25.9 (1.7)	27.4 (1.9)	29.2 (2.4)	31.3 (3.3)	32.7 (3.4)	33.7 (3.8)	36.2 (3.7)	37.9 (4.7)

Panama

Birth of order i

Completed parity j	1	2	3	4	5	6	7	8	9	10	11	12	13	14	15
1	25.4 (6.7)														
2	22.8 (5.4)	25.7 (5.4)													
3	22.4 (4.1)	25.0 (4.1)	28.1 (4.6)												
4	21.0 (3.3)	23.7 (4.2)	26.6 (4.5)	29.3 (4.7)											
5	20.3 (3.1)	23.0 (3.4)	25.1 (3.8)	28.1 (4.2)	31.1 (4.3)										
6	19.1 (3.2)	21.2 (3.3)	23.9 (3.5)	26.6 (3.6)	28.9 (3.9)	31.6 (4.3)									
7	19.6 (3.4)	21.7 (3.4)	23.8 (3.5)	26.2 (3.5)	28.4 (3.7)	30.6 (3.9)	32.9 (4.1)								
8	19.3 (3.8)	21.2 (3.8)	23.3 (3.8)	25.3 (4.0)	27.4 (3.8)	29.4 (3.6)	31.9 (3.5)	34.8 (3.5)							
9	17.8 (2.2)	19.9 (2.4)	22.0 (2.3)	24.1 (2.6)	26.3 (2.8)	28.5 (2.9)	31.0 (3.1)	33.1 (3.0)	35.3 (2.9)						
10	17.4 (2.1)	19.7 (2.2)	21.8 (2.4)	23.8 (2.3)	26.2 (2.5)	28.4 (2.7)	30.4 (2.8)	32.6 (3.0)	34.6 (2.8)	36.7 (3.2)					
11	18.3 (2.7)	20.2 (2.8)	22.3 (2.8)	24.3 (2.7)	26.2 (2.6)	28.3 (2.8)	30.2 (3.1)	32.4 (3.3)	34.5 (3.2)	36.5 (3.1)	38.6 (3.2)				
12	17.0 (1.9)	19.0 (1.8)	20.4 (1.8)	22.0 (1.7)	23.8 (1.9)	25.8 (1.8)	27.8 (1.8)	29.8 (1.7)	31.8 (1.8)	33.7 (2.2)	36.0 (2.2)	38.0 (2.4)			
13	16.6 (.4)	18.5 (1.1)	19.9 (1.5)	21.3 (1.7)	22.7 (2.1)	25.1 (3.3)	28.2 (4.1)	30.1 (3.0)	31.9 (2.7)	33.6 (2.2)	34.6 (2.8)	36.4 (2.8)	38.8 (4.0)		
14	16.7 (1.2)	18.3 (1.2)	20.6 (1.3)	22.8 (1.4)	24.1 (1.7)	25.3 (1.9)	26.8 (1.9)	28.0 (2.2)	29.4 (2.3)	30.9 (2.8)	32.4 (2.8)	33.7 (2.6)	35.1 (2.8)	36.6 (2.9)	
15	.0 (.0)	.0 (.0)	.0 (.0)	.0 (.0)	.0 (.0)	.0 (.0)	.0 (.0)	.0 (.0)	.0 (.0)	.0 (.0)	.0 (.0)	.0 (.0)	.0 (.0)	.0 (.0)	.0 (.0)

Paraguay

Birth of order i

Completed parity j	1	2	3	4	5	6	7	8	9	10	11	12	13	14	15
1	27.6 (7.2)														
2	24.0 (5.2)	29.6 (6.6)													
3	23.6 (5.0)	26.5 (5.0)	30.8 (5.8)												
4	22.0 (3.7)	25.0 (3.5)	29.1 (4.6)	33.3 (5.6)											
5	22.6 (5.1)	25.0 (4.9)	28.0 (4.7)	31.2 (4.6)	34.8 (4.5)										
6	20.8 (3.7)	23.6 (3.8)	26.3 (4.0)	29.0 (4.1)	31.9 (4.4)	35.7 (4.3)									
7	21.0 (3.5)	23.4 (3.7)	25.8 (3.6)	28.5 (3.8)	30.8 (3.9)	33.5 (4.0)	36.5 (3.8)								
8	19.9 (2.9)	22.1 (2.9)	24.5 (2.8)	27.0 (2.9)	29.3 (3.1)	31.5 (3.2)	34.4 (3.3)	37.4 (3.2)							
9	20.7 (2.6)	22.7 (2.6)	25.0 (2.5)	27.3 (2.7)	29.5 (2.8)	31.9 (2.7)	34.4 (3.1)	36.8 (3.0)	39.8 (3.2)						
10	18.9 (2.5)	20.9 (2.7)	23.2 (2.9)	25.3 (2.8)	27.4 (2.9)	29.6 (2.8)	31.8 (2.8)	34.0 (2.7)	36.2 (2.7)	39.0 (2.7)					
11	18.6 (1.8)	20.9 (1.8)	22.8 (1.9)	25.0 (2.2)	27.1 (2.3)	29.3 (2.1)	31.5 (2.3)	33.7 (2.6)	35.8 (2.4)	37.9 (2.6)	40.5 (2.9)				
12	18.7 (2.2)	20.7 (1.9)	23.0 (1.8)	24.9 (1.8)	26.7 (1.7)	28.7 (1.8)	30.9 (2.0)	32.8 (2.2)	34.8 (2.4)	36.9 (2.7)	39.0 (2.6)	41.8 (2.7)			
13	18.0 (1.6)	19.9 (1.5)	21.8 (1.7)	23.8 (2.0)	26.2 (2.1)	28.2 (2.2)	29.9 (2.1)	31.9 (2.0)	33.9 (2.0)	35.8 (2.4)	37.7 (2.4)	39.5 (2.4)	42.0 (2.2)		
14	18.5 (1.5)	20.7 (2.2)	22.6 (2.1)	24.7 (2.2)	26.2 (2.3)	28.3 (2.2)	29.4 (1.6)	30.9 (1.2)	32.3 (1.0)	33.5 (.8)	34.6 (1.0)	37.0 (2.0)	39.1 (2.2)	41.3 (2.1)	
15	17.9 (1.9)	19.6 (1.9)	21.2 (2.1)	22.8 (2.1)	24.5 (2.1)	26.3 (2.8)	28.0 (2.9)	29.9 (2.7)	31.2 (2.6)	32.7 (2.5)	34.2 (2.6)	35.8 (2.3)	37.5 (2.4)	39.3 (2.5)	41.1 (2.7)

Peru

Birth of order i

Completed parity j	1	2	3	4	5	6	7	8	9	10	11	12	13	14	15
1	28.6 (7.3)														
2	24.7 (6.0)	29.0 (6.5)													
3	24.3 (5.0)	27.5 (5.2)	32.5 (5.6)												
4	23.2 (4.2)	26.3 (4.7)	29.9 (5.2)	34.2 (5.5)											
5	22.6 (3.9)	25.4 (4.1)	28.0 (4.3)	31.1 (4.4)	35.4 (4.7)										
6	21.6 (4.3)	24.3 (4.3)	27.0 (4.5)	29.5 (4.5)	32.5 (4.5)	35.9 (4.6)									
7	20.8 (3.5)	23.3 (3.6)	25.8 (3.7)	28.0 (4.0)	30.9 (4.3)	33.6 (4.4)	37.2 (4.2)								
8	20.5 (3.6)	23.0 (3.7)	25.3 (3.7)	27.5 (3.9)	30.0 (4.0)	32.5 (3.9)	35.0 (4.1)	38.4 (4.2)							
9	19.7 (2.9)	22.1 (2.9)	24.1 (2.8)	26.3 (2.8)	28.4 (2.8)	30.8 (2.8)	33.2 (3.0)	35.8 (3.0)	38.9 (3.1)						
10	19.5 (3.0)	21.7 (3.0)	23.6 (3.1)	25.7 (3.2)	27.6 (3.4)	29.7 (3.6)	31.7 (3.4)	34.0 (3.6)	36.4 (3.7)	39.7 (3.4)					
11	19.5 (2.7)	21.5 (2.8)	23.4 (2.9)	25.5 (3.0)	27.3 (3.1)	29.3 (3.2)	31.3 (3.2)	33.3 (3.1)	35.6 (3.0)	37.8 (3.1)	40.8 (3.0)				
12	18.2 (3.0)	20.1 (3.1)	22.2 (3.1)	24.2 (3.4)	26.0 (3.2)	27.8 (3.5)	29.7 (3.4)	31.7 (3.6)	33.9 (3.6)	35.8 (3.5)	38.1 (3.4)	40.9 (3.2)			
13	18.5 (2.7)	19.9 (2.6)	21.5 (2.7)	23.2 (2.7)	24.8 (2.8)	26.6 (2.9)	28.5 (2.8)	30.2 (2.9)	32.1 (3.3)	33.8 (3.4)	35.9 (3.3)	38.1 (3.0)	40.3 (3.3)		
14	17.1 (2.5)	18.9 (2.6)	20.9 (2.2)	23.2 (2.2)	25.0 (1.8)	26.6 (1.9)	28.3 (1.8)	29.8 (1.9)	31.8 (2.3)	33.2 (2.4)	34.7 (2.4)	36.2 (2.1)	37.9 (2.2)	40.2 (2.9)	
15	17.9 (2.5)	19.4 (2.3)	21.1 (2.4)	22.6 (2.5)	24.2 (2.7)	26.1 (2.6)	27.5 (2.8)	28.9 (2.7)	30.2 (2.8)	31.6 (2.8)	33.1 (2.8)	34.8 (2.8)	36.6 (2.6)	38.0 (2.9)	40.3 (3.2)

Philippines

Birth of order i

Completed parity j	1	2	3	4	5	6	7	8	9	10	11	12	13	14	15
1	30.4 (7.6)														
2	27.9 (6.0)	31.9 (6.1)													
3	26.5 (5.5)	29.2 (5.7)	33.3 (5.7)												
4	24.6 (4.7)	27.3 (4.9)	30.2 (4.9)	34.4 (5.0)											
5	24.1 (4.0)	26.5 (4.0)	29.1 (4.0)	32.0 (4.0)	35.2 (4.1)										
6	22.8 (3.8)	25.1 (3.7)	27.7 (3.6)	30.4 (3.8)	33.3 (3.8)	36.8 (3.9)									
7	22.1 (3.4)	24.2 (3.3)	26.5 (3.2)	28.9 (3.2)	31.4 (3.1)	34.2 (3.1)	37.7 (3.3)								
8	21.0 (3.1)	23.0 (3.1)	25.1 (3.2)	27.5 (3.1)	29.9 (3.2)	32.4 (3.2)	34.9 (3.2)	38.0 (3.2)							
9	20.2 (2.8)	22.3 (2.8)	24.6 (3.0)	27.0 (3.4)	29.3 (3.4)	31.6 (3.3)	34.0 (3.4)	36.4 (3.4)	39.6 (3.5)						
10	19.7 (2.6)	21.7 (2.6)	23.8 (2.6)	25.9 (2.7)	28.0 (2.6)	30.1 (2.7)	32.4 (2.8)	34.6 (2.7)	37.1 (2.8)	40.1 (2.8)					
11	19.2 (2.5)	21.0 (2.5)	23.1 (2.6)	25.3 (2.7)	27.3 (2.7)	29.4 (2.6)	31.5 (2.6)	33.6 (2.7)	35.7 (2.8)	37.8 (2.6)	40.6 (2.5)				
12	18.6 (2.2)	20.4 (2.1)	22.6 (2.0)	24.6 (2.0)	26.7 (1.9)	28.6 (1.9)	30.5 (2.0)	32.4 (2.0)	34.4 (2.1)	36.3 (2.3)	38.4 (2.0)	41.0 (2.5)			
13	18.6 (2.3)	20.5 (2.3)	22.1 (2.3)	24.0 (2.3)	25.9 (2.2)	27.7 (2.0)	29.3 (2.0)	31.2 (2.2)	33.1 (2.3)	35.2 (2.5)	37.3 (2.7)	39.3 (2.7)	41.7 (2.5)		
14	18.8 (2.3)	20.4 (2.1)	22.1 (2.0)	24.0 (2.0)	25.7 (1.8)	27.6 (2.4)	29.0 (2.4)	30.9 (2.1)	32.5 (2.2)	34.2 (2.1)	35.8 (2.3)	37.5 (2.3)	39.0 (2.5)	41.6 (2.4)	
15	17.8 (1.8)	19.3 (1.7)	20.5 (1.8)	22.4 (1.9)	24.1 (2.2)	25.4 (2.1)	27.2 (2.3)	29.1 (2.0)	30.7 (2.0)	32.1 (1.8)	33.8 (1.6)	35.7 (2.1)	37.3 (2.3)	38.7 (2.3)	40.8 (2.2)

Portugal

Birth of order i

Completed parity j	1	2	3	4	5	6	7	8	9	10	11	12	13	14	15
1	27.3														
	(5.2)														
2	25.2	30.0													
	(4.1)	(4.7)													
3	24.4	27.4	32.4												
	(3.8)	(4.0)	(4.8)												
4	24.1	26.4	29.4	33.9											
	(3.9)	(4.2)	(4.2)	(4.7)											
5	22.9	25.1	27.6	30.7	34.8										
	(3.6)	(3.5)	(3.6)	(3.8)	(4.1)										
6	23.4	25.4	27.6	30.2	33.0	36.5									
	(3.5)	(3.3)	(3.4)	(3.6)	(3.6)	(3.8)									
7	23.1	25.3	27.4	29.6	31.9	34.3	38.2								
	(3.7)	(3.7)	(3.6)	(3.5)	(3.4)	(3.2)	(3.1)								
8	21.8	24.0	26.2	28.7	31.2	33.4	35.9	39.0							
	(2.9)	(2.8)	(3.2)	(3.2)	(3.5)	(3.6)	(4.2)	(3.5)							
9	23.1	24.8	26.0	27.7	29.5	31.7	34.2	37.3	40.7						
	(3.1)	(2.9)	(2.9)	(2.9)	(3.0)	(2.8)	(2.7)	(2.7)	(2.9)						
10	22.4	24.2	25.9	28.3	30.3	32.3	34.1	36.3	38.2	41.2					
	(1.8)	(1.8)	(1.7)	(1.7)	(1.9)	(2.2)	(2.4)	(2.8)	(2.9)	(2.6)					
11	21.7	23.2	24.4	26.3	27.6	29.4	31.4	33.4	35.2	36.8	39.6				
	(2.4)	(2.4)	(2.4)	(2.7)	(2.8)	(2.8)	(3.0)	(2.9)	(3.2)	(3.5)	(3.4)				
12	22.4	24.0	25.6	27.3	29.8	31.4	32.5	34.4	36.0	37.0	39.1	41.8			
	(2.5)	(3.2)	(3.6)	(3.0)	(2.8)	(2.6)	(2.6)	(2.5)	(2.4)	(2.0)	(2.4)	(2.2)			
13	20.8	22.5	24.6	26.5	28.1	29.6	31.3	32.8	34.1	35.4	36.9	38.8	40.6		
	(1.8)	(1.3)	(1.0)	(1.0)	(1.2)	(1.5)	(1.5)	(1.3)	(1.2)	(1.0)	(.8)	(1.0)	(1.5)		
14	20.6	23.5	25.0	26.4	27.9	29.4	30.7	32.2	33.3	34.2	35.7	36.5	37.6	39.9	
	(2.6)	(1.8)	(1.9)	(1.4)	(1.2)	(1.4)	(1.7)	(2.2)	(2.5)	(2.6)	(3.2)	(3.3)	(3.6)	(5.0)	
15	18.8	20.3	21.9	23.3	24.8	26.2	27.8	28.4	29.4	30.4	32.8	34.2	36.1	38.2	41.7
	(.4)	(1.2)	(1.7)	(2.0)	(2.3)	(1.9)	(2.5)	(2.2)	(2.4)	(3.3)	(3.1)	(2.8)	(2.5)	(2.9)	(2.7)

Senegal

Birth of order i

Completed parity j	1	2	3	4	5	6	7	8	9	10	11	12	13	14
1	22.1													
	(6.8)													
2	21.0	27.4												
	(5.8)	(7.3)												
3	20.6	24.2	28.6											
	(4.2)	(5.0)	(6.5)											
4	19.6	23.3	27.6	32.8										
	(4.3)	(4.7)	(5.0)	(5.5)										
5	19.7	23.3	26.1	29.6	33.5									
	(3.4)	(3.8)	(3.8)	(3.9)	(4.4)									
6	19.1	22.9	26.0	29.2	32.6	36.4								
	(3.3)	(3.9)	(4.0)	(4.0)	(4.1)	(4.0)								
7	19.6	22.6	25.8	28.6	31.4	34.4	37.7							
	(3.1)	(3.4)	(3.7)	(3.6)	(3.6)	(3.5)	(3.6)							
8	18.4	21.2	24.1	26.8	29.6	32.2	35.1	38.2						
	(2.2)	(2.5)	(2.6)	(2.7)	(2.7)	(2.9)	(3.0)	(3.1)						
9	18.4	21.0	23.6	26.2	28.8	31.3	33.9	36.6	39.6					
	(2.5)	(2.6)	(2.7)	(2.8)	(2.7)	(2.6)	(2.7)	(2.7)	(2.9)					
10	17.5	20.2	22.5	24.9	27.4	29.8	32.3	34.9	37.4	40.3				
	(2.2)	(2.2)	(2.3)	(2.6)	(2.7)	(2.9)	(3.1)	(3.3)	(3.3)	(2.9)				
11	17.4	19.8	22.2	24.5	27.0	29.3	31.5	33.9	36.2	38.7	41.5			
	(2.3)	(2.4)	(2.5)	(2.5)	(2.5)	(2.6)	(2.6)	(2.6)	(2.6)	(2.6)	(2.7)			
12	17.7	20.4	22.9	25.0	27.2	29.5	31.3	33.4	35.8	37.4	39.9	42.1		
	(1.7)	(1.7)	(1.6)	(1.7)	(1.7)	(1.8)	(1.9)	(1.9)	(1.9)	(2.1)	(2.5)	(2.8)		
13	16.7	18.5	20.9	22.5	24.5	26.4	28.5	30.4	32.3	34.3	36.4	38.4	40.8	
	(1.1)	(.7)	(1.0)	(.9)	(1.4)	(2.2)	(2.0)	(2.6)	(2.4)	(2.5)	(2.9)	(3.1)	(2.8)	
14	17.5	19.1	20.1	21.0	22.8	24.7	26.5	28.8	30.6	33.2	34.4	36.6	38.8	40.6
	(1.8)	(1.6)	(.2)	(.2)	(.2)	(.4)	(1.2)	(1.6)	(2.2)	(1.0)	(.6)	(.9)	(.2)	(.5)

Sri Lanka

Birth of order i

Completed parity j	1	2	3	4	5	6	7	8	9	10	11	12	13	14	15
1	27.9 (6.6)														
2	25.7 (6.5)	30.1 (6.3)													
3	23.5 (5.5)	27.0 (5.5)	31.0 (5.6)												
4	22.5 (5.1)	25.5 (4.9)	29.0 (4.8)	33.3 (4.8)											
5	21.4 (4.4)	24.0 (4.4)	27.0 (4.5)	30.2 (4.5)	34.4 (5.0)										
6	20.9 (3.8)	23.4 (3.6)	25.9 (3.6)	28.6 (3.8)	31.7 (4.0)	35.7 (4.3)									
7	19.7 (3.3)	21.9 (3.2)	24.5 (3.1)	27.0 (3.4)	29.8 (3.4)	32.7 (3.5)	36.0 (3.7)								
8	19.4 (3.8)	21.6 (3.9)	23.8 (3.9)	26.3 (3.9)	28.6 (4.0)	31.0 (4.0)	33.7 (4.2)	36.8 (4.3)							
9	18.4 (2.5)	20.4 (2.6)	22.6 (2.6)	25.0 (2.9)	27.5 (2.9)	30.0 (3.0)	32.2 (2.9)	34.9 (3.1)	38.2 (3.3)						
10	18.9 (3.3)	20.9 (3.2)	23.1 (3.1)	25.1 (3.0)	27.2 (3.0)	29.3 (3.0)	31.5 (3.0)	33.8 (3.1)	36.3 (3.2)	38.7 (3.4)					
11	17.9 (3.1)	19.8 (3.0)	21.8 (3.0)	23.7 (3.0)	25.9 (3.2)	28.0 (3.2)	30.2 (3.4)	32.2 (3.4)	34.5 (3.4)	36.9 (3.4)	39.8 (3.6)				
12	16.7 (3.0)	18.8 (3.1)	20.7 (2.9)	22.6 (2.9)	24.5 (3.3)	26.2 (3.2)	28.2 (3.1)	30.0 (3.1)	31.9 (3.1)	33.8 (3.2)	36.0 (3.2)	39.2 (3.5)			
13	18.0 (2.9)	19.7 (2.8)	21.5 (3.0)	23.2 (3.1)	25.1 (3.3)	26.8 (3.3)	28.8 (3.2)	30.7 (2.9)	32.5 (3.1)	34.0 (3.3)	36.2 (3.0)	38.0 (3.1)	40.4 (3.5)		
14	17.5 (1.8)	19.0 (2.0)	21.1 (2.2)	22.4 (2.5)	23.9 (3.0)	25.3 (3.2)	26.9 (3.4)	29.3 (3.5)	30.9 (3.6)	32.6 (3.8)	35.0 (4.2)	36.6 (4.4)	38.7 (4.1)	40.5 (4.1)	
15	14.9 (1.4)	16.5 (1.7)	18.2 (1.3)	20.0 (.8))	21.6 (.8))	23.2 (.8))	24.6 (1.3)	26.5 (1.6)	28.2 (2.0)	29.7 (2.4)	30.8 (2.2)	32.1 (2.2)	33.3 (1.9)	35.9 (2.0)	37.6 (1.5)

Sudan

Birth of order i

Completed parity j	1	2	3	4	5	6	7	8	9	10	11	12	13
1	24.4 (7.2)												
2	24.9 (7.7)	28.9 (7.8)											
3	22.6 (6.5)	26.5 (6.5)	30.3 (7.0)										
4	22.3 (6.1)	26.2 (6.5)	29.9 (6.6)	33.2 (6.8)									
5	22.5 (5.9)	25.1 (5.7)	28.2 (5.9)	31.3 (5.3)	35.2 (4.9)								
6	20.6 (5.0)	23.1 (5.1)	25.7 (5.1)	29.1 (4.7)	31.9 (4.8)	34.9 (5.1)							
7	21.4 (4.9)	23.7 (4.7)	26.5 (4.8)	29.3 (4.9)	31.5 (5.0)	33.8 (5.0)	36.7 (4.7)						
8	19.2 (3.6)	21.9 (4.0)	24.7 (4.4)	26.9 (4.4)	29.2 (4.3)	31.2 (4.3)	33.5 (4.4)	37.0 (4.3)					
9	18.7 (3.5)	20.8 (3.6)	23.2 (3.5)	25.5 (3.8)	27.6 (4.0)	29.8 (4.1)	31.9 (4.2)	34.9 (4.8)	37.7 (5.1)				
10	19.2 (4.0)	21.6 (4.3)	23.9 (4.3)	26.0 (4.3)	27.9 (4.3)	30.1 (4.4)	32.2 (4.3)	34.6 (4.1)	36.8 (4.3)	39.5 (4.3)			
11	17.8 (4.5)	19.4 (4.2)	21.8 (4.7)	23.7 (4.7)	26.0 (4.8)	27.6 (4.7)	29.7 (4.3)	31.6 (4.1)	33.8 (4.0)	36.0 (3.6)	38.9 (4.1)		
12	16.4 (3.1)	18.6 (4.2)	20.7 (3.9)	23.4 (3.6)	25.1 (3.8)	26.7 (3.8)	28.7 (3.4)	30.6 (3.3)	32.0 (3.6)	34.2 (3.7)	36.1 (3.6)	38.2 (3.8)	
13	16.1 (2.5)	17.8 (2.9)	18.9 (3.1)	21.9 (5.8)	23.4 (5.8)	24.8 (5.9)	26.2 (6.4)	27.9 (6.1)	30.2 (4.9)	32.4 (4.0)	33.9 (4.2)	36.0 (3.7)	36.9 (4.2)

Syria

Birth of order i

Completed parity j	1	2	3	4	5	6	7	8	9	10	11	12	13	14	15
1	27.5 (6.7)														
2	29.6 (7.4)	32.6 (7.7)													
3	25.2 (6.0)	28.5 (5.7)	32.3 (5.7)												
4	25.7 (5.6)	28.3 (5.8)	31.1 (5.7)	34.3 (5.4)											
5	23.8 (5.1)	26.2 (5.2)	28.9 (5.4)	32.0 (5.4)	35.3 (5.5)										
6	22.8 (4.3)	25.3 (4.1)	27.9 (4.3)	30.3 (4.5)	33.4 (4.4)	36.8 (4.4)									
7	22.0 (4.1)	24.2 (4.0)	26.9 (4.0)	29.4 (3.8)	31.9 (3.7)	34.8 (3.7)	37.8 (3.7)								
8	21.5 (3.8)	23.7 (3.8)	25.9 (3.9)	28.1 (3.9)	30.4 (3.9)	32.8 (4.0)	35.3 (3.9)	38.5 (3.7)							
9	20.8 (3.5)	22.8 (3.6)	25.0 (3.6)	27.2 (3.8)	29.4 (3.8)	31.8 (3.8)	34.2 (3.9)	36.7 (4.0)	39.6 (3.7)						
10	19.9 (3.0)	21.9 (3.2)	23.9 (3.2)	26.0 (3.3)	28.1 (3.3)	30.1 (3.2)	32.1 (3.5)	34.3 (3.4)	36.6 (3.4)	39.3 (3.3)					
11	19.2 (3.4)	20.9 (3.4)	23.0 (3.5)	25.0 (3.4)	27.1 (3.4)	29.3 (3.4)	31.3 (3.6)	33.3 (3.6)	35.5 (3.7)	37.9 (3.6)	40.5 (3.6)				
12	18.7 (2.7)	20.6 (2.7)	22.5 (2.9)	24.2 (2.9)	26.3 (2.9)	28.4 (2.9)	30.2 (2.9)	32.0 (2.9)	34.1 (3.0)	36.1 (3.1)	38.4 (2.7)	40.8 (3.1)			
13	18.2 (3.0)	19.8 (3.1)	21.6 (3.0)	23.3 (2.8)	25.0 (3.1)	27.1 (3.5)	28.5 (3.8)	30.2 (4.0)	32.2 (4.0)	34.1 (3.8)	35.5 (4.0)	37.5 (3.4)	39.7 (3.3)		
14	19.3 (3.2)	20.8 (2.9)	22.2 (3.0)	24.1 (2.7)	25.8 (2.8)	27.7 (2.8)	29.5 (2.9)	30.7 (2.4)	32.1 (2.5)	33.9 (2.7)	35.6 (2.4)	37.7 (2.5)	39.4 (2.3)	41.8 (2.5)	
15	18.0 (2.4)	19.5 (2.3)	21.2 (2.0)	22.7 (2.0)	24.4 (2.3)	26.1 (2.1)	28.0 (2.1)	29.4 (2.1)	31.1 (2.6)	32.7 (2.6)	34.4 (2.5)	36.2 (2.8)	37.8 (2.8)	39.5 (3.0)	41.5 (3.1)

Thailand

Birth of order i

Completed parity j	1	2	3	4	5	6	7	8	9	10	11	12	13	14	15
1	28.9 (6.4)														
2	25.6 (5.8)	30.3 (5.9)													
3	23.8 (4.8)	26.8 (4.9)	31.3 (5.4)												
4	23.8 (4.6)	26.9 (4.8)	29.7 (5.3)	32.8 (5.4)											
5	22.8 (3.1)	25.4 (3.2)	28.1 (3.6)	31.1 (3.9)	34.5 (4.3)										
6	22.1 (3.6)	24.5 (3.7)	27.0 (3.7)	29.7 (3.8)	32.4 (3.9)	36.0 (4.3)									
7	21.5 (3.0)	24.0 (2.9)	26.5 (3.0)	28.8 (2.9)	31.6 (3.2)	34.4 (3.2)	37.4 (3.7)								
8	21.0 (2.9)	23.4 (2.9)	25.6 (2.9)	28.2 (3.0)	30.8 (3.0)	33.3 (3.0)	35.8 (3.2)	39.1 (3.5)							
9	20.4 (2.6)	22.5 (2.6)	24.6 (2.7)	26.9 (2.8)	29.3 (2.8)	31.4 (2.7)	33.7 (2.8)	36.1 (2.8)	38.9 (3.2)						
10	20.2 (2.4)	22.3 (2.2)	24.5 (2.3)	26.6 (2.5)	28.8 (2.5)	30.7 (2.4)	32.7 (2.4)	34.9 (2.3)	37.4 (2.3)	40.2 (2.5)					
11	19.7 (3.0)	22.0 (2.7)	24.1 (2.6)	25.7 (2.6)	27.5 (2.7)	29.4 (2.5)	31.5 (2.5)	33.5 (2.5)	35.4 (2.5)	37.9 (2.6)	40.7 (2.8)				
12	19.1 (2.5)	21.0 (2.3)	23.0 (2.5)	24.9 (2.6)	26.7 (2.7)	28.5 (2.8)	30.4 (2.9)	32.3 (3.0)	33.9 (3.1)	35.9 (3.5)	37.9 (3.9)	40.5 (3.5)			
13	19.0 (2.3)	20.5 (2.4)	22.0 (2.2)	23.8 (2.2)	25.5 (1.9)	27.6 (1.6)	29.3 (1.5)	31.3 (2.2)	33.0 (2.4)	35.1 (2.3)	37.0 (2.2)	39.5 (1.6)	41.8 (1.5)		
14	19.3 (3.0)	20.7 (2.7)	22.2 (2.4)	23.9 (2.1)	25.1 (2.1)	26.8 (2.3)	29.7 (2.7)	31.7 (2.9)	32.9 (3.4)	33.9 (3.2)	35.9 (2.6)	37.6 (2.6)	39.7 (1.7)	41.9 (2.0)	
15	19.4 (1.0)	20.8 (1.3)	22.1 (1.7)	24.1 (1.8)	25.8 (2.0)	27.3 (2.3)	29.3 (2.7)	30.1 (2.9)	32.1 (3.0)	33.5 (2.8)	35.1 (2.8)	37.1 (2.7)	39.0 (2.5)	40.4 (2.6)	41.9 (2.6)

236

Trinidad and Tobago

Completed parity j	Birth of order i														
	1	2	3	4	5	6	7	8	9	10	11	12	13	14	15
1	22.1 (6.5)														
2	24.4 (6.6)	28.2 (6.7)													
3	22.8 (4.2)	26.1 (4.3)	29.9 (4.9)												
4	22.4 (4.9)	25.0 (4.8)	27.5 (4.8)	31.1 (5.5)											
5	21.0 (3.6)	23.4 (3.8)	25.7 (3.9)	28.3 (4.0)	31.9 (4.5)										
6	20.5 (3.7)	22.8 (3.9)	25.0 (3.9)	27.3 (4.1)	30.3 (4.5)	33.4 (5.1)									
7	19.2 (3.0)	21.6 (3.3)	24.0 (3.9)	26.0 (4.0)	28.4 (4.3)	31.1 (4.3)	34.6 (4.8)								
8	18.1 (2.8)	20.3 (2.8)	22.2 (2.8)	24.1 (2.8)	26.3 (3.2)	28.5 (3.3)	31.2 (3.8)	35.6 (4.4)							
9	18.4 (2.9)	20.4 (2.9)	22.6 (2.9)	24.4 (2.7)	26.2 (2.8)	28.3 (3.0)	31.0 (3.6)	33.7 (3.0)	36.8 (3.5)						
10	18.5 (3.4)	20.5 (3.3)	22.2 (3.2)	24.2 (3.3)	25.9 (3.3)	27.8 (3.2)	29.6 (3.3)	31.4 (2.8)	33.8 (3.3)	36.8 (3.4)					
11	17.6 (2.6)	19.4 (2.6)	21.2 (2.6)	23.0 (2.8)	25.2 (2.9)	26.9 (2.9)	28.8 (2.7)	30.8 (2.8)	32.9 (3.4)	35.0 (3.4)	37.8 (3.7)				
12	18.5 (2.7)	20.6 (2.5)	22.3 (2.4)	24.1 (2.3)	25.8 (2.3)	27.5 (2.2)	29.3 (2.3)	31.0 (2.3)	32.8 (2.4)	34.7 (2.0)	36.9 (2.2)	39.5 (3.0)			
13	17.1 (3.3)	18.9 (3.1)	20.5 (2.8)	22.4 (2.6)	23.9 (2.6)	25.4 (2.8)	26.7 (2.6)	28.5 (2.4)	30.1 (2.7)	31.9 (2.6)	33.5 (2.8)	36.2 (2.4)	38.8 (3.2)		
14	18.4 (.3)	19.7 (.4)	21.5 (.4)	23.4 (.8)	24.6 (.3)	26.1 (.9)	27.3 (1.0)	28.6 (1.3)	29.8 (1.5)	31.1 (1.4)	32.5 (1.5)	33.6 (1.4)	34.9 (1.3)	36.8 (2.2)	
15	16.5 (1.8)	18.2 (1.5)	19.7 (1.7)	21.5 (1.4)	23.1 (1.9)	24.4 (2.1)	26.1 (2.3)	27.4 (2.4)	28.8 (2.6)	30.2 (2.9)	31.5 (2.9)	32.9 (3.3)	34.7 (3.3)	36.8 (4.0)	38.7 (3.8)

Tunisia

Completed parity j	Birth of order i													
	1	2	3	4	5	6	7	8	9	10	11	12	13	14
1	26.2 (6.5)													
2	28.6 (7.1)	32.3 (7.7)												
3	25.6 (6.1)	28.8 (5.9)	32.5 (5.7)											
4	24.4 (4.6)	27.5 (4.9)	30.7 (5.3)	34.4 (5.4)										
5	23.8 (4.2)	26.5 (4.2)	29.3 (4.4)	32.0 (4.5)	35.8 (4.5)									
6	22.5 (3.8)	25.0 (3.8)	27.5 (4.0)	30.2 (4.2)	33.1 (4.6)	36.6 (4.7)								
7	21.7 (3.9)	24.0 (3.9)	26.3 (4.0)	29.1 (4.0)	31.7 (4.2)	34.4 (4.6)	37.8 (4.3)							
8	20.8 (3.5)	23.0 (3.4)	25.2 (3.5)	27.6 (3.6)	29.7 (3.7)	32.2 (3.9)	34.9 (3.8)	37.9 (3.8)						
9	20.5 (3.3)	22.4 (3.3)	24.6 (3.3)	26.8 (3.4)	28.9 (3.4)	31.2 (3.5)	33.8 (3.5)	36.4 (3.6)	39.0 (3.7)					
10	18.9 (3.1)	20.8 (3.3)	22.8 (3.3)	24.9 (3.4)	27.0 (3.6)	29.1 (3.6)	31.4 (3.5)	34.0 (3.5)	36.6 (3.5)	39.1 (3.5)				
11	19.0 (3.2)	20.7 (3.4)	22.5 (3.4)	24.6 (3.6)	26.7 (3.7)	28.5 (3.7)	30.5 (3.9)	32.4 (4.2)	34.5 (4.3)	36.7 (4.2)	39.0 (4.0)			
12	19.5 (3.4)	21.3 (3.6)	23.1 (3.2)	24.9 (3.3)	26.8 (3.5)	28.6 (3.4)	30.6 (3.6)	32.5 (4.0)	34.4 (3.9)	36.2 (3.8)	38.1 (3.6)	40.8 (3.5)		
13	18.0 (2.8)	19.5 (2.9)	21.1 (2.7)	22.7 (2.5)	24.4 (2.4)	25.7 (2.6)	27.4 (3.0)	29.4 (3.2)	31.1 (3.0)	33.6 (3.4)	35.3 (3.4)	37.6 (2.9)	40.4 (2.8)	
14	18.6 (2.2)	20.5 (2.5)	22.9 (2.7)	24.8 (2.5)	26.4 (2.6)	28.2 (2.8)	31.0 (3.3)	32.7 (3.2)	34.1 (2.8)	35.4 (2.9)	36.9 (3.3)	38.4 (3.5)	39.9 (3.6)	41.9 (3.9)

Turkey

Birth of order i

Completed parity j	1	2	3	4	5	6	7	8	9	10	11	12	13	14	15
1	27.4 (8.1)														
2	22.8 (4.8)	27.0 (5.0)													
3	22.0 (4.5)	25.3 (4.9)	29.3 (4.8)												
4	20.4 (3.3)	23.0 (3.3)	26.3 (3.8)	30.4 (4.2)											
5	20.4 (3.3)	23.0 (3.5)	25.5 (3.6)	28.4 (3.8)	32.4 (4.3)										
6	20.0 (3.5)	22.2 (3.6)	24.6 (3.7)	27.1 (3.8)	30.3 (4.0)	34.2 (4.4)									
7	19.7 (3.1)	22.1 (3.4)	24.3 (3.6)	26.5 (3.6)	29.2 (3.5)	32.0 (3.9)	35.6 (3.8)								
8	20.0 (3.4)	22.0 (3.4)	23.8 (3.4)	25.9 (3.6)	28.3 (3.6)	30.5 (3.7)	33.2 (4.1)	36.5 (4.4)							
9	18.8 (2.9)	20.8 (2.9)	23.1 (3.0)	25.3 (3.0)	27.2 (3.1)	29.2 (3.1)	31.6 (3.4)	34.2 (3.7)	37.3 (3.5)						
10	19.5 (2.9)	21.5 (3.0)	23.4 (3.2)	25.4 (3.4)	27.3 (3.2)	29.3 (3.3)	31.4 (3.3)	33.5 (3.3)	36.0 (2.7)	38.9 (2.8)					
11	18.0 (2.8)	20.0 (2.6)	21.5 (2.5)	23.3 (2.8)	25.1 (2.9)	27.1 (3.1)	29.1 (3.1)	30.9 (3.1)	33.0 (3.4)	35.7 (3.3)	38.2 (3.6)				
12	18.1 (2.0)	20.3 (2.9)	22.1 (3.1)	23.6 (3.2)	25.2 (3.4)	26.6 (3.3)	28.2 (3.6)	30.0 (3.4)	31.9 (3.2)	34.0 (2.9)	35.9 (2.8)	38.5 (3.0)			
13	18.1 (3.3)	20.0 (3.2)	21.6 (3.0)	23.1 (3.1)	24.5 (3.1)	26.0 (3.1)	27.5 (3.3)	28.8 (3.5)	30.4 (3.6)	32.4 (3.4)	34.6 (3.5)	36.6 (3.3)	39.6 (3.2)		
14	16.6 (3.1)	18.5 (3.8)	20.0 (3.8)	21.2 (3.5)	22.7 (3.7)	24.4 (3.5)	26.6 (4.1)	28.3 (4.0)	29.9 (4.0)	31.5 (4.0)	33.1 (4.2)	34.9 (4.2)	36.2 (4.3)	38.5 (4.4)	
15	17.3 (3.2)	18.7 (3.1)	20.0 (3.1)	21.7 (2.7)	22.9 (3.0)	24.3 (3.2)	25.4 (3.3)	27.3 (3.9)	28.3 (3.9)	29.2 (4.4)	30.5 (4.4)	31.8 (3.8)	33.8 (3.3)	35.6 (3.0)	37.3 (2.6)

Venezuela

Birth of order i

Completed parity j	1	2	3	4	5	6	7	8	9	10	11	12	13	14	15
1	29.6 (6.2)														
2	25.7 (6.6)	30.1 (6.1)													
3	24.3 (4.8)	26.9 (5.2)	31.2 (6.0)												
4	22.1 (5.7)	24.5 (5.4)	27.3 (5.4)	32.0 (5.8)											
5	20.3 (3.0)	22.3 (3.3)	24.8 (4.0)	27.8 (3.6)	31.8 (5.3)										
6	20.0 (2.6)	22.6 (3.2)	25.0 (4.0)	27.5 (4.4)	30.4 (4.3)	34.0 (4.6)									
7	21.5 (3.6)	23.4 (3.5)	25.5 (3.8)	27.4 (3.5)	29.8 (3.4)	32.2 (3.1)	35.1 (3.3)								
8	18.9 (2.3)	20.8 (2.1)	23.0 (2.2)	25.5 (1.8)	27.8 (2.0)	30.3 (2.3)	32.6 (2.6)	36.0 (2.9)							
9	19.0 (2.5)	21.0 (3.0)	23.3 (3.2)	25.4 (3.2)	27.6 (3.2)	29.8 (3.3)	31.9 (3.3)	34.7 (2.3)	37.3 (2.7)						
10	19.1 (3.2)	21.6 (3.2)	23.3 (3.1)	25.6 (3.1)	27.6 (2.9)	29.1 (3.0)	31.4 (3.4)	33.5 (3.4)	35.6 (3.3)	37.8 (3.6)					
11	17.7 (2.8)	20.1 (3.0)	21.8 (3.2)	23.9 (3.3)	25.8 (3.4)	27.5 (3.4)	29.2 (3.3)	31.2 (3.5)	33.1 (3.6)	34.6 (3.5)	37.4 (3.3)				
12	17.4 (2.7)	19.2 (2.6)	21.4 (3.5)	23.2 (3.6)	25.0 (3.7)	26.6 (3.3)	28.2 (3.2)	29.8 (3.8)	31.5 (3.4)	33.7 (3.9)	35.7 (3.7)	38.7 (2.9)			
13	18.9 (2.5)	20.8 (2.5)	22.8 (2.7)	24.2 (2.9)	25.9 (2.6)	28.0 (3.0)	29.3 (3.1)	30.5 (3.1)	32.8 (2.8)	34.2 (2.8)	35.7 (2.7)	37.6 (2.1)	39.9 (2.5)		
14	16.6 (2.2)	18.1 (2.5)	20.4 (3.6)	21.5 (4.2)	23.2 (4.0)	25.7 (3.4)	26.8 (3.3)	28.0 (3.6)	29.5 (3.8)	31.4 (3.2)	32.6 (3.8)	35.0 (3.2)	37.3 (3.0)	39.7 (2.8)	
15	17.9 (.8)	19.3 (1.0)	20.2 (.8)	21.5 (.8)	22.5 (.7)	23.6 (.5)	25.6 (1.1)	27.1 (.9)	28.8 (1.4)	30.1 (1.2)	31.2 (1.1)	32.8 (1.4)	33.9 (1.4)	34.7 (1.2)	37.7 (1.9)

Yemen Arab Republic

Completed parity j	Birth of order i												
	1	2	3	4	5	6	7	8	9	10	11	12	13
1	33.0 (9.9)												
2	31.8 (7.2)	35.3 (5.2)											
3	26.4 (5.7)	29.8 (6.2)	34.3 (7.1)										
4	24.6 (6.8)	27.6 (6.5)	31.6 (6.3)	35.4 (6.3)									
5	27.4 (7.1)	30.2 (6.7)	32.5 (6.6)	35.2 (6.1)	38.4 (5.6)								
6	25.0 (7.0)	27.2 (7.3)	30.4 (6.9)	33.1 (6.7)	35.6 (6.4)	38.5 (6.2)							
7	22.1 (4.7)	24.7 (5.0)	27.2 (4.9)	30.1 (4.5)	33.5 (4.3)	35.9 (4.7)	39.1 (4.7)						
8	20.6 (4.9)	22.9 (4.9)	25.6 (4.9)	27.9 (4.7)	30.4 (4.9)	33.0 (5.0)	35.4 (5.1)	38.2 (5.1)					
9	20.7 (5.1)	23.5 (5.5)	25.8 (5.6)	28.1 (5.3)	30.5 (5.4)	32.4 (5.3)	35.0 (5.3)	37.7 (4.9)	40.9 (4.1)				
10	21.6 (5.1)	23.4 (5.1)	25.1 (5.0)	27.0 (5.0)	28.8 (5.2)	31.4 (5.2)	33.7 (5.1)	35.9 (4.7)	38.6 (4.3)	40.8 (4.4)			
11	19.6 (5.6)	21.6 (5.4)	23.4 (5.1)	24.9 (5.0)	27.0 (4.9)	28.9 (5.0)	31.3 (4.9)	33.7 (4.3)	35.7 (4.3)	37.8 (4.2)	40.5 (4.2)		
12	20.9 (7.7)	23.4 (8.0)	24.7 (7.6)	26.1 (7.5)	27.3 (7.5)	29.4 (7.7)	31.0 (7.7)	32.4 (7.6)	34.1 (7.7)	36.5 (7.7)	38.3 (7.4)	41.0 (6.3)	
13	18.0 (3.9)	20.0 (3.5)	21.8 (3.8)	23.9 (4.1)	26.1 (4.1)	27.9 (4.0)	29.9 (3.6)	31.8 (4.1)	34.1 (5.1)	35.7 (5.4)	39.4 (4.7)	41.9 (3.1)	43.1 (3.2)

Appendix C

Current parity distributions and mean parities for five-year age and marital duration groups for all ever-married women included in the sample for 41 LDC-World Fertility Surveys (including Portugal) and 14 European World Fertility Surveys (including USA). For details see discussion in Section 2.4.

Bangladesh

Children ever born	Age group							Marital duration (in years)						
	15-19	20-24	25-29	30-34	35-39	40-44	45-49	0-4	5-9	10-14	15-19	20-24	25-29	30+
0	49.7	8.5	3.0	1.8	2.2	2.5	2.6	59.0	10.4	4.9	2.2	1.9	2.2	2.5
1	33.9	19.1	3.8	1.7	1.3	2.0	3.6	33.4	26.3	7.9	2.9	1.9	1.5	3.1
2	13.2	27.5	9.6	4.8	2.7	3.8	4.5	6.5	35.6	14.2	5.6	4.7	3.9	4.0
3	2.5	22.7	17.6	7.0	4.2	4.8	6.4	.9	17.5	22.1	11.6	6.1	3.6	6.4
4	.7	15.1	21.2	12.2	7.7	4.4	5.8	.0	7.7	23.1	16.3	10.6	6.0	5.0
5	.0	5.7	21.2	17.7	10.2	8.9	8.5	.0	1.5	17.8	19.4	12.1	9.0	9.9
6	.0	1.2	13.3	20.6	15.8	10.4	12.4	.1	.4	6.1	20.2	17.6	14.8	10.2
7	.0	.3	6.7	14.0	17.6	15.5	15.2	.0	.1	3.0	11.5	15.6	15.2	15.9
8	.0	.0	2.7	9.6	16.4	14.5	10.9	.0	.0	.8	5.6	15.0	12.9	13.0
9	.0	.0	.8	7.6	8.7	15.2	9.7	.1	.1	.0	3.4	7.6	13.6	11.6
10	.0	.0	.1	2.8	6.6	7.8	9.9	.0	.2	.0	.9	4.4	8.4	8.3
11	.0	.0	.1	.2	3.8	6.2	3.9	.0	.1	.0	.4	1.4	5.0	4.7
12	.0	.0	.0	.0	1.7	2.4	3.8	.0	.0	.0	.0	.5	2.4	3.2
13	.0	.0	.0	.0	.9	1.1	.9	.0	.0	.0	.0	.2	1.2	1.0
14	.0	.0	.0	.2	.0	.4	1.1	.0	.0	.0	.0	.2	.4	.7
15	.0	.0	.0	.0	.2	.2	.7	.0	.0	.0	.0	.2	.0	.6
(N=100%)	1462	1335	1124	784	679	630	494	1173	1090	1167	858	758	613	851
Mean	.71	2.40	4.24	5.67	6.72	7.07	6.79	.51	1.96	3.49	5.02	6.09	6.98	6.85

Benin

Children ever born	Age group							Marital duration (in years)						
	15-19	20-24	25-29	30-34	35-39	40-44	45-49	0-4	5-9	10-14	15-19	20-24	25-29	30+
0	45.1	11.8	4.8	3.2	3.9	2.9	3.5	25.3	4.5	3.5	2.4	2.6	3.3	2.5
1	47.0	36.0	8.8	4.0	2.2	2.6	2.5	46.8	10.0	2.6	2.2	2.8	1.2	3.8
2	7.5	32.5	22.2	6.7	5.2	5.0	7.8	20.8	32.3	10.0	3.6	5.6	5.8	2.5
3	.4	13.7	24.1	11.8	6.9	6.6	7.4	4.4	31.1	14.0	6.1	6.3	6.2	2.5
4	.0	4.7	20.9	18.5	10.1	11.8	8.5	1.2	14.9	26.3	12.9	7.7	7.9	10.1
5	.0	1.0	12.6	19.4	15.1	10.0	7.4	.5	5.1	21.9	17.2	11.7	6.6	7.6
6	.0	.1	4.0	16.7	18.9	14.7	8.2	.4	1.3	12.3	19.4	16.7	10.0	11.4
7	.0	.1	1.8	12.1	13.5	14.2	16.0	.0	.3	7.2	17.2	14.3	16.2	13.9
8	.0	.0	.6	4.7	10.3	15.0	12.8	.1	.1	1.4	10.7	13.8	16.6	11.4
9	.0	.0	.2	2.0	8.6	8.1	13.8	.1	.0	.6	6.7	10.3	12.0	15.2
10	.0	.0	.0	.8	2.2	4.5	6.0	.4	.0	.3	1.2	3.5	7.5	6.3
11	.0	.0	.0	.0	1.7	3.7	3.9	.0	.3	.0	.4	2.3	4.1	11.4
12	.0	.0	.0	.0	1.3	.8	1.1	.0	.1	.0	.0	1.6	1.7	.0
13	.0	.0	.0	.0	.2	.0	.7	.0	.0	.0	.0	.5	.4	.0
14	.0	.0	.0	.0	.0	.3	.0	.0	.0	.0	.0	.0	.4	.0
15	.0	.0	.0	.0	.0	.0	.4	.0	.0	.0	.0	.0	.0	1.3
(N=100%)	266	769	820	594	465	381	282	854	779	693	505	426	241	79
Mean	.63	1.68	3.16	4.73	5.76	6.08	6.29	1.17	2.68	4.23	5.65	6.14	6.62	6.96

Cameroon

Children ever born	Age group							Marital duration (in years)						
	15-19	20-24	25-29	30-34	35-39	40-44	45-49	0-4	5-9	10-14	15-19	20-24	25-29	30+
0	46.4	16.7	11.0	9.6	11.3	10.8	13.7	34.4	12.2	11.2	8.6	11.2	13.6	22.5
1	39.6	28.7	12.1	8.9	8.8	9.4	9.3	39.7	15.7	10.2	7.5	8.7	10.3	8.2
2	11.3	28.4	15.0	7.8	6.9	8.1	4.4	17.9	24.0	8.9	8.2	5.7	9.2	5.8
3	2.3	19.2	19.7	9.3	7.8	7.2	8.8	5.6	24.8	13.3	8.5	7.6	5.8	8.8
4	.5	5.3	20.6	16.3	8.3	6.5	7.0	1.4	14.4	18.5	11.0	8.4	5.3	5.4
5	.0	1.6	11.6	17.5	8.9	7.7	7.6	.5	6.0	16.4	14.0	6.0	6.9	5.8
6	.0	.0	7.0	13.3	13.7	9.6	10.1	.4	2.0	12.0	13.7	12.3	7.6	7.3
7	.0	.0	2.3	8.8	11.7	12.5	7.7	.0	.6	5.6	11.4	12.2	9.0	10.0
8	.0	.0	.6	5.2	10.5	9.1	10.1	.1	.3	2.5	9.7	10.5	10.2	6.0
9	.0	.0	.1	2.5	7.0	8.2	7.9	.2	.1	.8	4.3	8.7	10.0	6.4
10	.0	.0	.0	.8	2.6	4.4	4.9	.0	.0	.2	1.8	4.2	4.8	5.8
11	.0	.0	.0	.0	2.2	3.6	4.3	.0	.0	.3	1.1	2.9	3.9	4.1
12	.0	.0	.0	.0	.4	1.4	2.9	.0	.1	.0	.0	1.3	2.3	2.0
13	.0	.0	.0	.0	.0	.9	.5	.0	.0	.0	.3	.2	.3	1.3
14	.0	.0	.0	.0	.0	.4	.7	.0	.0	.0	.0	.1	.8	.4
15	.0	.0	.0	.0	.0	.0	.0	.0	.0	.0	.0	.0	.0	.3
(N=100%)	787	1339	1250	1112	951	867	588	1479	1396	1242	1085	868	667	530
Mean	.71	1.73	3.05	4.19	4.89	5.23	5.25	1.04	2.46	3.69	4.76	5.21	5.17	4.71

Costa Rica

Children ever born	Age group							Marital duration (in years)						
	15-19	20-24	25-29	30-34	35-39	40-44	45-49	0-4	5-9	10-14	15-19	20-24	25-29	30+
0	.0	14.0	7.2	3.7	4.3	2.0	3.6	21.0	4.2	2.3	1.1	1.3	1.5	1.4
1	.0	36.5	22.7	9.9	3.7	3.5	3.6	43.5	17.9	4.6	2.6	3.5	.4	4.1
2	.0	31.1	26.7	18.2	10.6	8.8	5.5	25.5	34.2	16.2	11.0	3.0	3.1	5.4
3	.0	12.7	20.5	18.3	11.0	9.5	11.7	7.3	25.2	22.6	9.2	9.8	6.2	6.8
4	.0	4.6	9.7	12.6	15.4	10.3	7.5	1.3	11.3	18.3	14.3	9.0	6.2	4.1
5	.0	.7	7.8	12.6	10.6	10.0	4.4	.5	3.5	16.0	15.4	9.3	4.2	2.7
6	.0	.4	4.0	10.3	11.0	9.3	8.3	.0	2.9	10.0	13.2	11.0	9.6	9.5
7	.0	.0	.6	7.9	8.3	6.8	8.6	.5	.5	5.7	11.4	9.0	8.1	5.4
8	.0	.0	.3	3.5	5.9	7.5	8.6	.2	.3	2.3	6.6	11.0	6.5	10.8
9	.0	.0	.2	1.4	7.9	7.5	7.0	.3	.2	.5	7.3	9.3	8.8	9.5
10	.0	.0	.3	1.2	4.3	7.0	6.8	.0	.0	.5	4.4	8.0	8.8	9.5
11	.0	.0	.0	.5	3.3	4.8	6.2	.0	.0	.5	2.2	5.3	9.6	5.4
12	.0	.0	.0	.0	2.0	4.3	7.5	.0	.0	.0	.9	4.8	10.4	8.1
13	.0	.0	.0	.0	.8	3.8	4.7	.0	.0	.0	.2	3.0	7.7	5.4
14	.0	.0	.0	.0	.4	2.3	1.8	.0	.0	.2	.2	1.0	3.8	2.7
15	.0	.0	.0	.0	.4	2.8	4.2	.0	.0	.2	.0	2.0	5.0	9.5
(N=100%)	0	543	629	573	508	399	385	620	666	562	455	400	260	74
Mean	1.61	2.51	3.90	5.40	6.67	7.18	2.48	3.98	5.48	6.99	8.65	8.32	.00	

Dominican Republic

Children ever born	Age group							Marital duration (in years)						
	15-19	20-24	25-29	30-34	35-39	40-44	45-49	0-4	5-9	10-14	15-19	20-24	25-29	30+
0	43.1	17.4	6.2	3.8	2.6	6.0	3.5	35.5	7.3	4.1	1.6	3.5	3.0	4.0
1	39.7	29.2	12.6	6.0	2.3	4.7	7.1	41.5	15.0	6.6	3.2	4.6	4.5	4.0
2	15.1	24.4	10.9	9.5	7.2	5.6	5.8	19.8	27.1	8.1	6.4	5.0	4.5	4.0
3	2.2	16.4	18.6	13.7	6.9	6.4	8.8	2.6	25.6	17.0	10.5	6.0	5.6	3.0
4	.0	8.7	16.9	10.8	11.5	10.7	10.6	.6	16.7	14.7	11.8	11.7	8.6	10.0
5	.0	3.1	15.7	16.8	9.2	8.1	7.5	.0	6.4	22.3	12.7	6.4	9.1	8.0
6	.0	.8	6.9	14.3	10.7	12.4	7.5	.0	1.3	14.0	14.3	11.3	7.1	9.0
7	.0	.0	4.0	11.4	9.5	4.7	6.6	.0	.4	10.2	9.2	8.2	7.6	3.0
8	.0	.0	1.0	5.7	12.4	9.4	7.1	.0	.0	2.0	13.1	10.6	10.1	4.0
9	.0	.0	.5	3.8	8.6	8.1	6.2	.0	.0	.8	8.3	8.9	9.1	5.0
10	.0	.0	.7	1.9	8.6	4.3	8.4	.0	.2	.3	5.7	7.8	6.1	14.0
11	.0	.0	.0	1.3	5.5	6.4	8.4	.0	.0	.0	2.2	8.2	6.6	14.0
12	.0	.0	.0	.3	2.9	6.0	5.3	.0	.0	.0	.6	3.5	8.6	8.0
13	.0	.0	.0	.6	1.4	4.7	2.7	.0	.0	.0	.3	2.8	6.1	3.0
14	.0	.0	.0	.0	.3	.4	1.3	.0	.0	.0	.0	.7	.5	2.0
15	.0	.0	.0	.0	.3	2.1	3.1	.0	.0	.0	.0	.7	3.0	5.0
(N=100%)	232	483	420	315	347	234	226	501	468	394	314	282	198	100
Mean	.76	1.82	3.37	4.84	6.46	6.58	6.69	.91	2.58	4.25	5.82	6.69	7.35	7.85

Ecuador

Children ever born	Age group							Marital duration (in years)						
	15-19	20-24	25-29	30-34	35-39	40-44	45-49	0-4	5-9	10-14	15-19	20-24	25-29	30+
0	35.5	10.2	4.8	2.7	2.1	2.0	1.6	21.4	3.8	2.4	.3	1.0	1.3	.7
1	46.1	31.7	14.9	8.0	3.6	2.4	2.9	45.4	11.1	4.4	2.8	1.9	1.3	2.1
2	15.8	29.4	25.6	12.4	6.8	6.3	5.3	26.2	29.2	10.6	4.8	5.2	3.1	4.3
3	2.3	18.1	18.8	18.1	10.4	7.4	7.5	5.3	29.5	18.6	10.5	5.6	5.0	2.9
4	.3	7.4	16.1	12.9	12.2	8.9	10.0	1.5	16.8	18.4	12.2	7.8	10.0	2.9
5	.0	2.7	9.3	12.3	13.3	10.4	8.9	.0	5.9	18.1	13.1	13.8	6.8	5.7
6	.0	.5	7.0	10.9	13.7	10.6	8.4	.0	2.7	14.0	15.9	12.0	10.2	1.4
7	.0	.0	2.3	9.7	10.4	9.7	9.5	.1	.6	7.0	14.4	12.0	10.0	6.4
8	.0	.0	.6	7.2	9.0	8.4	11.3	.1	.1	4.8	11.4	9.9	9.2	15.0
9	.0	.0	.6	3.7	6.8	11.3	7.5	.0	.2	1.2	8.3	11.6	9.7	9.3
10	.0	.0	.1	1.1	4.8	6.9	7.8	.0	.0	.4	3.3	7.0	10.5	10.0
11	.0	.0	.0	.5	2.7	5.0	6.7	.0	.0	.1	1.7	5.2	6.0	12.1
12	.0	.0	.0	.3	3.0	5.2	4.9	.0	.0	.0	.8	4.8	7.3	10.0
13	.0	.0	.0	.3	.3	3.0	3.5	.0	.0	.0	.3	1.4	4.2	7.9
14	.0	.0	.0	.0	.5	1.3	1.6	.0	.0	.0	.2	.2	2.6	3.6
15	.0	.0	.0	.0	.5	1.1	2.7	.0	.0	.0	.0	.6	2.6	5.7
(N=100%)	310	792	863	790	664	538	451	1014	965	752	640	516	381	140
Mean	.86	1.91	3.02	4.48	5.83	6.85	7.13	1.21	2.78	4.33	5.88	6.84	7.79	9.08

Egypt

Children ever born	Age group							Marital duration (in years)						
	15-19	20-24	25-29	30-34	35-39	40-44	45-49	0-4	5-9	10-14	15-19	20-24	25-29	30+
0	52.5	18.1	8.5	4.1	3.2	4.1	3.7	37.1	6.7	3.8	2.3	2.4	2.7	2.9
1	36.1	26.2	12.9	5.5	3.8	2.5	4.1	38.6	10.3	4.9	3.1	2.6	2.4	1.9
2	8.1	25.9	18.9	10.5	5.9	4.9	4.2	20.7	26.4	9.1	5.6	3.8	3.5	2.1
3	2.4	18.9	20.5	12.7	8.7	5.8	3.7	3.4	33.4	17.3	7.2	5.9	4.5	1.9
4	.7	8.7	17.5	15.3	10.0	7.3	7.2	.2	17.2	23.8	13.0	6.6	6.7	4.8
5	.1	1.6	10.6	16.8	12.1	11.4	9.4	.0	4.6	19.1	17.0	12.1	10.6	6.7
6	.0	.3	7.0	13.9	14.4	13.4	10.1	.1	1.3	13.2	18.9	13.4	12.1	9.8
7	.0	.3	3.0	9.7	14.1	13.3	13.0	.0	.1	6.2	14.9	16.4	13.0	13.3
8	.0	.1	.8	6.4	12.6	11.8	12.0	.0	.0	1.7	10.5	14.7	13.5	13.3
9	.0	.0	.4	3.2	6.9	9.6	11.2	.0	.0	.6	4.7	10.4	11.4	12.3
10	.0	.0	.0	1.4	4.3	8.4	10.1	.0	.0	.1	1.8	6.5	10.8	12.5
11	.0	.0	.0	.4	2.0	3.3	4.5	.0	.0	.1	.8	2.3	4.0	6.7
12	.0	.0	.0	.2	.8	2.4	4.1	.0	.0	.0	.2	1.5	3.1	5.8
13	.0	.0	.0	.0	.5	.9	1.3	.0	.0	.0	.0	.7	.7	2.9
14	.0	.0	.0	.0	.2	.6	1.0	.0	.0	.0	.0	.3	.7	1.5
15	.0	.0	.0	.0	.2	.5	.6	.0	.0	.0	.0	.3	.3	1.3
(N=100%)	678	1598	1696	1523	1329	1061	903	1916	1664	1390	1308	1108	883	519
Mean	.63	1.81	3.07	4.61	5.79	6.46	6.86	.91	2.64	4.11	5.46	6.48	6.89	7.82

Fiji

Children ever born	Age group							Marital duration (in years)						
	15-19	20-24	25-29	30-34	35-39	40-44	45-49	0-4	5-9	10-14	15-19	20-24	25-29	30+
0	58.3	22.4	8.6	5.0	4.4	4.2	6.4	35.3	6.4	4.8	4.1	3.3	4.3	4.5
1	33.8	33.7	14.6	5.5	5.2	3.6	4.5	39.5	12.1	5.8	4.5	4.5	3.4	2.4
2	6.6	25.8	24.0	9.8	7.1	6.0	5.0	20.1	30.6	10.7	5.4	6.2	4.8	2.4
3	1.3	12.7	22.3	16.7	10.7	7.6	5.9	4.8	29.4	19.4	8.3	10.5	6.1	4.5
4	.0	4.1	17.3	17.7	10.9	8.3	5.0	.3	15.3	22.5	15.2	8.1	4.5	6.5
5	.0	1.2	8.0	19.2	15.5	11.2	8.4	.0	5.0	18.6	20.8	13.5	8.6	6.5
6	.0	.1	3.5	13.0	12.9	11.5	10.7	.1	.8	11.3	16.4	11.4	10.6	12.2
7	.0	.0	1.1	6.9	15.2	12.8	11.8	.0	.2	4.9	12.9	15.1	14.3	9.8
8	.0	.0	.5	3.4	8.6	10.7	12.5	.0	.1	1.4	7.1	11.1	12.4	12.7
9	.0	.0	.1	1.9	4.8	8.4	10.9	.0	.0	.1	3.4	7.6	12.0	11.0
10	.0	.0	.0	.6	2.9	8.4	6.8	.0	.0	.4	1.4	4.8	9.7	9.4
11	.0	.0	.0	.1	1.0	4.1	5.2	.0	.0	.0	.3	2.1	4.3	9.0
12	.0	.0	.0	.2	.7	1.8	2.7	.0	.1	.0	.3	1.3	2.5	3.3
13	.0	.0	.0	.0	.3	.5	1.4	.0	.0	.0	.0	.3	1.1	1.6
14	.0	.0	.0	.0	.0	.6	.9	.0	.0	.0	.0	.2	.9	1.2
15	.0	.0	.0	.0	.0	.2	1.8	.0	.0	.0	.0	.0	.5	2.9
(N=100%)	228	907	1049	953	735	616	440	1067	960	849	736	629	442	245
Mean	.51	1.46	2.72	4.22	5.19	6.17	6.55	.96	2.56	3.87	5.01	5.73	6.72	7.35

Ghana

Children ever born	Age group							Marital duration (in years)						
	15-19	20-24	25-29	30-34	35-39	40-44	45-49	0-4	5-9	10-14	15-19	20-24	25-29	30+
0	37.3	12.3	5.8	4.2	1.0	2.6	2.1	27.2	4.3	2.9	1.4	2.1	1.7	.6
1	54.5	39.2	13.5	5.7	2.3	1.9	2.1	53.5	16.1	4.6	1.7	2.4	1.5	3.0
2	8.0	31.4	26.7	10.1	6.3	5.6	4.6	16.8	37.9	11.2	7.1	5.2	3.2	4.8
3	.2	12.0	25.6	19.2	10.2	6.8	6.4	1.4	28.0	23.5	10.7	8.3	3.9	5.5
4	.0	4.3	15.9	21.8	16.5	10.2	8.4	.6	11.3	25.6	18.0	12.4	6.6	6.7
5	.0	.8	8.4	16.0	16.4	12.5	6.6	.1	2.2	18.5	19.6	10.6	9.5	4.8
6	.0	.0	3.1	11.6	15.5	13.5	13.2	.2	.1	8.5	18.5	15.1	13.0	7.3
7	.0	.0	.7	8.1	14.2	14.2	13.2	.0	.0	3.7	14.8	14.6	13.4	16.4
8	.0	.0	.4	2.5	9.9	12.8	14.4	.1	.0	.7	5.8	13.7	18.1	12.7
9	.0	.0	.0	.8	4.3	9.9	12.6	.0	.0	.5	1.8	8.9	13.7	11.5
10	.0	.0	.0	.3	2.4	6.6	9.4	.0	.0	.1	.3	5.1	9.8	13.9
11	.0	.0	.0	.0	.9	2.1	4.8	.0	.0	.0	.3	1.6	3.4	7.9
12	.0	.0	.0	.0	.1	.2	1.1	.0	.0	.0	.0	.0	.7	2.4
13	.0	.0	.0	.0	.0	1.0	.9	.0	.0	.0	.0	.2	1.5	1.8
14	.0	.0	.0	.0	.0	.0	.2	.0	.0	.0	.0	.0	.0	.6
15	.0	.0	.0	.0	.0	.0	.0	.0	.0	.0	.0	.0	.0	.0
(N=100%)	424	1032	981	795	697	576	438	1117	1084	820	718	630	409	165
Mean	.71	1.59	2.76	4.06	5.39	6.14	6.73	.96	2.33	3.81	5.02	5.93	6.97	7.31

Guyana

Children ever born	15-19	20-24	25-29	30-34	35-39	40-44	45-49
	Age group						
0	41.3	21.6	9.8	3.7	3.5	6.9	3.9
1	41.0	27.3	14.0	4.6	4.3	6.0	7.0
2	14.9	22.3	19.6	9.2	7.0	4.5	4.7
3	2.0	15.5	18.3	12.5	9.4	7.2	7.5
4	.8	8.6	17.0	16.8	9.4	.6.7	6.5
5	.0	3.3	11.3	12.5	11.7	8.6	8.3
6	.0	1.1	7.0	16.9	12.3	10.7	9.6
7	.0	.1	1.8	9.9	13.1	7.9	11.9
8	.0	.0	.3	6.1	10.1	9.3	11.4
9	.0	.0	.4	3.1	6.2	10.3	8.3
10	.0	.0	.4	1.8	6.4	8.1	7.3
11	.0	.0	.0	1.8	3.5	5.3	4.2
12	.0	.0	.0	.4	2.1	5.0	4.4
13	.0	.0	.0	.4	.8	2.6	1.8
14	.0	.0	.0	.2	.0	.2	2.3
15	.0	.0	.0	.0	.2	.7	.8
(N=100%)	356	721	705	543	487	419	385
Mean	.80	1.77	2.98	4.89	5.85	6.40	6.54

Children ever born	0-4	5-9	10-14	15-19	20-24	25-29	30+
	Marital duration (in years)						
0	38.3	8.8	5.2	3.8	3.7	2.2	2.9
1	38.4	16.3	6.8	4.4	3.5	5.4	6.3
2	17.5	24.8	13.0	6.3	3.3	4.9	3.4
3	5.0	23.8	15.3	10.1	7.7	4.9	6.3
4	.7	17.2	20.4	12.2	7.2	6.0	4.6
5	.0	6.2	18.2	12.2	10.3	7.4	8.0
6	.0	2.9	12.8	16.2	14.0	11.2	6.9
7	.0	.0	4.9	12.2	14.5	12.0	8.0
8	.0	.0	1.4	10.5	10.7	10.4	11.4
9	.0	.0	.9	5.3	7.9	10.6	10.9
10	.0	.0	.7	4.2	7.9	7.9	9.7
11	.0	.0	.4	1.7	5.8	4.6	6.9
12	.0	.0	.0	.2	2.6	7.6	5.7
13	.0	.0	.0	.4	.7	3.0	4.6
14	.1	.0	.0	.2	.0	1.1	2.9
15	.0	.0	.0	.0	.2	.8	1.7
(N=100%)	805	761	555	524	429	367	175
Mean	.93	2.54	3.93	5.43	6.42	7.08	7.43

Haiti

Children ever born	15-19	20-24	25-29	30-34	35-39	40-44	45-49
	Age group						
0	47.0	25.5	11.6	4.9	5.6	4.1	2.6
1	43.3	39.7	22.9	12.9	9.4	6.7	5.4
2	6.9	20.0	24.6	16.8	12.8	6.3	5.8
3	2.0	10.1	18.4	18.4	9.5	8.8	8.6
4	.8	3.9	10.7	15.0	12.2	9.4	10.6
5	.0	.6	7.1	13.5	10.7	10.2	11.8
6	.0	.2	3.8	8.2	12.5	12.6	10.0
7	.0	.0	.9	7.8	10.4	11.2	10.6
8	.0	.0	.0	1.7	7.4	10.8	11.2
9	.0	.0	.0	.8	4.8	10.0	9.2
10	.0	.0	.0	.0	2.9	5.7	6.8
11	.0	.0	.0	.0	1.2	2.6	4.4
12	.0	.0	.0	.0	.6	1.2	1.2
13	.0	.0	.0	.0	.0	.4	.4
14	.0	.0	.0	.0	.0	.0	.4
15	.0	.0	.0	.0	.0	.0	.8
(N=100%)	129	424	471	375	346	266	260
Mean	.66	1.30	2.34	3.54	4.66	5.69	6.06

Children ever born	0-4	5-9	10-14	15-19	20-24	25-29	30+
	Marital duration (in years)						
0	37.5	10.4	3.7	2.1	4.3	.8	.0
1	47.3	20.5	10.6	7.6	5.4	5.6	12.4
2	13.8	28.4	14.6	10.7	8.9	2.3	8.2
3	1.3	25.4	17.2	11.3	8.8	3.1	3.1
4	.2	11.7	19.9	10.5	9.5	8.5	6.2
5	.0	2.8	19.4	12.9	7.9	14.4	6.2
6	.0	.8	10.1	18.7	9.6	9.3	10.3
7	.0	.0	3.7	15.5	12.5	11.5	10.3
8	.0	.0	.6	7.1	13.6	10.1	12.4
9	.0	.0	.3	2.9	11.6	11.8	8.2
10	.0	.0	.0	.3	4.8	11.5	12.4
11	.0	.0	.0	.3	2.3	6.8	4.1
12	.0	.0	.0	.0	.9	2.5	2.1
13	.0	.0	.0	.0	.0	.6	2.1
14	.0	.0	.0	.0	.0	.0	2.1
15	.0	.0	.0	.0	.0	1.1	.0
(N=100%)	497	555	368	323	292	185	51
Mean	.79	2.19	3.61	4.80	5.69	6.94	6.51

Indonesia

Children ever born	15-19	20-24	25-29	30-34	35-39	40-44	45-49
	Age group						
0	53.2	16.0	7.8	6.3	5.9	4.8	9.0
1	37.4	32.8	14.4	9.9	8.5	9.1	7.6
2	7.3	30.0	21.8	11.9	8.7	6.7	10.5
3	1.7	14.1	23.0	13.9	8.9	10.2	7.7
4	.4	5.1	17.5	14.9	11.2	9.6	9.2
5	.0	1.5	9.8	15.4	14.4	11.0	8.3
6	.0	.2	3.9	13.4	15.5	12.7	9.8
7	.0	.1	1.3	7.1	10.8	11.2	9.8
8	.0	.1	.4	5.1	6.8	8.9	10.8
9	.0	.0	.0	1.1	4.4	6.5	6.2
10	.0	.0	.0	.9	3.2	3.9	5.0
11	.0	.0	.0	.1	.7	3.3	3.2
12	.0	.0	.0	.0	.7	1.7	1.9
13	.0	.0	.0	.0	.3	.2	.4
14	.0	.0	.0	.0	.0	.1	.2
15	.0	.0	.0	.0	.0	.0	.4
(N=100%)	994	1624	1501	1414	1408	1250	964
Mean	.59	1.66	2.82	4.03	4.83	5.31	5.22

Children ever born	0-4	5-9	10-14	15-19	20-24	25-29	30+
	Marital duration (in years)						
0	43.8	8.5	6.0	6.3	4.9	5.5	8.0
1	41.1	23.6	9.7	9.8	9.0	6.5	8.6
2	13.5	33.2	17.1	9.9	9.0	8.1	8.6
3	1.6	23.9	21.5	11.9	7.8	10.6	7.5
4	.0	8.6	21.7	14.1	10.1	8.3	10.4
5	.0	1.9	15.9	14.7	12.7	11.3	8.8
6	.0	.3	6.0	14.6	16.5	13.6	8.5
7	.0	.0	1.4	10.3	11.6	10.4	9.6
8	.0	.0	.6	5.6	8.2	9.5	10.8
9	.0	.0	.1	1.6	5.0	6.4	6.7
10	.0	.0	.0	1.2	3.4	4.3	5.3
11	.0	.0	.0	.2	.9	3.2	4.0
12	.0	.0	.0	.0	.7	1.8	2.2
13	.0	.0	.0	.0	.2	.3	.5
14	.0	.0	.0	.0	.0	.1	.2
15	.0	.0	.0	.0	.0	.0	.4
(N=100%)	1686	1460	1372	1320	1327	1107	883
Mean	.73	2.07	3.26	4.27	5.00	5.38	5.37

244

Ivory Coast

Children ever born	Age group							Marital duration (in years)						
	15-19	20-24	25-29	30-34	35-39	40-44	45-49	0-4	5-9	10-14	15-19	20-24	25-29	30+
0	40.1	9.9	5.1	4.9	3.1	3.3	5.0	31.2	4.7	3.7	4.1	2.8	4.5	3.4
1	45.3	25.0	9.1	4.4	4.6	5.9	4.3	41.3	13.8	5.8	3.6	5.0	4.2	4.9
2	13.5	34.2	15.0	6.1	5.1	3.9	4.8	20.9	29.2	7.2	5.2	4.1	3.1	5.9
3	.8	19.3	23.0	11.3	7.4	4.3	4.5	4.2	27.3	15.2	9.8	3.5	5.0	4.9
4	.1	8.6	23.2	13.8	7.9	6.9	5.5	1.0	15.8	23.5	9.9	5.4	6.4	6.4
5	.1	2.9	13.7	21.3	11.8	6.1	9.5	.6	6.2	23.1	14.1	9.8	7.5	6.9
6	.0	.1	6.6	15.7	14.4	10.0	9.3	.3	1.5	11.3	16.9	13.0	8.1	10.8
7	.0	.0	2.8	13.6	16.6	13.0	8.0	.2	.7	6.3	18.2	16.0	9.5	6.9
8	.0	.0	1.1	5.3	13.4	14.6	12.3	.1	.4	2.2	9.5	15.2	15.6	10.8
9	.0	.0	.3	2.0	9.1	15.9	13.1	.2	.2	.9	4.0	15.4	15.6	11.8
10	.0	.0	.0	1.2	4.1	6.9	9.8	.1	.2	.4	2.8	4.8	9.2	10.8
11	.0	.0	.0	.3	1.9	6.1	8.5	.0	.0	.2	1.3	3.3	7.8	9.9
12	.0	.0	.0	.0	.3	1.8	2.8	.0	.0	.0	.4	.7	2.2	3.4
13	.0	.0	.0	.0	.0	1.2	.8	.0	.0	.0	.1	.6	.8	1.0
14	.0	.0	.0	.0	.2	.0	1.5	.0	.0	.0	.1	.4	.3	1.5
15	.0	.0	.0	.0	.0	.2	.3	.0	.0	.0	.0	.0	.3	.5
(N=100%)	740	1125	919	733	583	492	398	1268	1141	804	676	539	359	203
Mean	.76	2.01	3.41	4.78	5.88	6.72	6.85	1.09	2.69	4.20	5.45	6.51	6.92	6.97

Jamaica

Children ever born	Age group							Marital duration (in years)						
	15-19	20-24	25-29	30-34	35-39	40-44	45-49	0-4	5-9	10-14	15-19	20-24	25-29	30+
0	36.6	18.4	7.6	4.9	4.8	6.3	8.4	34.8	9.4	4.8	4.4	5.5	6.6	3.3
1	44.6	27.1	18.1	10.2	7.8	8.7	8.7	43.0	20.0	10.0	8.5	7.2	5.8	11.0
2	14.2	27.3	19.6	13.3	11.8	10.8	7.4	17.2	29.4	13.6	11.2	8.3	9.7	5.5
3	4.0	16.1	18.4	15.1	8.6	7.5	7.1	4.2	21.3	17.7	11.9	7.2	5.4	5.5
4	.3	8.3	14.0	16.4	8.9	10.8	10.5	.2	12.2	20.3	9.5	12.7	8.9	5.5
5	.3	2.5	12.6	11.2	12.6	9.0	7.4	.0	5.4	14.5	14.1	8.9	8.9	7.7
6	.0	.2	5.8	11.2	13.7	7.2	7.7	.2	1.5	9.3	12.7	11.9	7.0	6.6
7	.0	.2	3.1	7.6	6.7	9.0	11.5	.0	.3	5.8	10.5	8.0	8.9	14.3
8	.0	.0	.6	4.2	8.9	10.5	9.0	.0	.3	1.9	7.3	10.0	11.7	9.9
9	.0	.0	.2	3.1	7.5	6.0	6.2	.5	.2	.9	5.1	8.0	6.2	7.7
10	.0	.0	.0	2.6	3.5	6.3	5.9	.0	.0	.9	3.6	5.3	7.4	6.6
11	.0	.0	.0	.0	2.2	3.9	4.0	.0	.0	.2	.7	3.6	4.3	6.6
12	.0	.0	.0	.3	1.9	1.8	3.1	.0	.0	.0	.2	1.9	5.8	1.1
13	.0	.0	.0	.0	.8	.9	1.5	.0	.0	.0	.2	1.1	1.6	2.2
14	.0	.0	.0	.0	.3	.9	1.2	.0	.0	.0	.0	.0	1.2	5.5
15	.0	.0	.0	.0	.0	.6	.3	.0	.0	.0	.0	.3	.4	1.1
(N=100%)	303	565	485	384	372	334	323	575	609	462	411	361	257	91
Mean	.88	1.78	2.94	4.14	5.19	5.45	5.61	.96	2.34	3.76	4.79	5.55	6.10	6.60

Jordan

Children ever born	Age group							Marital duration (in years)						
	15-19	20-24	25-29	30-34	35-39	40-44	45-49	0-4	5-9	10-14	15-19	20-24	25-29	30+
0	42.2	11.3	2.9	3.2	2.4	2.4	2.3	29.8	3.5	1.9	1.5	1.0	2.8	2.0
1	32.7	17.0	6.8	3.9	2.8	.8	1.2	34.9	2.5	2.1	1.7	1.1	1.0	1.4
2	19.9	23.3	12.0	4.4	2.2	2.9	1.1	23.6	18.1	3.7	1.7	1.6	2.1	.5
3	4.7	23.7	14.8	6.5	4.4	3.0	2.4	10.5	26.7	7.6	2.8	4.0	.8	1.3
4	.6	17.2	19.5	10.6	6.0	4.1	4.5	1.2	29.5	16.1	4.7	4.5	4.3	1.9
5	.0	4.3	15.7	11.6	7.7	4.0	4.5	.0	11.8	18.0	11.0	3.2	4.2	2.2
6	.0	3.0	14.1	15.7	11.5	7.5	7.2	.0	6.8	22.0	16.8	7.2	5.0	5.7
7	.0	.2	8.9	16.8	15.3	8.0	10.1	.0	.9	15.9	21.4	12.0	9.3	6.3
8	.0	.0	3.6	11.9	12.5	9.4	8.1	.0	.0	7.7	15.2	12.9	7.6	9.1
9	.0	.0	1.6	8.8	10.5	15.2	12.9	.0	.1	3.3	10.6	19.0	11.6	12.8
10	.0	.0	.0	4.0	11.7	16.0	11.0	.0	.0	.7	6.8	16.9	14.6	12.5
11	.0	.0	.1	2.4	6.6	7.8	15.0	.0	.0	.9	3.5	7.7	12.2	18.3
12	.0	.0	.0	.4	2.2	6.6	8.1	.0	.0	.0	1.1	3.8	8.4	9.6
13	.0	.0	.0	.1	2.8	7.3	4.8	.0	.0	.0	1.0	3.1	8.2	8.1
14	.0	.0	.0	.0	1.3	3.1	3.4	.0	.0	.0	.2	1.7	4.3	4.6
15	.0	.0	.0	.0	.3	1.8	3.2	.0	.0	.0	.0	.2	3.5	3.8
(N=100%)	329	596	709	628	543	435	372	725	696	596	574	471	333	216
Mean	.89	2.45	4.23	5.89	7.28	8.56	8.78	1.18	3.44	5.39	6.90	8.19	9.08	9.59

Kenya

Children ever born	Age group							Marital duration (in years)						
	15-19	20-24	25-29	30-34	35-39	40-44	45-49	0-4	5-9	10-14	15-19	20-24	25-29	30+
0	34.8	8.8	4.5	2.4	1.6	3.5	2.7	21.9	3.0	3.7	1.9	1.8	3.1	3.3
1	43.2	25.4	6.0	2.7	3.1	2.8	2.1	36.2	8.6	4.0	2.6	2.2	2.0	2.1
2	15.9	29.2	13.2	3.6	3.5	2.0	2.5	27.7	17.0	5.4	2.9	2.5	2.4	1.8
3	5.8	21.3	17.3	8.0	5.2	2.2	4.3	11.3	26.3	9.3	5.5	3.4	3.7	2.5
4	.3	10.5	22.4	10.3	5.1	3.7	3.4	1.9	26.1	15.5	6.2	4.5	2.0	1.8
5	.0	3.7	20.1	16.5	7.7	5.3	5.6	.6	12.6	24.9	11.0	5.7	4.6	5.8
6	.0	.7	10.1	20.6	13.0	11.2	6.4	.2	4.3	19.8	16.8	11.7	6.1	7.6
7	.0	.5	4.1	17.2	15.6	13.2	10.7	.2	1.2	10.7	19.8	13.4	12.9	7.6
8	.0	.0	1.7	11.2	17.8	13.2	15.3	.0	.4	4.1	18.2	16.9	13.2	18.0
9	.0	.0	.4	4.8	12.4	17.4	13.5	.0	.3	1.8	8.8	15.6	16.7	13.1
10	.0	.0	.1	1.7	7.8	11.0	15.0	.0	.1	.3	3.7	11.4	15.5	14.2
11	.0	.0	.1	.8	4.4	7.9	8.0	.0	.0	.6	1.4	6.4	9.1	8.7
12	.0	.0	.0	.3	2.0	4.3	5.6	.0	.0	.0	.9	3.3	4.6	7.1
13	.0	.0	.1	.0	.5	1.3	3.0	.0	.0	.0	.3	.9	1.8	4.9
14	.0	.0	.0	.0	.1	.7	1.1	.0	.0	.0	.0	.2	1.3	1.4
15	.0	.0	.0	.0	.1	.2	.8	.0	.0	.0	.0	.0	1.1	.2
(N=100%)	521	1130	1425	1003	912	616	634	1307	1237	1110	990	737	633	305
Mean	.94	2.16	3.84	5.62	6.86	7.55	7.90	1.39	3.31	4.82	6.36	7.42	7.99	8.18

Republic of Korea

Children ever born	Age group							Marital duration (in years)						
	15-19	20-24	25-29	30-34	35-39	40-44	45-49	0-4	5-9	10-14	15-19	20-24	25-29	30+
0	54.5	29.6	7.7	2.8	1.3	1.5	1.6	24.1	1.8	1.8	1.2	.5	2.6	1.0
1	43.6	42.7	25.4	5.8	3.0	4.5	3.1	44.5	7.5	3.7	2.8	2.8	4.7	2.0
2	1.8	23.3	32.9	15.5	7.1	5.2	4.4	29.0	28.9	9.0	5.7	4.7	4.3	4.0
3	.0	3.9	25.0	30.0	18.4	8.7	6.4	2.3	44.9	26.4	16.2	8.5	5.8	5.7
4	.0	.4	7.5	27.2	24.8	16.2	12.7	.1	14.4	33.5	26.9	18.6	12.7	9.2
5	.0	.0	1.3	13.0	20.6	20.9	15.9	.0	2.0	19.0	23.1	21.9	17.8	13.9
6	.0	.0	.2	4.4	14.5	17.0	16.3	.0	.5	5.3	15.2	21.7	16.1	14.4
7	.0	.0	.0	1.2	6.7	13.5	16.7	.0	.0	1.2	6.3	11.9	18.0	19.3
8	.0	.0	.0	.1	2.3	7.7	12.0	.0	.0	.0	1.5	6.2	10.9	15.6
9	.0	.0	.0	.1	1.0	2.9	5.3	.0	.0	.0	.9	2.6	3.7	6.9
10	.0	.0	.0	.0	.3	1.3	3.0	.0	.0	.0	.1	.6	2.1	4.5
11	.0	.0	.0	.0	.0	.3	1.6	.0	.0	.0	.0	.0	.7	2.5
12	.0	.0	.0	.0	.0	.2	.4	.0	.0	.0	.0	.0	.4	.7
13	.0	.0	.0	.0	.0	.0	.3	.0	.0	.0	.0	.0	.2	.2
14	.0	.0	.0	.0	.0	.0	.1	.0	.0	.0	.0	.0	.0	.2
15	.0	.0	.0	.0	.0	.0	.0	.0	.0	.0	.0	.0	.0	.0
(N=100%)	55	557	1172	1078	1024	869	675	1197	1028	814	808	645	534	404
Mean	.47	1.03	2.04	3.37	4.39	5.14	5.79	1.10	2.71	3.71	4.42	5.15	5.49	6.29

Lesotho

Children ever born	Age group							Marital duration (in years)						
	15-19	20-24	25-29	30-34	35-39	40-44	45-49	0-4	5-9	10-14	15-19	20-24	25-29	30+
0	56.1	18.3	5.9	3.7	3.9	5.9	4.0	37.7	6.4	2.4	3.7	4.6	5.3	3.9
1	38.4	39.0	13.2	7.3	7.2	6.9	7.4	45.2	14.5	7.0	6.1	7.4	7.8	8.0
2	5.5	30.0	27.2	9.9	7.3	9.3	9.7	15.2	36.9	11.6	9.2	6.1	8.5	7.9
3	.0	8.3	29.2	18.7	11.9	10.1	9.6	1.2	29.4	21.6	11.4	9.2	9.5	9.8
4	.0	2.9	17.8	21.3	14.3	10.3	10.3	.5	10.0	31.2	12.5	11.6	8.3	9.2
5	.0	1.4	4.9	21.0	15.9	9.9	10.6	.1	2.5	17.7	20.3	10.2	8.4	15.0
6	.0	.0	1.3	10.4	15.4	12.1	11.4	.0	.0	7.6	16.3	13.9	11.1	9.9
7	.0	.0	.3	4.6	12.6	12.0	10.5	.0	.3	.7	13.1	12.6	11.1	13.1
8	.0	.0	.1	1.9	7.2	10.4	8.8	.0	.0	.2	5.2	14.1	9.8	5.5
9	.0	.0	.0	.8	2.6	7.4	7.3	.0	.0	.0	1.0	6.5	10.8	5.1
10	.0	.0	.0	.2	1.2	3.6	4.8	.0	.0	.0	.8	1.5	6.0	6.2
11	.0	.0	.0	.0	.2	.9	2.7	.0	.0	.0	.2	.6	1.8	3.2
12	.0	.0	.0	.2	.2	.8	2.0	.0	.0	.0	.2	1.3	.8	2.3
13	.0	.0	.0	.0	.0	.4	.7	.0	.0	.0	.0	.3	.8	.0
14	.0	.0	.0	.0	.0	.0	.3	.0	.0	.0	.0	.0	.0	.8
15	.0	.0	.0	.0	.0	.0	.0	.0	.0	.0	.0	.0	.0	.0
(N=100%)	372	773	676	514	482	494	293	920	763	552	512	378	352	126
Mean	.49	1.43	2.62	3.95	4.73	5.14	5.42	.82	2.31	3.61	4.63	5.28	5.49	5.42

Malaysia

Children ever born	Age group							Marital duration (in years)						
	15-19	20-24	25-29	30-34	35-39	40-44	45-49	0-4	5-9	10-14	15-19	20-24	25-29	30+
0	42.1	18.2	8.6	2.6	2.0	2.6	3.2	29.3	2.5	2.8	.9	2.0	1.4	3.7
1	39.8	30.9	15.2	6.7	4.7	4.9	5.1	40.1	10.6	4.9	3.1	3.1	3.6	5.6
2	14.3	27.4	21.5	12.4	7.9	6.4	7.4	25.4	26.3	10.8	6.8	5.1	3.3	8.1
3	2.7	16.4	21.8	17.0	10.9	9.8	7.9	5.0	33.8	18.3	11.7	8.1	6.8	8.0
4	.8	5.5	16.4	15.5	12.3	9.5	9.5	.3	17.7	22.0	13.9	8.8	8.6	9.1
5	.0	1.0	9.6	17.4	13.5	11.0	9.7	.0	7.0	20.7	15.0	13.9	10.1	8.5
6	.4	.6	4.9	12.6	12.6	9.8	10.9	.0	1.9	13.4	15.7	12.2	11.9	9.0
7	.0	.1	1.3	9.0	12.5	12.4	9.5	.0	.1	4.5	16.1	13.9	12.8	9.3
8	.0	.0	.5	4.9	9.6	10.3	9.9	.0	.0	1.6	10.8	10.9	11.7	10.3
9	.0	.0	.3	1.2	6.4	7.6	9.4	.0	.0	.8	3.6	8.9	9.9	8.8
10	.0	.0	.0	.4	4.7	7.9	6.2	.0	.0	.2	1.8	7.0	9.0	7.0
11	.0	.0	.0	.2	1.5	3.7	5.8	.0	.0	.0	.1	3.5	5.1	6.3
12	.0	.0	.0	.2	.7	2.8	2.9	.0	.0	.0	.2	1.6	3.6	3.3
13	.0	.0	.0	.0	.3	.3	1.3	.0	.0	.0	.1	.3	.8	1.5
14	.0	.0	.0	.0	.2	.5	.6	.0	.0	.0	.0	.3	.6	.7
15	.0	.0	.0	.0	.3	.5	.7	.0	.0	.0	.0	.3	.8	.8
(N=100%)	259	909	1192	1089	1115	860	897	1250	1108	956	878	863	664	602
Mean	.82	1.66	2.82	4.28	5.49	6.08	6.22	1.07	2.83	4.07	5.32	6.22	6.79	6.26

Mauritania

Children ever born	Age group							Marital duration (in years)						
	15-19	20-24	25-29	30-34	35-39	40-44	45-49	0-4	5-9	10-14	15-19	20-24	25-29	30+
0	36.0	13.7	6.3	4.3	4.0	5.8	3.7	39.5	9.8	4.7	3.9	3.7	3.4	3.0
1	40.5	23.3	11.0	5.1	4.2	2.9	6.8	41.1	20.6	8.7	6.9	3.3	3.4	4.8
2	16.7	25.0	11.6	7.8	5.5	5.8	8.4	14.9	27.4	12.6	6.4	4.2	6.0	6.9
3	4.1	20.3	17.9	11.5	9.2	10.1	6.5	3.0	24.1	19.3	9.0	8.1	9.1	6.6
4	1.6	10.4	16.9	13.0	12.4	8.7	9.2	.7	11.7	19.4	12.9	11.6	8.6	7.5
5	1.0	4.4	17.1	18.0	13.0	10.8	9.4	.1	4.8	17.3	17.3	17.3	11.2	7.8
6	.0	1.9	9.3	11.5	11.3	10.6	9.4	.3	1.0	9.8	14.4	9.9	8.8	11.9
7	.0	.9	5.4	11.5	11.3	13.2	11.8	.0	.2	4.5	13.6	14.0	11.9	11.9
8	.2	.1	3.2	9.0	8.6	8.5	6.8	.1	.2	2.6	8.6	10.3	8.6	7.5
9	.0	.0	1.0	3.6	7.8	10.3	11.0	.0	.1	.7	3.2	7.9	10.6	13.1
10	.0	.0	.3	3.0	6.9	5.6	5.5	.3	.0	.3	2.0	6.3	7.3	6.3
11	.0	.0	.1	1.1	3.4	3.2	5.2	.0	.0	.1	1.5	2.2	4.7	5.4
12	.0	.0	.0	.6	1.0	3.2	4.2	.0	.0	.0	.2	.7	4.2	4.8
13	.0	.0	.0	.0	1.1	.8	1.3	.0	.0	.0	.0	.4	1.8	1.5
14	.0	.0	.0	.0	.2	.3	.5	.0	.0	.0	.0	.0	.5	.6
15	.0	.0	.0	.0	.0	.3	.3	.0	.0	.0	.0	.0	.0	.6
(N=100%)	518	711	657	540	439	317	320	614	694	639	495	456	323	281
Mean	.99	2.17	3.73	5.00	5.79	5.97	6.10	.89	2.29	3.77	5.03	5.81	6.39	6.56

Mexico

Children ever born	Age group							Marital duration (in years)						
	15-19	20-24	25-29	30-34	35-39	40-44	45-49	0-4	5-9	10-14	15-19	20-24	25-29	30+
0	32.1	13.1	6.2	3.2	2.3	3.1	4.5	25.6	3.3	2.1	2.0	1.9	2.5	2.9
1	39.7	26.8	10.4	4.9	3.6	2.7	4.9	38.3	7.8	3.7	2.2	3.3	2.8	2.5
2	22.3	26.7	17.6	10.5	5.3	6.9	4.0	26.9	24.2	7.1	4.2	3.1	4.9	1.2
3	5.1	20.3	20.0	11.9	8.6	6.0	6.5	8.2	31.3	14.0	6.8	5.5	3.7	3.3
4	.8	8.7	16.6	14.6	9.6	7.3	8.2	.8	19.8	18.1	11.0	7.5	5.4	7.4
5	.0	3.4	14.6	14.1	8.9	8.7	7.7	.1	9.1	22.0	11.8	6.3	8.4	5.8
6	.0	.7	8.6	12.8	12.6	10.1	8.0	.0	3.0	17.6	15.1	10.4	7.7	5.3
7	.0	.4	3.8	11.2	13.3	9.6	9.8	.0	1.0	9.3	16.9	11.7	9.6	9.9
8	.0	.0	1.3	8.2	11.0	10.6	8.0	.1	.2	4.0	13.9	11.3	11.2	7.8
9	.0	.0	.5	4.2	8.7	9.6	12.0	.0	.2	1.4	7.2	13.7	12.1	11.9
10	.0	.0	.2	2.6	7.3	7.0	8.2	.0	.0	.6	5.4	10.1	8.4	10.7
11	.0	.0	.1	1.3	4.3	6.6	5.7	.0	.0	.2	2.3	6.7	9.3	7.0
12	.0	.0	.0	.1	2.5	4.8	4.5	.0	.0	.0	.8	3.8	6.0	8.6
13	.0	.0	.0	.1	1.0	3.9	3.5	.0	.0	.0	.3	2.6	4.0	7.0
14	.0	.0	.0	.1	.7	1.3	2.0	.0	.1	.0	.2	1.1	1.6	4.1
15	.0	.0	.0	.1	.1	1.7	2.6	.0	.0	.0	.0	.9	2.5	4.5
(N=100%)	471	1120	1202	1047	995	770	650	1429	1250	1059	908	795	571	243
Mean	1.03	1.99	3.41	4.95	6.34	7.02	7.03	1.21	3.04	4.65	6.14	7.29	7.68	8.49

Morocco

Children ever born	Age group							Marital duration (in years)						
	15-19	20-24	25-29	30-34	35-39	40-44	45-49	0-4	5-9	10-14	15-19	20-24	25-29	30+
0	45.7	15.9	9.9	5.6	6.0	5.4	8.5	33.5	7.0	6.0	5.6	6.0	5.2	9.2
1	36.7	27.9	11.4	6.8	4.9	3.1	4.3	39.3	12.4	4.8	5.6	3.6	3.2	5.1
2	14.4	25.4	13.9	6.8	4.4	3.6	4.3	22.6	20.6	6.3	4.5	4.3	3.6	4.4
3	1.6	17.2	20.0	9.0	5.4	4.5	3.6	4.0	31.1	12.7	5.8	4.0	4.8	2.5
4	1.3	8.7	18.9	14.1	6.5	5.3	4.2	.4	21.1	18.3	9.1	5.7	6.3	3.4
5	.3	3.7	13.2	13.4	8.9	6.0	5.4	.1	6.6	22.3	11.1	7.1	3.8	6.7
6	.0	.4	7.3	15.3	13.8	10.7	8.5	.0	1.0	15.2	16.0	13.3	10.9	7.1
7	.0	.1	2.5	14.8	13.0	11.3	8.3	.0	.0	8.0	18.1	13.4	9.2	8.3
8	.0	.5	1.9	7.8	13.0	12.0	13.0	.0	.1	4.5	12.1	14.5	11.8	12.0
9	.0	.1	.7	4.0	12.0	13.4	10.5	.0	.0	1.3	7.8	14.0	13.2	9.7
10	.0	.0	.1	1.5	7.4	9.6	12.1	.0	.0	.3	3.1	8.1	11.5	12.2
11	.0	.0	.0	.3	3.0	6.7	6.0	.0	.0	.2	.6	3.4	7.1	6.9
12	.0	.0	.0	.5	1.3	5.4	6.0	.0	.0	.0	.6	1.7	5.9	6.9
13	.0	.0	.0	.2	.3	1.3	2.9	.0	.0	.0	.0	.5	1.7	3.2
14	.0	.0	.0	.0	.0	.9	1.4	.0	.0	.0	.0	.2	.8	1.8
15	.0	.0	.0	.0	.0	.7	1.1	.0	.0	.0	.0	.2	1.1	.7
(N=100%)	313	728	725	603	631	551	554	796	684	600	486	580	524	435
Mean	.77	1.92	3.25	4.91	6.13	7.10	7.07	.99	2.71	4.41	5.59	6.49	7.25	7.10

Nepal

Children ever born	Age group							Marital duration (in years)						
	15-19	20-24	25-29	30-34	35-39	40-44	45-49	0-4	5-9	10-14	15-19	20-24	25-29	30+
0	74.4	25.1	7.5	4.9	3.0	3.9	4.1	63.8	17.1	5.7	4.0	2.9	3.1	4.0
1	19.8	31.6	12.6	6.3	5.6	3.8	3.3	28.9	25.4	9.2	4.9	4.2	3.8	2.2
2	5.4	24.3	20.8	10.9	6.7	7.4	7.9	5.9	32.4	17.2	8.0	7.3	7.1	6.3
3	.4	14.1	23.8	16.2	10.9	6.4	8.8	.8	19.0	25.9	13.4	8.7	7.0	8.0
4	.0	3.6	19.2	17.8	14.8	14.6	10.2	.1	5.2	22.9	18.2	14.7	12.3	9.4
5	.0	1.0	10.1	19.2	13.4	12.8	11.6	.2	.7	12.4	20.9	13.9	11.4	11.7
6	.0	.2	4.3	13.6	17.3	12.6	11.0	.0	.1	5.1	17.2	16.5	11.2	11.3
7	.0	.0	1.3	7.1	11.6	14.0	11.9	.1	.0	1.3	8.6	13.7	13.2	13.0
8	.0	.0	.1	2.8	8.1	9.0	13.1	.0	.0	.2	3.3	7.9	13.5	12.1
9	.0	.0	.1	1.2	4.8	9.1	8.1	.0	.0	.0	1.1	6.3	10.8	8.6
10	.0	.0	.0	.0	1.9	3.8	4.8	.1	.0	.0	.1	2.6	3.3	6.1
11	.0	.0	.0	.1	1.6	1.4	3.2	.0	.0	.0	.3	.7	2.3	4.4
12	.0	.0	.0	.0	.1	.7	1.4	.0	.0	.0	.0	.1	.5	2.3
13	.0	.0	.0	.0	.2	.3	.4	.0	.0	.0	.0	.4	.3	.2
14	.0	.0	.0	.0	.0	.1	.0	.0	.0	.0	.0	.0	.0	.2
15	.0	.0	.0	.0	.0	.0	.2	.0	.0	.0	.0	.0	.0	.3
(N=100%)	748	1216	1138	864	734	725	516	1114	1153	1042	875	787	539	431
Mean	.32	1.43	2.91	4.10	5.11	5.56	5.81	.47	1.72	3.17	4.42	5.29	5.79	6.14

Nigeria

Children ever born	Age group							Marital duration (in years)						
	15-19	20-24	25-29	30-34	35-39	40-44	45-49	0-4	5-9	10-14	15-19	20-24	25-29	30+
0	41.6	12.7	7.4	5.1	5.2	6.9	8.0	32.3	9.8	5.5	4.0	6.0	8.3	7.9
1	40.8	25.5	11.0	6.0	6.6	6.8	3.9	43.4	14.9	6.3	4.8	7.0	4.7	4.5
2	12.3	26.7	18.3	10.4	7.1	7.3	7.0	17.9	26.3	13.3	8.8	5.9	6.5	5.8
3	3.9	18.5	19.7	14.0	11.1	10.8	6.9	4.6	25.3	17.2	11.2	10.3	8.3	8.2
4	1.4	10.4	18.5	19.5	10.8	12.5	9.6	1.1	15.6	20.8	16.1	12.5	9.7	8.0
5	.1	4.1	11.7	15.0	15.5	11.9	9.0	.4	4.9	16.8	16.4	13.6	6.5	10.1
6	.0	1.3	7.6	13.2	12.6	10.3	12.3	.1	2.3	11.7	14.9	10.0	10.9	12.0
7	.0	.3	3.1	8.5	11.1	9.7	11.5	.2	.7	5.7	10.0	10.8	12.9	8.0
8	.0	.2	1.4	4.4	8.3	8.2	9.0	.0	.0	2.0	7.8	9.3	7.5	8.3
9	.0	.2	.9	1.0	4.8	7.2	7.0	.0	.1	.4	2.7	6.2	9.3	7.6
10	.0	.0	.1	1.5	4.0	4.6	6.4	.0	.0	.3	1.6	4.3	8.9	6.5
11	.0	.0	.3	.1	1.3	1.4	4.0	.0	.0	.0	.8	1.1	3.2	5.3
12	.0	.0	.0	.2	.7	1.3	2.9	.0	.0	.0	.2	1.4	1.7	3.5
13	.0	.0	.0	.5	.8	1.1	1.9	.0	.0	.0	.1	1.6	1.4	3.1
14	.0	.0	.0	.4	.0	.0	.3	.0	.0	.0	.4	.0	.1	.6
15	.0	.0	.0	.0	.0	.0	.3	.0	.0	.0	.0	.0	.1	.6
(N=100%)	85	145	171	153	110	90	59	143	159	177	134	109	58	32
Mean	.83	2.10	3.31	4.36	5.12	5.15	5.87	1.02	2.50	3.85	4.85	5.26	5.79	6.08

Pakistan

Age group

Children ever born	15-19	20-24	25-29	30-34	35-39	40-44	45-49
0	55.9	19.6	8.4	4.4	4.5	4.3	2.8
1	31.5	23.6	8.9	4.1	3.6	2.2	3.7
2	11.0	24.6	15.2	8.7	4.2	3.4	3.8
3	1.2	19.1	19.7	8.3	6.9	3.7	6.7
4	.2	7.7	19.5	14.8	7.6	6.5	4.7
5	.0	3.6	14.5	15.0	11.8	8.1	9.5
6	.0	1.2	8.2	18.1	14.2	9.4	10.2
7	.0	.7	4.3	13.1	16.8	15.9	13.8
8	.0	.0	1.2	7.6	11.5	15.0	13.2
9	.0	.0	.1	3.9	7.7	11.8	11.7
10	.0	.0	.1	1.0	7.3	9.6	9.5
11	.0	.0	.0	.9	2.5	4.3	5.4
12	.0	.0	.0	.0	.5	3.7	2.8
13	.0	.0	.0	.0	.9	1.2	1.5
14	.0	.0	.0	.0	.0	.4	.7
15	.0	.0	.0	.0	.0	.4	.3
(N=100%)	631	848	912	818	623	618	502
Mean	.58	1.91	3.39	4.97	6.05	6.96	6.87

Marital duration (in years)

Children ever born	0-4	5-9	10-14	15-19	20-24	25-29	30+
0	51.6	8.9	5.1	3.8	2.6	4.4	2.3
1	34.8	14.1	4.0	3.4	3.0	3.1	2.7
2	12.2	29.1	9.8	6.4	3.4	2.8	3.2
3	1.5	27.1	15.8	6.6	6.6	3.9	6.1
4	.0	13.9	22.4	10.7	7.0	5.2	6.2
5	.0	5.1	21.5	14.4	8.5	10.3	5.9
6	.0	1.5	12.9	19.2	14.3	9.7	9.8
7	.0	.4	6.4	17.5	17.1	14.8	15.6
8	.0	.0	1.4	10.1	14.3	14.4	13.5
9	.0	.0	.6	5.4	8.4	12.6	11.4
10	.0	.0	.1	1.5	9.5	8.7	11.5
11	.0	.0	.0	.9	3.5	4.3	6.0
12	.0	.0	.0	.1	1.3	3.3	3.0
13	.0	.0	.0	.2	.3	2.0	1.3
14	.0	.0	.0	.0	.2	.0	1.2
15	.0	.0	.0	.0	.0	.4	.3
(N=100%)	974	903	804	729	513	620	411
Mean	.63	2.46	4.08	5.46	6.52	6.90	7.16

Panama

Age group

Children ever born	15-19	20-24	25-29	30-34	35-39	40-44	45-49
0	.0	15.3	6.6	3.2	1.6	2.6	4.2
1	.0	31.9	16.9	8.4	5.9	4.6	3.6
2	.0	28.6	21.9	14.6	10.9	9.2	9.0
3	.0	15.1	19.2	19.7	15.8	8.7	12.6
4	.0	6.8	15.5	16.8	10.5	11.5	8.7
5	.0	1.9	9.7	13.3	10.7	14.8	11.8
6	.0	.2	6.7	8.7	12.3	9.9	10.9
7	.0	.0	2.9	7.2	11.1	9.4	9.5
8	.0	.2	.6	4.0	7.3	8.9	7.6
9	.0	.0	.1	2.8	5.9	5.6	5.3
10	.0	.0	.0	.4	4.2	6.1	5.6
11	.0	.0	.0	.4	3.0	4.6	3.9
12	.0	.0	.0	.1	.6	2.3	3.9
13	.0	.0	.0	.3	.2	1.0	1.1
14	.0	.0	.0	.0	.2	.3	.6
15	.0	.0	.0	.0	.0	.5	1.7
(N=100%)	0	570	699	679	506	392	357
Mean	1.74	2.95	4.05	5.20	5.80	5.87	2.66

Marital duration (in years)

Children ever born	0-4	5-9	10-14	15-19	20-24	25-29	30+
0	24.6	3.1	1.4	1.7	1.8	2.4	3.0
1	43.9	12.7	7.8	4.9	3.6	1.7	1.5
2	23.1	32.9	15.0	8.8	7.0	4.5	5.2
3	5.8	27.9	20.9	13.2	11.1	10.7	9.0
4	1.3	16.5	19.2	14.9	9.3	8.7	4.5
5	.6	4.7	17.0	14.4	13.7	12.8	9.0
6	.6	1.2	11.9	12.3	12.2	10.7	11.9
7	.0	.6	4.8	13.2	10.1	11.8	12.7
8	.0	.4	1.6	7.6	11.4	7.3	9.0
9	.0	.0	.3	6.3	7.0	6.9	6.0
10	.0	.0	.2	1.3	6.2	8.3	9.0
11	.2	.0	.0	.9	3.6	8.0	5.2
12	.0	.0	.0	.2	1.8	3.5	6.7
13	.0	.0	.0	.2	.8	1.4	2.2
14	.0	.0	.0	.0	.3	.3	1.5
15	.0	.0	.0	.0	.0	1.0	3.7
(N=100%)	533	684	641	536	386	289	134
Mean	3.84	5.07	5.92	6.59	7.21	.00	

Paraguay

Age group

Children ever born	15-19	20-24	25-29	30-34	35-39	40-44	45-49
0	38.7	17.4	6.7	5.9	3.1	3.2	2.5
1	47.4	35.7	23.7	9.9	9.6	5.6	5.8
2	12.9	26.2	22.3	18.9	11.3	9.9	7.7
3	1.0	12.6	18.7	15.2	16.5	14.2	11.3
4	.0	6.6	12.8	12.2	10.6	7.0	7.7
5	.0	1.1	7.4	13.5	11.0	9.1	9.1
6	.0	.4	5.8	8.4	9.2	8.3	6.1
7	.0	.0	2.2	6.5	7.7	7.2	8.0
8	.0	.0	.4	5.1	8.3	8.6	9.1
9	.0	.0	.2	2.7	5.4	5.9	8.3
10	.0	.0	.0	.8	3.8	6.4	7.5
11	.0	.0	.0	.6	1.7	4.8	7.5
12	.0	.0	.0	.2	1.0	4.8	4.1
13	.0	.0	.0	.0	.4	2.1	2.8
14	.0	.0	.0	.0	.2	1.6	.3
15	.0	.0	.0	.0	.2	1.1	2.2
(N=100%)	194	557	556	475	480	373	362
Mean	.76	1.60	2.67	3.89	4.83	6.06	6.51

Marital duration (in years)

Children ever born	0-4	5-9	10-14	15-19	20-24	25-29	30+
0	27.8	5.0	3.0	3.3	1.1	1.1	3.1
1	45.5	20.3	7.4	6.8	5.3	3.8	2.1
2	21.8	25.0	17.6	11.1	7.5	9.1	1.0
3	3.7	24.9	22.2	14.2	10.3	9.4	4.2
4	.7	14.7	15.9	8.5	11.4	4.2	7.3
5	.0	6.4	14.4	13.2	12.5	4.9	7.3
6	.3	2.4	10.6	10.1	10.3	6.4	6.3
7	.3	.5	6.4	9.2	9.2	8.7	6.3
8	.0	.5	1.5	11.6	9.7	9.4	12.5
9	.0	.0	.6	7.1	6.1	11.3	7.3
10	.0	.2	.0	3.1	6.7	9.1	11.5
11	.0	.2	.2	1.4	3.6	7.5	15.6
12	.0	.0	.2	.2	3.6	6.8	6.3
13	.0	.0	.0	.0	.8	5.3	3.1
14	.0	.0	.0	.2	1.4	.4	1.0
15	.0	.0	.0	.0	.3	2.6	5.2
(N=100%)	726	655	472	424	359	265	96
Mean	1.06	2.60	3.75	5.05	6.04	7.37	8.24

Peru

Children ever born	Age group							Marital duration (in years)						
	15-19	20-24	25-29	30-34	35-39	40-44	45-49	0-4	5-9	10-14	15-19	20-24	25-29	30+
0	27.9	7.6	5.0	2.0	1.2	1.8	2.6	18.1	2.5	1.5	1.2	.8	1.0	.1
1	45.3	30.7	12.0	6.5	4.6	3.8	3.3	43.8	8.8	3.5	3.7	3.3	1.9	.0
2	21.9	31.4	19.2	12.9	6.8	4.2	6.2	29.5	25.6	8.5	5.4	4.5	2.5	5.8
3	4.7	19.5	20.9	16.5	11.1	9.7	6.8	7.5	32.1	17.6	8.7	7.7	5.3	4.1
4	.2	7.4	19.6	15.4	10.0	10.2	7.0	1.0	18.9	21.2	12.1	8.4	5.3	5.4
5	.0	2.7	12.7	14.4	12.0	9.0	9.7	.0	9.0	20.4	12.4	11.3	6.7	5.2
6	.0	.6	6.8	11.2	13.0	10.3	10.6	.2	2.1	13.7	16.4	10.3	11.8	7.1
7	.0	.0	2.7	10.7	11.2	11.1	10.4	.0	.5	8.6	14.5	11.3	12.6	11.6
8	.0	.1	.7	6.3	10.6	10.5	9.2	.0	.3	4.2	11.8	11.9	9.8	10.1
9	.0	.0	.3	2.8	8.6	10.3	9.1	.0	.0	.7	8.8	11.4	10.8	12.7
10	.0	.0	.0	.6	5.9	7.2	6.9	.0	.1	.1	3.3	8.1	10.1	9.3
11	.0	.0	.0	.4	3.0	5.5	6.5	.0	.0	.0	1.4	6.3	8.5	7.4
12	.0	.0	.0	.1	1.0	3.3	6.5	.0	.0	.0	.3	2.5	7.1	11.1
13	.0	.0	.0	.1	.5	1.7	2.2	.0	.0	.0	.3	1.3	3.1	3.2
14	.0	.0	.0	.1	.2	.8	1.3	.0	.0	.0	.0	.6	1.3	3.8
15	.0	.0	.0	.1	.2	.6	1.7	.0	.0	.0	.0	.2	2.2	3.2
(N=100%)	311	893	1056	928	922	804	726	1132	1132	972	862	795	554	192
Mean	1.04	2.00	3.23	4.49	5.88	6.58	6.96	1.30	2.97	4.44	5.78	6.73	7.83	8.40

Philippines

Children ever born	Age group							Marital duration (in years)						
	15-19	20-24	25-29	30-34	35-39	40-44	45-49	0-4	5-9	10-14	15-19	20-24	25-29	30+
0	36.8	8.9	5.3	2.4	2.4	2.3	2.6	18.5	2.8	1.5	1.6	1.2	2.0	2.0
1	43.5	31.4	14.7	5.8	4.0	3.1	3.2	45.0	6.8	3.2	2.5	2.1	1.9	.6
2	17.7	33.1	20.7	12.7	5.8	4.7	4.0	31.0	24.7	6.9	4.5	2.7	2.5	1.0
3	2.1	17.5	23.5	17.4	10.0	6.8	6.5	4.9	35.1	15.9	8.4	4.4	3.4	3.4
4	.0	7.2	18.7	17.3	12.2	9.0	7.1	.4	21.4	23.0	10.9	7.1	5.4	4.6
5	.0	1.8	10.9	16.2	12.5	9.5	7.9	.1	7.3	22.6	14.9	9.7	5.7	2.9
6	.0	.2	4.5	13.3	14.1	11.8	10.5	.1	1.6	16.7	18.0	12.0	9.6	6.6
7	.0	.0	1.5	8.3	12.9	11.0	10.4	.1	.3	8.0	15.9	14.2	9.3	8.6
8	.0	.0	.2	4.1	12.0	11.3	11.2	.0	.0	1.6	13.1	15.7	12.9	11.2
9	.0	.0	.0	1.3	7.4	9.4	14.9	.0	.0	.3	6.0	13.0	15.6	19.9
10	.0	.0	.1	.6	4.0	8.8	9.3	.0	.0	.1	2.8	8.9	12.0	16.7
11	.0	.0	.0	.4	1.9	5.7	5.5	.0	.0	.0	1.2	5.5	8.0	8.9
12	.0	.0	.0	.0	.6	3.6	3.2	.0	.0	.0	.2	2.1	5.7	6.8
13	.0	.0	.0	.0	.2	1.8	2.3	.0	.0	.0	.1	.8	3.9	3.9
14	.0	.0	.0	.0	.1	.7	.6	.0	.0	.1	.0	.3	1.1	1.3
15	.0	.0	.0	.0	.0	.6	.7	.0	.0	.0	.0	.2	.9	1.6
(N=100%)	276	1222	1775	1711	1673	1410	1201	1650	2009	1661	1515	1253	854	325
Mean	.85	1.89	2.96	4.27	5.66	6.74	6.99	1.24	2.95	4.45	5.77	7.05	7.89	8.53

Portugal

Children ever born	Age group							Marital duration (in years)						
	15-19	20-24	25-29	30-34	35-39	40-44	45-49	0-4	5-9	10-14	15-19	20-24	25-29	30+
0	48.3	24.6	10.0	4.5	4.0	5.7	6.0	27.7	4.3	4.1	4.5	3.7	3.3	3.6
1	47.2	51.1	46.7	26.4	18.4	17.8	18.5	54.4	36.9	19.9	15.8	16.5	16.9	5.4
2	3.4	18.4	32.9	43.4	40.2	33.7	28.4	15.0	43.3	42.8	37.7	32.5	24.5	17.9
3	1.1	4.9	6.9	15.9	17.8	16.0	16.2	2.1	11.3	18.9	17.2	17.3	15.7	23.2
4	.0	.9	2.3	5.3	9.6	10.6	9.8	.6	3.0	8.1	10.9	10.0	12.4	8.9
5	.0	.0	.7	2.7	4.0	6.2	5.1	.0	.9	3.2	5.4	7.2	5.1	10.7
6	.0	.0	.4	.9	2.3	3.5	5.4	.0	.1	2.0	2.8	5.2	5.3	10.7
7	.0	.0	.1	.5	1.9	2.7	3.5	.1	.1	.7	3.2	2.4	5.1	7.1
8	.0	.0	.0	.1	1.1	2.0	1.9	.1	.0	.2	1.3	2.0	4.3	.0
9	.0	.0	.0	.0	.3	.3	1.5	.0	.0	.0	.3	1.1	2.3	.0
10	.0	.0	.0	.2	.3	.5	1.2	.0	.0	.0	.6	.8	1.8	3.6
11	.0	.0	.0	.0	.0	.3	1.2	.0	.0	.0	.0	.5	1.8	5.4
12	.0	.0	.0	.0	.0	.1	.7	.0	.0	.0	.1	.3	1.0	.0
13	.0	.0	.0	.0	.1	.3	.1	.0	.0	.0	.0	.5	.3	.0
14	.0	.0	.0	.0	.0	.1	.2	.0	.0	.0	.1	.0	.3	1.8
15	.0	.0	.0	.0	.0	.1	.2	.0	.0	.0	.0	.1	.3	1.8
(N=100%)	692	4262	6400	7186	7054	7388	7054	7761	7746	7761	7396	5856	3080	436
Mean	.57	1.06	1.49	2.08	2.54	2.83	3.16	.95	1.75	2.29	2.75	3.08	3.69	4.61

Senegal

Children ever born	Age group							Marital duration (in years)						
	15-19	20-24	25-29	30-34	35-39	40-44	45-49	0-4	5-9	10-14	15-19	20-24	25-29	30+
0	44.1	10.4	4.7	4.0	3.6	3.8	3.1	34.5	6.8	4.3	3.9	2.5	3.1	3.3
1	42.4	29.1	10.1	3.6	5.8	4.6	3.1	45.1	15.8	4.9	3.9	5.7	4.2	2.8
2	12.1	29.2	13.9	6.2	5.6	4.3	4.3	17.4	29.5	8.2	5.4	5.3	3.3	4.4
3	1.1	20.8	18.1	7.2	6.9	5.1	3.9	2.3	29.8	16.4	6.4	4.6	4.2	3.9
4	.2	7.5	24.3	9.3	7.5	6.9	7.4	.5	13.0	27.1	6.2	8.4	6.7	7.8
5	.0	2.6	16.8	16.5	7.9	7.7	5.4	.0	4.1	21.6	15.1	7.8	6.7	6.1
6	.0	.3	8.4	23.3	14.1	8.2	8.9	.0	.9	12.7	22.1	13.0	9.2	8.3
7	.0	.0	2.3	16.7	15.1	12.0	11.3	.0	.2	3.2	19.8	16.0	8.9	11.7
8	.0	.0	.9	8.5	15.3	14.3	13.2	.0	.0	.9	10.9	16.2	15.6	11.1
9	.0	.0	.3	2.8	9.1	13.0	12.5	.0	.0	.6	3.7	10.1	15.3	10.6
10	.0	.0	.2	1.4	5.4	8.9	10.5	.0	.0	.2	1.7	6.3	9.2	13.3
11	.0	.0	.0	.4	2.6	6.9	11.7	.1	.0	.0	.8	2.7	9.2	11.7
12	.0	.0	.0	.0	.8	3.1	4.3	.0	.0	.0	.2	1.3	3.3	4.4
13	.0	.0	.0	.0	.2	1.0	.0	.0	.0	.0	.0	.2	.8	.6
14	.0	.0	.0	.0	.0	.3	.4	.0	.0	.0	.0	.0	.6	.0
15	.0	.0	.0	.0	.0	.0	.0	.0	.0	.0	.0	.0	.0	.0
(N=100%)	535	653	642	497	496	392	257	820	584	536	516	476	360	180
Mean	.71	1.95	3.52	5.26	5.97	6.77	7.21	.90	2.43	4.00	5.53	6.24	7.14	7.23

Sri Lanka

Children ever born	Age group							Marital duration (in years)						
	15-19	20-24	25-29	30-34	35-39	40-44	45-49	0-4	5-9	10-14	15-19	20-24	25-29	30+
0	43.4	19.9	10.1	5.5	3.8	4.2	3.2	31.3	6.2	2.7	2.8	1.2	2.6	1.8
1	48.9	35.7	21.7	10.5	5.9	5.3	5.2	47.9	15.4	5.6	5.8	3.8	3.2	2.6
2	5.4	24.4	21.6	12.9	11.1	7.8	7.6	18.0	31.2	12.6	7.8	6.9	5.2	3.4
3	1.8	12.9	19.0	17.5	13.2	10.5	7.5	2.8	28.6	23.0	12.5	8.0	6.1	5.2
4	.5	5.5	13.8	17.3	13.5	11.2	8.6	.1	13.8	24.4	15.3	11.1	8.2	7.3
5	.0	1.2	8.4	15.9	12.3	10.4	10.5	.0	4.4	18.6	15.6	13.0	11.0	9.2
6	.0	.3	3.5	9.2	10.9	14.4	13.6	.0	.5	7.8	16.3	15.5	13.8	13.5
7	.0	.0	1.3	5.8	9.9	12.1	11.4	.0	.0	3.8	10.5	14.0	13.0	13.8
8	.0	.0	.6	3.6	9.9	8.4	9.6	.0	.0	1.2	9.3	12.3	10.9	10.0
9	.0	.0	.0	1.1	5.8	5.3	10.3	.0	.0	.2	2.6	7.3	10.0	15.3
10	.0	.0	.0	.5	2.2	4.5	5.7	.0	.0	.0	.9	4.6	7.4	5.7
11	.0	.0	.0	.2	.6	3.2	3.9	.0	.0	.0	.6	1.5	4.5	5.8
12	.0	.0	.0	.0	.5	1.4	1.5	.0	.0	.0	.0	.6	1.5	4.0
13	.0	.0	.0	.1	.2	.9	.8	.0	.0	.0	.1	.2	1.7	1.1
14	.0	.0	.0	.0	.1	.3	.4	.0	.0	.0	.0	.0	.6	.8
15	.0	.0	.0	.0	.1	.2	.1	.0	.0	.0	.0	.0	.2	.4
(N=100%)	176	912	1295	1221	1203	968	1035	1280	1231	1118	1057	893	795	436
Mean	.67	1.54	2.54	3.80	4.89	5.51	5.97	.92	2.44	3.76	4.84	5.79	6.47	6.97

Sudan

Children ever born	Age group							Marital duration (in years)						
	15-19	20-24	25-29	30-34	35-39	40-44	45-49	0-4	5-9	10-14	15-19	20-24	25-29	30+
0	52.2	14.4	7.5	5.4	5.3	6.5	8.6	41.8	6.2	6.1	3.7	4.2	7.3	8.7
1	29.8	21.2	10.0	4.8	4.5	5.0	4.9	35.9	10.2	5.8	4.3	3.6	3.0	6.7
2	14.2	25.2	16.8	7.4	5.8	7.1	6.4	18.7	29.0	7.4	5.8	3.7	6.9	7.5
3	3.8	19.0	18.7	9.3	8.0	6.5	6.6	3.2	29.5	13.7	8.0	5.3	4.1	8.7
4	.0	13.1	18.0	13.2	7.0	6.7	7.1	.0	17.2	21.1	8.4	8.9	7.6	2.4
5	.0	4.9	13.2	16.1	9.4	8.0	7.4	.3	6.7	20.8	12.9	6.2	8.0	5.9
6	.0	1.5	9.6	16.1	14.3	8.8	10.5	.1	1.0	16.9	16.7	13.3	8.0	9.9
7	.0	.7	3.6	12.0	11.4	14.0	9.1	.0	.2	4.9	16.0	14.8	10.4	8.7
8	.0	.0	1.7	9.4	13.2	12.8	13.2	.0	.0	2.6	14.2	12.6	15.6	11.9
9	.0	.0	.4	2.9	11.7	9.9	7.4	.1	.0	.6	5.4	13.6	12.3	6.3
10	.0	.0	.4	1.9	5.2	8.6	9.3	.0	.0	.1	2.7	8.3	9.3	10.3
11	.0	.0	.0	1.0	2.8	3.6	5.6	.0	.0	.0	1.6	3.4	4.5	6.7
12	.0	.0	.0	.3	.9	2.3	2.0	.0	.0	.0	.2	1.2	2.4	3.2
13	.0	.0	.0	.3	.5	.2	1.0	.0	.0	.0	.0	.8	.6	1.6
14	.0	.0	.0	.0	.0	.0	.5	.0	.0	.0	.0	.0	.0	.8
15	.0	.0	.0	.0	.0	.0	.5	.0	.0	.0	.0	.0	.0	.8
(N=100%)	232	515	715	501	589	303	259	483	609	615	545	407	294	161
Mean	.70	2.19	3.42	4.99	5.91	6.03	6.07	.86	2.67	4.13	5.60	6.46	6.35	6.17

Syria

	Age group								Marital duration (in years)						
Children ever born	15-19	20-24	25-29	30-34	35-39	40-44	45-49		0-4	5-9	10-14	15-19	20-24	25-29	30+
0	42.3	13.0	6.7	4.9	2.5	3.8	3.5		32.0	3.6	4.0	3.0	2.0	1.1	2.2
1	33.9	22.8	8.0	2.4	1.7	1.4	1.3		35.3	4.8	1.8	1.2	1.1	.6	1.8
2	17.6	25.2	14.2	6.3	2.7	2.5	2.1		24.9	18.5	5.1	1.4	1.7	1.1	.4
3	5.2	22.2	17.9	9.0	6.1	3.8	4.6		7.0	34.1	8.3	3.9	3.2	2.5	2.6
4	.9	10.7	17.9	15.3	9.2	4.0	5.0		.8	24.2	18.3	7.1	3.9	3.9	4.0
5	.0	4.0	16.0	16.1	11.3	8.3	6.2		.0	10.5	23.1	13.7	7.3	4.5	5.7
6	.0	1.3	11.6	16.9	13.1	12.9	8.7		.0	3.8	21.0	19.4	8.9	11.1	5.7
7	.0	.5	4.8	10.7	14.2	11.1	9.8		.0	.4	10.9	16.6	13.2	7.8	10.1
8	.0	.2	1.6	9.3	13.1	13.6	14.4		.0	.1	5.6	15.2	15.6	14.5	13.7
9	.0	.0	1.0	6.0	10.8	10.7	12.3		.0	.0	1.1	10.4	16.2	14.2	10.6
10	.0	.0	.1	2.1	8.6	11.8	9.4		.0	.0	.4	5.4	12.3	15.0	11.0
11	.0	.0	.1	.6	4.2	6.3	10.6		.0	.0	.3	1.4	7.6	10.9	13.2
12	.0	.0	.0	.4	1.4	4.7	6.2		.0	.0	.1	.9	3.7	6.4	8.8
13	.0	.0	.0	.0	.5	2.5	2.7		.0	.0	.0	.0	1.7	2.5	5.7
14	.0	.0	.0	.0	.2	1.1	2.3		.0	.0	.0	.1	1.1	1.4	3.1
15	.0	.0	.0	.0	.3	1.4	1.0		.0	.0	.0	.1	.4	2.5	1.3
(N=100%)	442	824	810	700	639	552	520		1047	894	732	691	537	359	227
Mean	.88	2.16	3.70	5.21	6.62	7.49	7.83		1.09	3.20	4.92	6.45	7.78	8.50	8.63

Thailand

	Age group								Marital duration (in years)						
Children ever born	15-19	20-24	25-29	30-34	35-39	40-44	45-49		0-4	5-9	10-14	15-19	20-24	25-29	30+
0	41.0	18.6	7.1	2.5	1.5	2.5	2.6		30.0	3.4	1.8	1.2	1.8	1.4	3.0
1	49.0	34.3	17.3	9.2	6.3	4.5	3.5		47.4	14.0	5.5	4.6	3.0	3.0	.8
2	9.5	30.5	24.7	15.7	8.7	6.5	4.7		20.6	34.4	13.8	7.7	4.5	3.8	3.6
3	.4	12.6	22.4	16.0	13.3	8.6	4.8		2.0	28.3	21.7	11.9	7.6	4.2	3.3
4	.0	3.3	17.3	19.0	14.0	9.1	11.0		.0	15.0	23.6	15.0	11.8	7.3	9.9
5	.0	.6	8.6	15.2	15.9	10.5	9.9		.0	4.3	19.5	16.4	13.1	9.1	5.3
6	.0	.2	1.8	13.1	14.1	12.0	11.2		.0	.6	9.3	18.4	12.4	12.7	11.8
7	.0	.0	.5	4.3	10.4	13.9	9.1		.0	.0	4.1	11.1	12.9	11.3	9.6
8	.0	.0	.1	3.0	9.9	10.1	11.4		.0	.0	.5	8.5	14.2	10.4	16.8
9	.0	.0	.1	1.6	3.2	8.9	11.6		.0	.0	.2	3.5	8.9	13.1	11.3
10	.0	.0	.0	.3	1.8	7.1	8.4		.0	.0	.0	1.1	6.0	10.9	7.6
11	.0	.0	.0	.0	.9	2.9	4.6		.0	.0	.0	.6	2.8	3.8	7.6
12	.0	.0	.0	.0	.0	1.9	4.0		.0	.0	.0	.0	.7	5.7	2.3
13	.0	.0	.0	.0	.0	.9	1.5		.0	.0	.0	.0	.2	2.0	2.3
14	.0	.0	.0	.0	.0	.5	.7		.0	.0	.0	.0	.2	.7	1.6
15	.0	.0	.0	.0	.0	.1	1.1		.0	.0	.0	.0	.0	.5	3.1
(N=100%)	217	609	746	607	601	580	460		813	740	642	558	538	397	132
Mean	.69	1.50	2.63	3.91	4.93	6.08	6.75		.95	2.53	3.80	5.02	6.09	7.17	7.45

Trinidad and Tobago

	Age group								Marital duration (in years)						
Children ever born	15-19	20-24	25-29	30-34	35-39	40-44	45-49		0-4	5-9	10-14	15-19	20-24	25-29	30+
0	56.5	34.9	18.4	9.8	6.0	5.6	6.1		53.4	18.7	6.5	6.4	3.7	4.4	2.8
1	33.9	29.0	19.1	11.9	8.7	6.4	6.7		33.1	22.3	12.1	7.6	5.6	5.5	8.1
2	8.0	19.7	27.0	20.3	17.5	8.6	6.8		11.1	31.7	24.3	15.3	7.9	6.2	5.4
3	1.2	11.1	14.1	15.2	11.2	11.9	8.4		1.9	16.9	19.5	12.6	12.1	8.7	3.3
4	.4	3.0	10.8	14.9	11.8	11.8	10.2		.3	6.8	17.2	16.5	11.3	10.6	8.5
5	.0	1.8	6.2	11.3	11.4	11.5	7.7		.1	2.8	10.7	13.7	15.4	9.7	5.2
6	.0	.3	2.4	7.0	9.1	12.3	10.9		.0	.5	5.6	10.3	12.0	14.2	8.4
7	.0	.1	1.7	3.9	9.0	6.6	11.7		.0	.2	2.1	7.9	10.1	10.1	12.2
8	.0	.0	.5	1.9	5.4	9.4	7.5		.0	.0	1.2	3.9	7.9	8.3	11.9
9	.0	.0	.0	1.7	3.5	4.7	5.3		.0	.0	.6	2.3	5.5	5.0	6.7
10	.0	.0	.0	1.1	3.1	4.8	4.6		.0	.0	.2	1.3	4.9	5.6	7.1
11	.0	.0	.0	.6	1.1	2.0	5.2		.0	.0	.0	1.2	.9	4.2	7.4
12	.0	.0	.0	.2	.9	1.4	4.6		.0	.0	.0	.4	1.2	3.6	5.6
13	.0	.0	.0	.2	.9	1.0	3.1		.0	.0	.0	.4	.8	2.0	4.9
14	.0	.0	.0	.0	.2	.3	.6		.0	.0	.0	.0	.3	.4	1.1
15	.0	.0	.0	.0	.2	1.5	.6		.0	.0	.0	.0	.5	1.5	1.3
(N=100%)	282	699	652	605	490	398	358		764	791	538	492	417	288	193
Mean	.55	1.26	2.19	3.37	4.46	5.29	5.96		.63	1.83	3.07	4.17	5.29	6.02	6.99

Tunisia

Children ever born	Age group								Marital duration (in years)					
	15-19	20-24	25-29	30-34	35-39	40-44	45-49	0-4	5-9	10-14	15-19	20-24	25-29	30+
0	46.9	20.8	6.6	4.5	4.1	3.6	3.7	28.4	4.2	3.6	2.5	3.0	2.2	3.5
1	46.2	32.0	15.7	4.0	3.5	1.9	2.5	40.6	7.8	2.3	2.3	2.7	1.8	2.0
2	3.8	26.7	18.8	9.2	3.8	3.4	2.3	24.7	21.6	6.2	2.3	2.1	2.2	1.5
3	3.1	15.7	23.3	12.4	5.7	4.2	5.8	5.9	33.9	14.4	6.9	3.2	2.8	3.5
4	.0	3.9	20.3	17.9	10.9	8.2	5.8	.3	22.4	22.7	13.7	8.0	3.5	4.0
5	.0	.6	10.2	20.1	13.3	12.4	8.4	.0	8.1	25.7	16.8	11.0	7.4	6.5
6	.0	.2	3.5	14.9	18.1	13.8	11.1	.0	1.8	15.2	19.6	16.2	11.6	10.0
7	.0	.0	1.0	8.8	14.7	13.8	12.6	.0	.3	6.1	16.2	17.0	12.7	10.9
8	.0	.0	.5	4.7	13.1	11.6	13.2	.0	.0	2.5	11.6	15.4	14.4	11.4
9	.0	.0	.0	2.5	6.3	12.5	14.6	.0	.0	.7	5.4	12.5	14.7	18.9
10	.0	.0	.0	.9	3.9	7.2	7.4	.0	.0	.7	1.5	5.1	11.4	11.4
11	.0	.0	.0	.1	1.3	4.7	4.9	.0	.0	.0	.6	2.4	7.9	6.5
12	.0	.0	.0	.0	.4	1.4	5.3	.0	.0	.0	.5	.6	4.6	6.0
13	.0	.0	.0	.0	.4	.6	1.4	.0	.0	.0	.0	.5	1.3	2.5
14	.0	.0	.0	.0	.3	.6	1.0	.0	.0	.0	.0	.3	1.5	1.0
15	.0	.0	.0	.0	.0	.1	.0	.0	.0	.0	.0	.0	.0	.5
(N=100%)	130	643	772	683	685	696	514	862	719	611	648	625	457	201
Mean	.63	1.52	2.88	4.53	5.81	6.60	7.04	1.09	2.95	4.43	5.67	6.51	7.66	7.73

Turkey

Children ever born	Age group							Marital duration (in years)						
	15-19	20-24	25-29	30-34	35-39	40-44	45-49	0-4	5-9	10-14	15-19	20-24	25-29	30+
0	49.3	16.4	6.1	4.1	2.0	2.9	2.4	35.2	5.4	3.7	1.5	2.6	1.3	3.1
1	38.0	27.7	12.1	4.8	2.8	1.6	1.8	40.7	12.1	3.5	2.7	1.8	1.2	1.3
2	9.6	28.6	25.5	14.8	9.2	7.5	7.8	18.5	34.5	15.5	10.6	7.2	6.7	4.4
3	2.9	17.4	20.2	18.9	13.2	11.0	9.4	4.9	26.8	22.2	15.3	10.9	8.7	6.6
4	.3	6.7	17.5	15.2	13.4	12.4	10.8	.7	13.4	21.4	15.3	12.7	11.6	9.2
5	.0	2.2	10.2	13.0	14.4	14.2	11.4	.0	4.8	16.5	14.1	15.8	13.1	9.2
6	.0	.9	5.5	10.7	10.6	9.7	10.6	.0	2.5	9.7	11.1	11.8	9.4	11.4
7	.0	.1	2.1	8.1	8.5	11.3	11.2	.0	.5	3.8	12.6	9.2 ·	10.8	14.4
8	.0	.0	.2	5.4	11.2	7.7	8.6	.0	.0	2.5	8.1	8.9	11.4	8.3
9	.0	.0	.5	2.5	5.7	7.9	8.8	.0	.0	1.2	5.0	6.0	9.1	11.4
10	.0	.0	.0	1.8	4.3	5.4	6.0	.0	.0	.0	2.7	6.1	6.4	6.1
11	.0	.0	.0	.3	2.8	3.8	4.4	.0	.0	.0	.8	3.1	4.8	6.6
12	.0	.0	.0	.3	1.1	1.8	3.4	.0	.0	.0	.3	2.2	2.7	3.1
13	.0	.0	.0	.0	.5	1.0	1.6	.0	.0	.0	.0	.9	.8	3.1
14	.0	.0	.0	.0	.3	1.3	.8	.0	.0	.0	.0	.6	1.5	.9
15	.0	.0	.0	.0	.0	.5	.6	.0	.0	.0	.0	.0	.6	1.3
(N=100%)	345	811	840	682	644	611	498	890	867	679	596	651	519	229
Mean	.67	1.81	2.99	4.28	5.48	5.95	6.29	.95	2.58	3.85	5.06	5.81	6.46	6.91

Venezuela

Children ever born	Age group							Marital duration (in years)						
	15-19	20-24	25-29	30-34	35-39	40-44	45-49	0-4	5-9	10-14	15-19	20-24	25-29	30+
0	35.6	13.4	5.9	4.0	2.5	2.0	.0	27.1	3.6	.4	2.8	1.0	.0	.0
1	46.6	30.9	18.2	8.5	5.8	4.3	.0	45.3	14.8	5.4	4.4	2.6	1.5	.0
2	14.0	26.8	22.7	17.9	9.7	10.1	.0	21.8	30.8	16.5	7.7	4.6	6.0	.0
3	3.4	16.5	18.0	16.5	13.1	8.4	.0	5.1	26.9	20.8	9.3	8.8	4.5	.0
4	.4	7.7	14.5	12.5	15.2	9.8	.0	.7	13.3	21.9	15.7	8.2	9.7	.0
5	.0	3.6	11.1	10.1	11.3	10.4	.0	.0	7.3	15.4	12.1	13.4	9.0	16.7
6	.0	1.0	4.4	9.5	11.8	9.2	.0	.0	2.3	8.3	15.9	8.2	14.9	.0
7	.0	.0	3.5	8.3	7.8	9.8	.0	.0	.9	5.8	12.3	11.4	9.0	16.7
8	.0	.0	1.5	5.6	7.6	6.6	.0	.0	.0	3.5	9.0	10.8	5.2	16.7
9	.0	.0	.0	4.8	6.5	7.8	.0	.0	.0	1.0	5.7	12.4	10.4	.0
10	.0	.0	.2	1.8	3.7	8.1	.0	.0	.0	.6	2.8	10.5	4.5	33.3
11	.0	.0	.0	.2	2.1	6.1	.0	.0	.0	.0	1.0	4.2	9.7	16.7
12	.0	.0	.0	.2	1.8	3.5	.0	.0	.0	.2	.8	1.6	9.0	.0
13	.0	.0	.0	.0	.2	1.7	.0	.0	.0	.0	.3	1.0	2.2	.0
14	.0	.0	.0	.0	.7	1.2	.0	.0	.0	.0	.3	1.3	1.5	.0
15	.0	.0	.0	.0	.2	.9	.0	.0	.0	.0	.0	.0	3.0	.0
(N=100%)	264	582	594	496	434	346	0	761	640	480	389	306	134	6
Mean	.86	1.89	2.96	4.21	5.24	6.30	.00	1.07	2.68	4.03	5.31	6.67	7.52	8.50

Yemen Arab Republic

Children ever born	Age group							Marital duration (in years)						
	15-19	20-24	25-29	30-34	35-39	40-44	45-49	0-4	5-9	10-14	15-19	20-24	25-29	30+
0	59.6	21.2	5.7	4.7	1.6	2.3	1.7	52.2	9.7	4.1	2.1	1.4	.0	3.8
1	25.3	28.4	14.4	4.5	2.0	1.5	3.1	33.3	19.6	6.0	1.2	1.3	1.4	2.9
2	11.3	20.8	17.8	8.2	6.0	4.8	3.0	11.8	27.1	11.0	4.6	6.8	5.6	1.8
3	3.2	17.1	15.7	10.5	6.3	8.5	5.8	2.0	25.3	15.1	6.9	6.6	6.9	5.0
4	.3	7.0	20.2	14.2	12.5	10.5	8.1	.2	12.3	24.7	13.4	9.5	8.6	8.8
5	.2	3.0	11.7	14.6	13.8	11.5	10.1	.0	4.9	16.1	17.9	11.0	9.8	8.5
6	.0	1.8	7.6	15.7	13.4	9.2	12.1	.1	.8	12.5	19.6	9.9	9.7	12.2
7	.0	.2	3.9	10.2	14.9	12.3	12.6	.0	.4	5.4	11.3	18.5	14.4	11.1
8	.0	.6	1.8	7.9	10.7	14.2	11.2	.1	.0	3.1	10.5	10.5	16.2	12.4
9	.0	.0	.4	4.2	9.4	10.2	9.4	.0	.0	1.3	6.2	9.2	10.4	10.7
10	.0	.0	.8	2.8	3.7	3.5	9.1	.2	.0	.4	2.7	7.3	6.1	6.2
11	.0	.0	.0	1.9	3.6	5.5	5.9	.0	.0	.3	2.5	4.5	5.6	6.5
12	.0	.0	.0	.7	1.4	3.4	2.1	.0	.0	.0	1.2	2.7	2.2	2.0
13	.0	.0	.0	.0	.4	.9	2.5	.0	.0	.0	.0	.8	.5	3.4
14	.0	.0	.0	.0	.3	.0	.7	.0	.0	.0	.0	.0	1.4	.0
15	.0	.0	.0	.0	.0	1.6	2.7	.0	.0	.0	.0	.0	.9	4.8
(N=100%)	442	511	526	388	306	203	228	664	534	410	397	273	159	167
Mean	.60	1.81	3.36	5.05	6.09	6.56	7.08	.68	2.31	4.09	5.79	6.48	6.90	7.18

Colombia

Children ever born	Age group							Marital duration (in years)						
	15-19	20-24	25-29	30-34	35-39	40-44	45-49	0-4	5-9	10-14	15-19	20-24	25-29	30+
0	36.7	12.9	7.0	2.4	3.9	3.2	2.4	26.5	3.6	1.9	2.8	.7	2.7	.0
1	36.3	29.7	15.1	6.6	4.9	4.1	3.5	41.1	10.5	4.4	4.0	2.6	2.7	1.0
2	21.4	30.7	22.2	11.3	8.5	6.7	4.3	24.2	31.0	12.0	4.6	4.6	3.0	5.1
3	4.2	17.0	19.7	18.5	12.0	9.4	7.8	6.2	29.0	17.8	12.4	9.0	4.5	5.1
4	.9	6.8	13.8	15.1	11.2	7.6	9.4	.5	16.1	18.6	11.8	9.3	4.2	5.1
5	.5	2.2	10.1	16.9	10.2	9.2	9.2	.9	6.3	19.0	13.4	10.4	5.7	10.1
6	.0	.7	6.6	9.8	8.9	8.1	8.6	.1	2.2	12.5	10.6	8.1	11.0	7.1
7	.0	.0	3.4	7.0	12.6	10.8	7.8	.4	1.0	7.0	11.8	13.7	9.8	5.1
8	.0	.0	1.5	5.6	9.3	9.9	8.6	.0	.0	3.9	11.8	11.6	9.5	6.1
9	.0	.0	.2	4.0	6.5	7.6	7.8	.0	.1	1.8	7.4	9.3	8.3	7.1
10	.0	.0	.3	1.1	3.5	7.6	8.6	.0	.1	.5	4.2	6.5	11.0	9.1
11	.0	.0	.0	1.1	3.5	6.7	7.5	.0	.0	.5	2.8	6.3	11.7	6.1
12	.0	.0	.2	.2	2.4	3.9	4.0	.0	.0	.0	1.4	3.5	5.7	9.1
13	.0	.0	.0	.4	1.6	2.1	4.0	.0	.0	.2	.4	2.6	4.5	8.1
14	.0	.0	.0	.0	.8	2.1	3.2	.0	.0	.0	.2	1.4	3.4	9.1
15	.0	.0	.0	.0	.2	.9	3.0	.0	.0	.0	.2	.5	2.3	7.1
(N=100%)	215	589	654	531	508	434	371	744	696	569	499	431	264	99
Mean	.98	1.84	3.06	4.49	5.65	6.61	7.25	1.19	2.78	4.35	5.74	6.84	8.01	8.92

Belgium

	Age group							Marital duration (in years)				
Children ever born	15-19	20-24	25-29	30-34	35-39	40-44		0-4	5-9	10-14	15-19	20-24
0	41.9	49.1	18.9	8.2	7.6	7.4		45.1	12.2	6.5	5.7	6.4
1	50.4	37.0	37.7	26.2	21.2	21.2		43.0	31.5	24.1	21.0	21.3
2	7.4	13.0	31.9	38.3	29.3	29.2		11.0	40.0	35.1	29.0	27.5
3	0.3	0.6	9.2	19.9	21.8	19.6		0.8	13.7	20.3	22.4	20.3
4	0.0	0.2	1.7	5.3	12.4	10.6		0.2	2.0	9.9	11.8	9.9
5	0.0	0.0	0.6	1.4	4.9	5.2		0.0	0.5	3.3	5.6	4.5
6	0.0	0.0	0.0	0.5	1.9	3.8		0.0	0.0	0.6	3.2	4.7
7	0.0	0.0	0.0	0.2	0.9	1.8		0.0	0.0	0.3	1.1	2.7
8	0.0	0.0	0.0	0.0	0.0	0.4		0.0	0.0	0.0	0.0	0.7
9	0.0	0.0	0.0	0.0	0.0	0.5		0.0	0.0	0.0	0.0	1.0
10	0.0	0.0	0.0	0.0	0.0	0.3		0.0	0.0	0.0	0.1	0.2
(N=100%)	353	462	774	814	801	792		1056	859	883	789	404
Mean	0.66	0.66	1.39	1.95	2.37	2.53		0.68	1.63	2.17	2.50	2.72

Czechoslovakia

	Age group							Marital duration (in years)				
Children ever born	15-19	20-24	25-29	30-34	35-39	40-44		0-4	5-9	10-14	15-19	20-24
0	21.1	13.1	4.9	1.8	2.0	3.9		13.1	3.3	2.4	2.3	1.4
1	78.9	48.1	26.4	18.6	15.2	16.5		51.9	21.4	14.8	16.4	11.4
2	0.0	34.3	52.3	54.8	49.1	45.0		31.8	56.5	55.1	47.1	46.9
3	0.0	4.2	13.6	20.1	24.3	21.1		2.7	15.4	22.1	24.4	24.5
4	0.0	0.2	2.4	3.2	4.7	8.5		0.5	2.4	3.6	4.9	10.2
5	0.0	0.0	0.4	0.9	2.7	3.0		0.0	0.8	0.8	4.0	2.1
6	0.0	0.0	0.0	0.2	1.9	1.3		0.0	0.1	0.8	0.9	1.9
7	0.0	0.0	0.0	0.5	0.2	0.2		0.0	0.0	0.5	0.0	0.5
8	0.0	0.0	0.0	0.0	0.0	0.4		0.0	0.0	0.0	0.0	0.5
9	0.0	0.0	0.0	0.0	0.0	0.0		0.0	0.0	0.0	0.0	0.0
10	0.0	0.0	0.0	0.0	0.0	0.2		0.0	0.0	0.0	0.0	0.2
(N=100%)	19	405	713	661	593	540		603	719	661	529	420
Mean	0.79	1.30	1.83	2.10	2.31	2.33		1.26	1.95	2.17	2.29	2.54

Denmark

	Age group							Marital duration (in years)				
Children ever born	15-19	20-24	25-29	30-34	35-39	40-44		0-4	5-9	10-14	15-19	20-24
0	55.0	33.3	11.6	5.2	6.0	6.1		28.5	7.0	4.8	3.3	2.5
1	45.0	47.0	32.2	15.0	9.6	11.6		48.3	20.8	9.2	10.0	8.3
2	0.0	16.7	44.0	50.2	40.0	37.1		19.2	54.5	49.7	36.9	33.2
3	0.0	2.7	9.8	24.6	30.3	24.1		2.6	15.2	29.0	31.7	27.1
4	0.0	0.3	2.0	3.9	9.2	14.6		1.2	2.1	5.2	13.5	17.7
5	0.0	0.0	0.4	0.6	3.3	3.2		0.1	0.1	1.6	3.3	5.4
6	0.0	0.0	0.0	0.4	1.6	1.9		0.1	0.3	0.4	1.3	3.2
7	0.0	0.0	0.0	0.0	0.0	0.8		0.0	0.0	0.0	0.0	1.4
8	0.0	0.0	0.0	0.0	0.0	0.4		0.0	0.0	0.0	0.0	0.7
9	0.0	0.0	0.0	0.0	0.0	0.0		0.0	0.0	0.0	0.0	0.0
10	0.0	0.0	0.0	0.0	0.0	0.2		0.0	0.0	0.0	0.0	0.4
(N=100%)	20	300	838	812	633	526		692	891	746	520	277
Mean	0.45	0.90	1.60	2.10	2.43	2.55		1.01	1.86	2.27	2.57	2.93

Finland

Children ever born	Age group							Marital duration (in years)				
	15-19	20-24	25-29	30-34	35-39	40-44		0-4	5-9	10-14	15-19	20-24
0	21.2	28.4	15.0	8.0	3.7	4.8		29.4	8.2	4.4	3.5	2.2
1	66.7	51.2	41.4	28.8	20.0	14.5		53.4	35.8	21.9	14.7	8.9
2	12.1	18.8	35.9	44.7	43.6	33.6		16.0	46.3	48.2	39.4	29.6
3	0.0	1.5	6.6	14.3	21.8	24.4		0.9	8.4	19.3	26.5	27.5
4	0.0	0.2	0.8	3.6	8.0	11.8		0.3	0.9	4.7	11.5	15.4
5	0.0	0.0	0.2	0.5	1.7	6.0		0.0	0.2	1.2	2.6	8.4
6	0.0	0.0	0.0	0.1	0.4	2.2		0.0	0.1	0.1	0.8	3.2
7	0.0	0.0	0.1	0.1	0.4	1.3		0.0	0.1	0.1	0.4	2.4
8	0.0	0.0	0.0	0.1	0.2	0.5		0.0	0.0	0.1	0.2	0.9
9	0.0	0.0	0.0	0.0	0.1	0.5		0.0	0.0	0.0	0.2	0.7
10	0.0	0.0	0.0	0.0	0.0	0.3		0.0	0.0	0.0	0.0	0.6
(N=100%)	33	602	1307	1318	1086	1000		1183	1479	1217	927	538
Mean	0.91	0.94	1.38	1.79	2.22	2.67		0.89	1.59	2.04	2.46	3.12

France

Children ever born	Age group							Marital duration (in years)				
	15-19	20-24	25-29	30-34	35-39	40-44		0-4	5-9	10-14	15-19	20-24
0	0.0	36.2	11.4	6.8	2.8	6.0		33.9	6.4	5.1	4.3	1.2
1	0.0	41.2	38.6	20.7	17.8	15.8		47.6	30.5	16.8	14.6	14.5
2	0.0	18.6	35.9	37.9	35.0	30.8		16.3	44.7	37.9	30.1	30.6
3	0.0	2.9	10.9	21.6	23.7	22.8		1.5	14.8	23.9	29.2	19.8
4	0.0	0.8	2.1	6.1	11.3	12.2		0.2	2.3	9.9	11.6	14.0
5	0.0	0.3	0.6	4.6	5.4	5.4		0.3	0.9	4.4	4.3	10.3
6	0.0	0.0	0.4	1.3	2.3	3.6		0.2	0.3	1.4	4.0	3.7
7	0.0	0.0	0.1	0.2	0.3	2.3		0.0	0.1	0.2	0.9	2.9
8	0.0	0.0	0.0	0.7	1.1	0.3		0.0	0.0	0.2	0.9	1.7
9	0.0	0.0	0.0	0.2	0.0	0.3		0.0	0.0	0.2	0.0	0.4
10	0.0	0.0	0.0	0.0	0.3	0.5		0.0	0.0	0.0	0.3	0.8
(N=100%)	0	381	708	459	354	386		590	689	435	329	242
Mean	0.00	0.92	1.58	2.25	2.58	2.69		0.88	1.81	2.40	2.70	3.11

Great Britain

Children ever born	Age group							Marital duration (in years)				
	15-19	20-24	25-29	30-34	35-39	40-44		0-4	5-9	10-14	15-19	20-24
0	44.3	46.9	22.1	9.8	7.8	6.0		51.2	11.8	5.7	4.3	4.7
1	51.4	30.1	29.7	16.7	15.0	13.8		36.0	25.0	14.1	13.5	11.5
2	4.3	17.8	35.5	44.5	37.9	35.3		10.7	48.3	45.5	36.8	31.6
3	0.0	4.3	10.2	20.3	23.0	21.6		1.8	12.5	24.7	25.9	19.9
4	0.0	0.9	2.1	6.5	10.5	13.5		0.2	2.1	7.2	12.9	17.8
5	0.0	0.0	0.5	1.3	2.7	4.9		0.0	0.2	2.1	3.3	6.3
6	0.0	0.0	0.1	0.7	2.1	2.8		0.0	0.1	0.5	2.3	4.9
7	0.0	0.0	0.0	0.1	0.7	1.3		0.0	0.0	0.1	0.8	1.9
8	0.0	0.0	0.0	0.0	0.4	0.4		0.0	0.0	0.0	0.3	0.9
9	0.0	0.0	0.0	0.0	0.0	0.0		0.0	0.0	0.0	0.0	0.0
10	0.0	0.0	0.0	0.0	0.0	0.1		0.0	0.0	0.0	0.0	0.2
(N=100%)	70	465	866	818	745	716		812	920	773	750	427
Mean	0.60	0.82	1.42	2.05	2.36	2.60		0.64	1.69	2.23	2.54	2.92

Hungary

Children ever born	Age group 15-19	20-24	25-29	30-34	35-39	40-44	Marital duration (in years) 0-4	5-9	10-14	15-19	20-24
0	35.3	19.5	6.0	5.2	4.9	0.0	22.8	4.4	4.2	3.3	0.0
1	54.3	52.1	34.3	26.8	26.2	0.0	54.3	31.0	24.1	25.8	20.4
2	7.8	24.5	45.6	53.2	50.3	0.0	20.2	51.3	55.0	50.2	46.9
3	2.6	3.6	11.5	10.4	13.5	0.0	2.4	10.9	12.7	13.8	22.4
4	0.0	0.2	1.5	2.3	3.0	0.0	0.1	1.7	1.7	4.1	4.1
5	0.0	0.0	0.4	1.0	1.2	0.0	0.1	0.1	1.1	1.3	4.1
6	0.0	0.0	0.4	0.9	0.4	0.0	0.0	0.3	0.7	0.6	2.0
7	0.0	0.0	0.1	0.1	0.4	0.0	0.0	0.1	0.2	0.3	0.0
8	0.0	0.0	0.1	0.1	0.0	0.0	0.0	0.1	0.0	0.2	0.0
9	0.0	0.0	0.0	0.1	0.1	0.0	0.0	0.0	0.1	0.2	0.0
10	0.0	0.0	0.0	0.0	0.1	0.0	0.0	0.0	0.0	0.2	0.0
(N-100%)	116	804	953	930	855	0	1064	1042	825	629	98
Mean	0.78	1.13	1.72	1.86	1.92	0.00	1.03	1.77	1.92	2.01	2.31

Italy

Children ever born	Age group 15-19	20-24	25-29	30-34	35-39	40-44	Marital duration (in years) 0-4	5-9	10-14	15-19	20-24
0	28.9	26.3	11.7	5.7	4.4	5.8	26.2	6.7	4.4	2.3	3.0
1	50.0	47.9	41.5	22.4	18.2	17.0	54.7	29.8	16.1	14.6	11.1
2	15.8	22.7	34.5	46.8	42.9	38.7	17.5	48.5	47.8	38.5	34.3
3	5.3	2.7	9.0	17.0	20.7	22.8	1.4	12.2	21.7	24.7	25.9
4	0.0	0.4	2.3	5.5	8.3	9.4	0.2	2.4	6.8	11.4	14.6
5	0.0	0.0	0.8	1.6	3.6	3.6	0.0	0.4	2.6	5.0	5.6
6	0.0	0.0	0.1	0.7	0.9	1.0	0.0	0.0	0.3	2.0	1.9
7	0.0	0.0	0.1	0.2	0.8	0.7	0.0	0.0	0.3	0.8	2.3
8	0.0	0.0	0.1	0.0	0.1	0.4	0.0	0.1	0.0	0.4	0.5
9	0.0	0.0	0.0	0.0	0.2	0.5	0.0	0.0	0.0	0.4	0.9
10	0.0	0.0	0.0	0.0	0.0	0.0	0.0	0.0	0.0	0.0	0.0
(N-100%)	38	551	1056	1253	1326	1135	1079	1397	1387	1045	432
Mean	0.97	1.03	1.52	2.03	2.30	2.38	0.95	1.75	2.21	2.60	2.83

Netherlands

Children ever born	Age group 15-19	20-24	25-29	30-34	35-39	40-44	Marital duration (in years) 0-4	5-9	10-14	15-19	20-24
0	33.3	40.2	17.1	8.9	10.3	17.1	38.7	7.6	4.7	0.0	0.0
1	66.7	39.7	30.7	15.2	12.4	28.9	41.4	20.4	10.2	0.0	0.0
2	0.0	18.3	43.7	53.5	41.8	30.3	18.6	56.6	47.4	0.0	0.0
3	0.0	1.4	7.2	18.1	27.0	18.4	1.3	13.0	28.1	0.0	0.0
4	0.0	0.4	1.0	3.9	7.4	3.9	0.1	1.9	8.6	0.0	0.0
5	0.0	0.0	0.2	0.2	0.8	1.3	0.0	0.3	0.6	0.0	0.0
6	0.0	0.0	0.1	0.2	0.0	0.0	0.0	0.1	0.3	0.0	0.0
7	0.0	0.0	0.0	0.0	0.3	0.0	0.0	0.0	0.1	0.0	0.0
8	0.0	0.0	0.0	0.0	0.0	0.0	0.0	0.0	0.0	0.0	0.0
9	0.0	0.0	0.0	0.0	0.0	0.0	0.0	0.0	0.0	0.0	0.0
10	0.0	0.0	0.0	0.0	0.0	0.0	0.0	0.0	0.0	0.0	0.0
(N-100%)	15	723	1819	1324	378	76	1504	2108	723	0	0
Mean	0.67	0.82	1.45	1.94	2.12	1.67	0.83	1.82	2.29	0.00	0.00

Norway

Children ever born	Age group							Marital duration (in years)				
	15-19	20-24	25-29	30-34	35-39	40-44		0-4	5-9	10-14	15-19	20-24
0	37.0	34.9	12.5	7.1	3.5	4.7		32.0	7.1	4.1	3.3	1.3
1	51.9	40.8	31.6	12.1	10.0	9.9		46.4	18.9	8.8	8.4	7.2
2	11.1	22.8	42.3	48.3	39.2	29.7		19.9	56.3	43.5	33.7	27.8
3	0.0	1.6	12.1	24.4	28.8	27.9		1.7	15.6	31.2	30.3	29.1
4	0.0	0.0	1.5	7.2	13.7	17.3		0.0	2.1	10.3	16.7	22.0
5	0.0	0.0	0.0	0.4	3.9	7.7		0.0	0.0	1.3	6.3	8.5
6	0.0	0.0	0.0	0.1	1.0	2.0		0.0	0.0	0.5	0.8	3.6
7	0.0	0.0	0.0	0.0	0.0	0.0		0.0	0.0	0.0	0.0	0.0
8	0.0	0.0	0.0	0.1	0.0	0.7		0.0	0.0	0.2	0.4	0.4
9	0.0	0.0	0.0	0.0	0.0	0.0		0.0	0.0	0.0	0.0	0.0
10	0.0	0.0	0.0	0.1	0.0	0.0		0.0	0.0	0.2	0.0	0.0
(N=100%)	27	373	743	718	518	444		694	794	634	478	223
Mean	0.74	0.91	1.58	2.16	2.55	2.78		0.91	1.87	2.43	2.73	3.06

Poland

Children ever born	Age group							Marital duration (in years)				
	15-19	20-24	25-29	30-34	35-39	40-44		0-4	5-9	10-14	15-19	20-24
0	40.7	20.6	6.2	4.0	2.8	3.1		20.0	4.2	1.8	2.1	1.8
1	52.9	55.9	38.4	22.7	14.0	14.0		57.0	29.6	16.7	13.1	9.6
2	5.7	20.4	39.5	43.8	40.2	35.8		20.2	45.7	45.7	39.4	33.5
3	0.7	2.8	11.8	19.9	24.0	22.3		2.6	15.2	22.6	24.8	24.7
4	0.0	0.3	3.2	5.9	10.3	12.5		0.2	4.2	7.6	10.9	15.1
5	0.0	0.0	0.7	2.5	4.6	5.8		0.0	0.9	3.7	5.2	6.4
6	0.0	0.0	0.2	0.7	2.2	3.3		0.0	0.2	1.3	2.3	4.4
7	0.0	0.0	0.0	0.3	1.2	1.4		0.0	0.0	0.2	1.2	2.3
8	0.0	0.0	0.1	0.1	0.5	0.7		0.0	0.0	0.2	0.6	0.9
9	0.0	0.0	0.0	0.1	0.1	0.8		0.0	0.0	0.1	0.4	0.9
10	0.0	0.0	0.0	0.1	0.1	0.1		0.0	0.0	0.1	0.1	0.1
(N=100%)	140	1730	2594	1906	1722	1705		2807	2476	1737	1704	1075
Mean	0.66	1.06	1.71	2.15	2.58	2.76		1.06	1.89	2.37	2.67	3.07

Spain

Children ever born	Age group							Marital duration (in years)				
	15-19	20-24	25-29	30-34	35-39	40-44		0-4	5-9	10-14	15-19	20-24
0	23.1	7.1	6.4	3.4	3.2	4.0		10.3	4.3	2.6	3.6	2.0
1	61.5	49.8	33.3	15.1	9.6	8.0		53.7	16.7	9.4	7.7	5.5
2	7.7	34.8	41.3	44.3	34.7	29.5		32.0	50.6	35.5	31.0	22.6
3	7.7	6.4	13.5	22.8	26.9	25.5		3.4	21.1	28.4	25.7	25.9
4	0.0	1.9	2.6	8.3	14.1	16.6		0.3	5.3	14.2	16.5	17.3
5	0.0	0.0	1.4	3.8	7.3	7.6		0.3	1.4	6.5	7.7	12.2
6	0.0	0.0	1.1	1.5	2.8	4.2		0.0	0.5	2.6	4.5	6.2
7	0.0	0.0	0.1	0.5	0.9	2.2		0.0	0.2	0.6	2.1	3.3
8	0.0	0.0	0.1	0.0	0.3	1.0		0.0	0.0	0.1	0.8	1.8
9	0.0	0.0	0.0	0.0	0.2	0.6		0.0	0.0	0.1	0.3	1.3
10	0.0	0.0	0.1	0.1	0.0	0.3		0.0	0.0	0.0	0.3	0.7
(N=100%)	13	267	843	1104	1085	1297		697	1218	1208	1032	452
Mean	1.00	1.46	1.83	2.38	2.80	3.09		1.31	2.13	2.76	3.04	3.67

United States

Children ever born	Age group							Marital duration (in years)				
	15-19	20-24	25-29	30-34	35-39	40-44		0-4	5-9	10-14	15-19	20-24
0	55.1	38.5	19.5	8.6	7.5	5.7		45.8	10.9	6.5	4.5	2.6
1	37.1	35.8	27.2	12.8	14.7	7.1		35.1	27.2	10.2	8.3	5.7
2	7.1	19.3	35.7	37.9	31.3	22.7		15.0	42.4	39.1	25.2	20.8
3	0.4	5.3	12.7	22.1	21.8	23.2		3.2	14.5	23.9	27.1	22.1
4	0.4	1.0	3.6	9.0	10.9	15.1		0.5	3.5	10.6	17.2	16.7
5	0.0	0.2	0.8	5.1	6.0	11.4		0.1	1.2	5.3	8.8	12.4
6	0.0	0.0	0.3	3.3	3.2	5.4		0.1	0.4	3.1	4.0	7.5
7	0.0	0.0	0.1	0.9	2.6	3.6		0.0	0.0	0.7	2.6	4.5
8	0.0	0.0	0.0	0.3	1.2	2.1		0.1	0.0	0.3	1.2	3.3
9	0.0	0.0	0.1	0.1	0.3	1.5		0.1	0.0	0.2	0.8	1.9
10	0.0	0.0	0.0	0.0	0.5	1.2		0.0	0.0	0.0	0.2	1.3
(N=100%)	267	1084	1424	1056	652	814		1644	1389	942	860	696
Mean	0.54	0.95	1.59	2.45	2.71	3.52		0.79	1.77	2.58	3.15	3.91

Yugoslavia

Children ever born	Age group							Marital duration (in years)				
	15-19	20-24	25-29	30-34	35-39	40-44		0-4	5-9	10-14	15-19	20-24
0	38.8	16.1	6.0	4.2	3.4	4.3		21.7	3.7	3.7	2.5	2.9
1	55.3	48.3	26.8	15.5	14.1	12.1		51.4	22.8	13.5	12.8	10.2
2	5.9	29.7	43.3	40.9	37.9	35.1		23.1	47.1	42.3	38.6	31.4
3	0.0	4.6	15.6	18.7	18.0	18.3		2.6	17.9	19.3	19.1	17.8
4	0.0	0.9	5.2	9.1	9.3	11.0		0.6	5.7	9.6	9.6	12.0
5	0.0	0.3	2.1	5.6	7.2	5.6		0.2	2.0	5.8	6.9	7.6
6	0.0	0.1	0.9	3.0	3.4	5.2		0.2	0.6	3.3	3.7	6.5
7	0.0	0.1	0.0	1.8	3.7	4.0		0.1	0.2	1.5	3.6	5.7
8	0.0	0.0	0.1	0.6	1.8	2.1		0.1	0.0	0.4	1.7	3.4
9	0.0	0.0	0.1	0.6	1.3	2.2		0.0	0.1	0.6	1.6	2.7
10	0.0	0.0	0.0	0.0	0.0	0.0		0.0	0.0	0.0	0.0	0.0
(N=100%)	219	1220	1475	1222	1303	1367		1643	1551	1410	1223	979
Mean	0.67	1.28	1.98	2.59	2.89	3.05		1.11	2.09	2.62	2.95	3.42

References

Allison, P.D., 1978, Measures of Inequality, *American Sociological Review* **43**: 865–880.

Anderton, D., Tsuya, N., Bean, L., and Mineau, G., 1987, Intergenerational Transmission of Relative Fertility and Life Course Patterns, *Demography* **24** (4): 467–480.

Ashurst, H., Balkaran, S., and Casterline, J.B., 1984, *Socio-Economic Differentials in Recent Fertility*, Comparative Studies No. 42, World Fertility Survey, London.

Berent, J., 1982, *Family Planning in Europe and USA in the 1970s*, Comparative Studies No. 20, World Fertility Survey, London.

Berent, J., 1983, *Family Size Preferences in Europe and USA: Ultimate Expected Number of Children*, Comparative Studies No. 26, World Fertility Survey, London.

Berent, J., Jones, E.F., and Khalid Siddiqui, M., 1982, *Basic Characteristics, Sample Designs and Questionnaires*, Comparative Studies No. 18, World Fertility Survey, London.

Bhrolchain, M.N., 1985, *Period Parity Progression Ratios and Birth, Intervals in England and Wales, 1941–1971: A Synthetic Life Table Analysis*, CPS Research Paper 85-4, Centre for Population Studies, London.

Birg, H., Huinink, J., Koch, H., and Vorholt, H., 1984, *Kohortenanalytische Darstellung der Geburtenentwicklung in der Bundesrepublik Deutschland*, Institut für Bevölkerungsforschung und Sozialpolitik, Bielefeld.

Bongaarts, J., 1978, A Framework for Analyzing the Proximate Determinants of Fertility, *Population and Development Review* **4** (1): 105–132.

Bongaarts, J. and Potter, R.G., 1983, *Fertility, Biology, and Behavior: An Analysis of the Proximate Determinants*, Academic Press, New York.

Brass, W. and Juárez, F., 1983, Censored Cohort Parity Progression Ratios from Birth Histories, *Asian and Pacific Census Forum* **10** (1): 5–13.

Bruckmann, G., 1969, Einige Bemerkungen zur statistischen Messung der Konzentration, *Metrika* **14**: 183–213.

Bruckmann, G., 1981, Kapitel 26: Konzentrationsmessung, in J. Bleymüller, G. Gehlert, and H. Gülicher, eds., *Statistik für Wirtschaftswissenschaftler*, 2nd ed., 185–190, Verlag Franz Vehlen, Munich.

Büttner, T., Lutz, W., and Speigner, W., 1987, *Some Demographic Aspects of Aging in the German Democratic Republic*, WP-87-116, International Institute for Applied Systems Analysis, Laxenburg, Austria.

Casterline, J.B., 1980, *Age at First Birth*, Comparative Studies No. 15, World Fertility Survey, London.

Chiang, C.L., 1984, *The Life Table and Its Applications*, Robert E. Krieger Publishing Co., Malabar, FL.

Chiang, C.L. and van den Berg, B.J., 1982, A Fertility Table for the Analysis of Human Reproduction, *Mathematical Biosciences* **62**: 237–251.

Cleland, J. and Hobcraft, J., eds., 1985, *Reproductive Change in Developing Countries: Insights from the World Fertility Survey*, Oxford University Press, New York.

Cleland, J. and Scott, C., eds., 1987, *The World Fertility Survey: An Assessment*, Oxford University Press, New York.

Coale, A., 1974, The Demographic Transition, *UN, The Population Debate, Dimensions and Perspectives: Papers of the World Population Conference*, 347–356, Bucharest.

Cochrane, S., O'Hara, D., and Leslie, J., 1980, *The Effects of Education on Health*, World Bank Working Paper No. 405, Washington, DC.

Crow, J.F., 1958, Some Possibilities for Measuring Selection Intensities in Man, *Human Biology* **30**: 1–13.

Davis, K. and Blake, J., 1956, Social Structure and Fertility: An Analytic Framework, *Economic Development and Cultural Change* **4**: 211–235.

Easterlin, R., 1978, The Economics and Sociology of Fertility: A Synthesis, in Ch. Tilly, ed., *Historical Studies of Changing Fertility*, Princeton University Press, Princeton, NJ.

Easterlin, R., 1980, *Birth and Fortune*, Basic Books, Inc., New York.

Espenshade, T.J., 1986, Markov Chain Models of Marital Event Histories, *Current Perspectives on Aging and the Life Cycle*, Vol. 2, 73–106.

Feeney, G., 1983, Population Dynamics based on Birth Intervals and Parity Progression, *Population Studies* **37** (1): 75–89.

Feeney, G. and Wijeyesekera, M., 1983, Parity Progression and Birth Interval Analysis in South Asia, paper presented at the Conference on Recent Population Trends in South Asia, New Delhi.

Feeney, G. and Yu, J., 1987, Period Parity Progression Measures of Fertility in China, *Population Studies* **41** (1): 77–102.

Feichtinger, G., 1978, Cohort Trends in the Timing of the Family Life Cycle in Austria and West Germany, *Zeitschrift für Bevölkerungswissenschaft* **4** (2): 149–159.

Feichtinger, G., 1987, The Statistical Measurement of the Family Life Cycle, in J. Bongaarts, T. Burch, and K. Wachter, eds., *Family Demography: Methods and their Applications*, 81–101, Oxford University Press, New York.

Feichtinger, G. and Lutz, W., 1983, Eine Fruchtbarkeitstafel auf Paritätsbasis, *Zeitschrift für Bevölkerungswissenschaft* **9** (3): 363–377.

Ford, K., 1984, *Timing and Spacing of Births*, Comparative Studies No. 38, World Fertility Survey, London.

Foster, J.E., 1985, Inequality Measurement, in H.P. Young, ed., *Fair Allocation: Proceedings of Symposia in Applied Mathematics*, Vol. 33, American Mathematical Society Press, Providence, RI.

Gilks, W., 1979, The Examination of a Model of Marital Fertility Depending on Both Age and Duration of Marriage, unpublished MSc dissertation, Department of Social Statistics, University of Southampton.

Gisser, R., 1985, Kinderwunsch und Kinderzahl (Desired and Actual Family Sizes), in R. Münz, ed., *Leben mit Kindern*, 37–70, Vienna.

Gisser, R., Lutz, W., and Münz, R., 1985, Kinderwunsch und Kinderzahl, in R. Münz, ed., *Leben mit Kindern*, 33–94, Vienna.

Glick, P., 1957, *American Families*, Wiley, New York.

Glick, P., 1977, Updating the Lifecycle of the Family, *Journal of Marriage* **39**: 5–12.

Goodman, L., Keyfitz, N., and Pullum, T., 1975, Addendum: Family Formation and the Frequency of Various Kinship Relationships, *Theoretical Population Biology* 8: 376–381.

Goodwin, D., Lutz, W., and Vaupel, J., 1986, Concentration and the Level of Fertility, unpublished draft paper, International Institute for Applied Systems Analysis, Laxenburg, Austria.

Goodwin, D. and Vaupel, J., 1985, *Concentration Curves and Have-Statistics for Ecological Analysis of Diversity, Part III: Comparison of Measures of Diversity*, WP-85-91, International Institute for Applied Systems Analysis, Laxenburg, Austria.

Hajnal, J., 1965, European Marriage Patterns in Perspective, in D.V. Glass and D.E.E. Eversley, eds., *Population in History: Essays in Historical Demography*, 101–143.

Haslinger, A., 1985, Fruchtbarkeitsentwicklung nach Heiratsjahrgängen: Ein Vergleich des Mikrozensus Juni 1981 mit der Longitudinalerhebung, in R. Münz, ed., *Leben mit Kindern*, 227–291, Vienna.

Henry, L., 1953, Fondements theoriques des mesures de la fécondité naturelle, *Review de l'Institut International de Statistique* 21 (3): 135–252.

Henry, L., 1961, Some Data on Natural Fertility, *Eugenics Quarterly* 18 (2): 81–91.

Herfindahl, O., 1950, Concentration in the Steel Industry, Dissertation, Columbia University, New York.

Heuser, R.L., 1976, Fertility Tables for Birth Cohorts by Color: United States, 1917–1973, DHEW Publication No. (HRS) 76–1152, US Dept. of HEW, Health Resources Administration, Rockville, MD.

Heuser, R.L., 1984, Fertility Tables for Birth Cohorts by Color, United States, 1917–1980, US Dept. of HEW, National Center for Health Statistics, Washington, DC.

Hobcraft, J. and Casterline, J.B., 1983, Speed of Reproduction, *WFS Comparative Studies* No. 25, International Statistical Institute, Voorburg, Netherlands.

Hobcraft, J. and McDonald, J., 1984, *Birth Intervals*, Comparative Studies No. 28, World Fertility Survey, London.

Höhn, Ch., 1982, Der Familienzyklus: Zur Notwendigkeit einer Konzepterweiterung, *Schriftenreihe des Bundesinstituts für Bevölkerungsforschung*, Vol. 12, FRG.

Howell, N., 1979, *Demography of the Dobe!Kung*, Academic Press, San Diego, CA.

Jones, E.F., 1982, *Socio-Economic Differentials in Achieved Fertility*, Comparative Studies No. 21, World Fertility Survey, London.

Keilman, N., 1986, Recent Trends in Family and Household Composition in Europe, unpublished manuscript, Netherlands Interuniversity Demographic Institute, The Hague.

Kendall, M.G. and Stuart, A., 1967, *The Advanced Theory of Statistics*, 2nd ed., Vol. 2, Griffin, London.

Keyfitz, N., 1985, *Applied Mathematical Demography*, 2nd ed., Springer-Verlag, New York.

King, M. and Lutz, W., 1988, *Beyond "The Average American Family": U.S. Cohort Parity Distributions and Fertility Concentration*, International Institute for Applied Systems Analysis, Laxenburg, Austria.

Koo, H.P. and Janowitz, B.K., 1983, Interrelationships Between Family and Marital Dissolution: Results of a Simultaneous Logit Model, *Demography* 20 (2): 129–146.

Krishnamoorthy, S., 1979, Classical Approach to Increment-Decrement Life Tables: An Application to the Study of the Marital Status of United States Females, 1970, *Mathematical Biosciences* 44: 139–154.

Kuijsten, A., 1986, *Advances in Family Demography*, The Hague.

Kytir, J. and Münz, R., 1986, Illegitimacy in Austria, *Demografische Informationen 1986*, 7–21.

Lorenz, M.O., 1905, Methods of Measuring the Concentration of Wealth, *Journal of American Statistical Association*, Vol. 9.

Lutz, W., 1984, Die Entwicklung paritätsspezifischer Fruchtbarkeitskontrolle, *Zeitschrift für Bevölkerungswissenschaft* 10 (4): 449–462.

Lutz, W., 1985a, Parity-Specific Fertility Analysis: A Comparative Analysis on 41 Countries Participating in the World Fertility Survey, Demographic Institute of the Austrian Academy of Sciences, Vienna.

Lutz, W., 1985b, Heiraten, Scheidungen und Kinderzahl: Demografische Tafeln zum Familien–Lebenszyklus in Österreich (Marriage, Divorce, and the Number of Children: A Life Table Approach to the Analysis of the Family Life Cycle in Austria), in *Demografische Informationen*, 3–21.

Lutz, W., 1985c, Ein Kind, zwei Kinder, drei Kinder? (One Child, Two Children, Three Children?), in R. Münz, ed., *Leben mit Kindern*, 77–81, Vienna.

Lutz, W., 1987a, *Finnish Fertility Since 1722*, Series D, No. 18, The Population Research Institute, Helsinki.

Lutz, W., 1987b, Factors Associated with the Finnish Fertility Decline Since 1776, *Population Studies* 41: 463–482.

Lutz, W., 1987c, Birth Control and the Concentration of Fertility: A Study of Eleven European Countries, paper prepared for the European Population Conference 1987, Jyväskylä, Finland.

Lutz, W. and Feichtinger, G., 1985, A Life Table Approach to Parity Progression and Marital Status Transitions, contributed paper to the IUSSP General Conference (Session F.13), Florence.

Lutz, W. and Pitkänen, K., 1986, *Tracing Back the Eighteenth Century "Nuptiality Transition" in Finland*, CP-86-1, International Institute for Applied Systems Analysis, Laxenburg, Austria.

Lutz, W. and Vaupel, J., 1987, The Division of Labor for Society's Reproduction: On the Concentration of Childbearing and Rearing in Austria, *Österreichische Zeitschrift für Statistik und Informatik* 17: 81–96.

Lutz, W. and Wolf, D., 1987, Fertility and Marital Status Changes over the Life Cycle: A Comparative Study of Finland and Austria, paper prepared for the European Population Conference 1987, Jyväskylä, Finland.

Lutz, W. and Yashin, A., 1987, *Comparative Anatomy of Fertility Trends: The Aging of the Baby Boom*, WP-87-12, International Institute for Applied Systems Analysis, Laxenburg, Austria.

Lutz, W., Pullum, T., and Wolf, D., 1988, How Does Cross-Generational Fertility Correlation Together with Heterogeneity in the Family Size Distribution Influence the Level of Fertility?, draft Working Paper, International Institute for Applied Systems Analysis, Laxenburg, Austria.

Marchal, F. and Rabut, O., 1972, Evolution recente de la fécondité en Europe Occidentale, *Population* 27: 838–874.

McCarthy, J., 1982, *Differentials in Age at First Marriage*, Comparative Studies No. 19, World Fertility Survey, London.

McDonald, P., 1984, *Nuptiality and Completed Fertility: A Study of Starting, Stopping and Spacing Behaviour*, Comparative Studies No. 35, World Fertility Survey, London.

Münz, R., ed., 1985, *Leben mit Kindern: Wunsch und Wirklichkeit* (Living with Children: Wish and Reality), Institute für Demographie, Vienna.

Münzner, H., 1963, Probleme der Konzentrationsmessung, *Allg. Stat. Archiv* 47: 1–9.

Page, H., 1977, Patterns Underlying Fertility Schedules: A Decomposition by Both Age and Marital Duration, *Population Studies* 31: 85–106.

Payne, C.D., ed., 1985, *The GLIM System Release 3.77*, GLIM Manual.

Piesch, W., 1975, *Statistische Konzentrationsmasse: Formale Eigenschaften und Verteilungstheoretische Zusammenhänge*, J.C.B. Mohr, Tübingen.

Pitkänen, K., 1982, The Educated People: The Precursors of the Fertility Transition in Finland, paper presented to the Scandinavian Demographic Conference.

Popper, K., 1972, *Objective Knowledge: An Evolutionary Approach*, Oxford University Press, London.

Preston, S., 1976, Family Sizes of Children and Family Sizes of Women, *Demography* 13 (1): 105–114.

Pullum, T., Tedrow, L., and Hertin, J., 1987, Change and Continuity in Completed Parity Distributions in the United States, Birth Cohorts of White Women: 1871–1935, submitted to *Demography*.

Rajulton, F., 1985, Heterogeneous Marital Behavior in Belgium, 1970 and 1977: An Application of the Semi-Markov Model to Period Data, *Mathematical Biosciences* 73: 197–225.

Rantakallio, P., 1971, The Effect of a Northern Climate on Seasonality of Births and the Outcome of Pregnancies, *Acta Paediatrica Scandinavica*, Supplement 218, Kirjapaino Osakeyhitiö Kaleva, Oulu, Finland.

Rogers, A. and Willekens, F., eds., 1986, *Migration and Settlement: A Multiregional Comparative Study*, D. Reidel Publishing Co., Dordrecht.

Rosenbluth, G., 1955, Measures of Concentration, in *Business Concentration and Price Policy*, National Bureau of Economic Research, Special Conference Series No. 5, 57–99, Princeton, NJ.

Ryder, N., 1982, *Progressive Fertility Analysis*, Technical Bulletins No. 8, World Fertility Survey, London.

Schoen, R., 1988, *Modeling Multigroup Populations*, Plenum Press, New York.

Singh, S., 1984, Assessment of Nuptiality Data, *World Fertility Survey 1972–1984*, Background Paper 3, Symposium, United Nations, New York.

Smith, D.P., 1980, *Age at First Marriage*, Comparative Studies No. 7, World Fertility Survey, London.

Spree, R., 1982, The German Petite Bourgeoisie and the Decline of Fertility: Some Statistical Evidence from the Late 19th and Early 20th Centuries, in *Historical Social Research – Quantum Information* 22: 15–49.

Spree, R., 1984, Der Geburtenrückgang in Deutschland vor 1939: Verlauf und schichtspezifische Ausprägung, *Demografische Informationen 1984*, 49–68.

Suchindran, C.M. and Koo, H., 1980, Divorce, Remarriage, and Fertility, paper presented at the annual meetings of the Population Association of America, Denver, CO.

Suchindran, C.M., Namboodiri, N.K., and West, K., 1977, Analyses of Fertility by Increment-Decrement Life Tables, *Proceedings of the American Statistical Association, Social Statistics Section 1*, 431–436, Washington, DC.

United Nations, 1955, *Handbook of Vital Statistics Methods: Studies in Methods*, Series F, No. 7, United Nations, New York.

United Nations, 1973, *The Determinants and Consequences of Population Trends*, Vol. 1, United Nations, New York.

United Nations, 1975, *UN Demographic Yearbook*, United Nations, New York.

United Nations, 1981, *UN Demographic Yearbook*, United Nations, New York.

United Nations, 1985, *World Population Prospects: Estimates and Projections as Assessed in 1982*, ST/ESA/SER.A/86, Department of International Economic and Social Affairs, United Nations, New York.

United Nations, 1987, *Fertility Behavior in the Context of Development: Evidence from the World Fertility Survey*, ST/ESA/SER.A/100, Department of International Economic and Social Affairs, United Nations, New York.

Vaupel, J. and Goodwin, D., 1986, A Division of Labor: The Concentration of Reproduction Among US Women, 1917–1980, submitted to *Demography* as a Research Note.

Vaupel, J., Gambill, B., and Yashin, A., 1987, *Thousands of Data at a Glance: Shaded Contour Maps of Demographic Surfaces*, RR-87-16, International Institute for Applied Systems Analysis, Laxenburg, Austria.

Wijewickrema, S. and Alli, 1984, Marital Status Trends in Belgium (1961–1977): Application of Multi-State Analysis, *Population and Family in the Low Countries, IV*, 47–72, Netherlands Interuniversity Demographic Institute, Voorburg, Netherlands.

Willekens, F., 1987, The Marital Status Life Table, in J. Bongaarts, T. Burch, and K. Wachter, eds., *Family Demography: Methods and their Applications*, 125–149, Kluwer, The Netherlands.

Willekens, F., Shah, I., Shah, J.M., and Ramachandran, P., 1982, Multi-State Analysis of Marital Status Life Tables: Theory and Application, *Population Studies* **36**: 129–144.

Wolf, D., 1986, Simulation Models for Analyzing Continuous-Time Event-History Models, in N. Tuma, ed., *Sociological Methodology 1986*, 283–308, Jossey-Bass, San Francisco, CA.

Wolf, D., 1987, The Multistate Life Table with Duration Dependence, WP-87-46, International Institute for Applied Systems Analysis, Laxenburg, Austria.

Index

Figures in *italic*, tables in **bold**

Abortion, 6, 7, 7, 14, 186
Absolute concentration, fertility,
    140–5, **141**, **143**, **144**
Abstinence, 6, 7, 23
Africa, **84**
  cohort analysis
    age of birth, **67**, **69**, 71, **74**
    birth interval, 76, **77**, **78**, **79**,
      80, **81**
    current parity distribution,
      84
    parity-progression, 48–9,
      49, 50, **54**, 55, **56**, 58, **206**,
      208, **210**, **212**, **214**
    total fertility rate, **60**, **62**, **98**
  concentration of reproduction,
    145, 170–1
  demographic dimensions, 16,
    16
  period analysis, **98**, **100**, 101,
    115, 117, **117**
  see also Benin, Cameroon,
    Egypt, Ethiopia, Ghana,
    Ivory Coast, Kenya,
    Lesotho, Libya,
Mauritania, Morocco,
    Nigeria, Senegal, Sudan,
    Tanzania, Tunisia, Zaire
Age, mother's
  cohort analysis, 65–75, **67**, *68*,
    69, *70*, *72*, *73*, **74**, **75**
  current parity distribution,
    82–3, **84**, **85**, 87, *88*, *89*, *90*
  methodology, 46, 47
  parity progression ratio, 50
  concentration of reproduction,
    150, 152–4, **153**, *153*, 175
  demographic dimension, 1, 2, 3
  birth interval, 24, *24*
  father, 27–8, *27*, *28*, *29*, 36,
    38, *39*
  marital duration, *20*, 21, *21*,
    22, 23
  modelling, 29–30, **32**, **33**, 34,
    34, 35, 36, 37
  mother, 6–12, *7*, *8*, *9*, *10*, *11*,
    27–8, *27*
  parity, 17, 18, *18*, 19, *19*
  time and age, 12–16, *13*, *14*,
    15